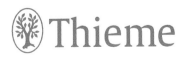

Brain Mapping

Indications and Techniques

Alfredo Quinones-Hinojosa, MD
Chair and the William J. and Charles H. Mayo Professor
Department of Neurosurgery
Mayo Clinic
Jacksonville, Florida, USA

Kaisorn L. Chaichana, MD
Consultant Neurosurgeon and Associate Professor of Neurosurgery
Department of Neurosurgery
Mayo Clinic
Jacksonville, Florida, USA

Deependra Mahato, DO, MS
Attending Neurosurgeon
Neurological Surgery Residency Program
Riverside University Health System
Moreno Valley, California, USA

120 illustrations

Thieme
New York • Stuttgart • Delhi • Rio de Janeiro

Library of Congress Cataloging-in-Publication Data

Names: Quiñones-Hinojosa, Alfredo, editor. | Chaichana, Kaisorn (Kaisorn L.), editor. | Mahato, Deependra, editor.
Title: Brain mapping : indications and techniques / [edited by] Alfredo Quiñones-Hinojosa, Kaisorn L. Chaichana, Deependra Mahato.
Other titles: Brain mapping (Quiñones-Hinojosa)
Description: New York : Thieme, [2020] | Includes bibliographical references and index. | Summary: "Despite advances in imaging techniques to identify eloquent cortical brain regions and subcortical white matter, brain mapping is the only method for obtaining real-time information with high sensitivity and specificity. This groundbreaking technology greatly enhances the neurosurgeon's ability to safely resect challenging lesions located in eloquent areas of the brain. The book starts with discussion of preoperative aspects, including the history of brain mapping and anatomy of eloquent cortical and eloquent white matter tracts. Subsequent chapters cover perioperative aspects of brain mapping including indirect and direct functional mapping, the role of neurophysiology, awake craniotomy operating room set-up and surgical instruments, and anesthetic considerations. Diverse awake and asleep brain mapping techniques are described for various intracranial pathologies, as well as advances in postoperative recovery of neurological function including physical and speech therapy"– Provided by publisher.
Identifiers: LCCN 2019027114 | ISBN 9781684200924 (hardback) | ISBN 9781684200931 (ebook)
Subjects: MESH: Brain Diseases–surgery | Brain Mapping–methods | Neurosurgical Procedures–methods
Classification: LCC RD593 | NLM WL 368 | DDC 617.4/81–dc23
LC record available at https://lccn.loc.gov/2019027114

Copyright © 2020 by Thieme Medical Publishers, Inc.

Thieme Publishers New York
333 Seventh Avenue, New York, NY 10001 USA
+1 800 782 3488, customerservice@thieme.com

Thieme Publishers Stuttgart
Rüdigerstrasse 14, 70469 Stuttgart, Germany
+49 [0]711 8931 421, customerservice@thieme.de

Thieme Publishers Delhi
A-12, Second Floor, Sector-2, Noida-201301
Uttar Pradesh, India
+91 120 45 566 00, customerservice@thieme.in

Thieme Revinter Publicações Ltda.
Rua do Matoso, 170 – Tijuca
Rio de Janeiro RJ 20270-135 - Brasil
+55 21 2563-9702
www.thiemerevinter.com.br

Cover design: Thieme Publishing Group
Typesetting by Thomson Digital, India

Printed in the United States of America
by King Printing Co., Inc.   5 4 3 2 1

ISBN 978-1-68420-092-4

Also available as an e-book:
eISBN 978-1-68420-093-1

Important note: Medicine is an ever-changing science undergoing continual development. Research and clinical experience are continually expanding our knowledge, in particular our knowledge of proper treatment and drug therapy. Insofar as this book mentions any dosage or application, readers may rest assured that the authors, editors, and publishers have made every effort to ensure that such references are in accordance with **the state of knowledge at the time of production of the book.**

Nevertheless, this does not involve, imply, or express any guarantee or responsibility on the part of the publishers in respect to any dosage instructions and forms of applications stated in the book. **Every user is requested to examine carefully** the manufacturers' leaflets accompanying each drug and to check, if necessary in consultation with a physician or specialist, whether the dosage schedules mentioned therein or the contraindications stated by the manufacturers differ from the statements made in the present book. Such examination is particularly important with drugs that are either rarely used or have been newly released on the market. Every dosage schedule or every form of application used is entirely at the user's own risk and responsibility. The authors and publishers request every user to report to the publishers any discrepancies or inaccuracies noticed. If errors in this work are found after publication, errata will be posted at www.thieme.com on the product description page.

Some of the product names, patents, and registered designs referred to in this book are in fact registered trademarks or proprietary names even though specific reference to this fact is not always made in the text. Therefore, the appearance of a name without designation as proprietary is not to be construed as a representation by the publisher that it is in the public domain.

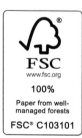

Contents

Section I: Preoperative Brain Mapping Features

Part 1: Brain Anatomy and Pathology

Part 2: Preoperative Mapping Adjuncts

Section II: Intraoperative Brain Mapping

Part 1: Awake

Contents

Foreword

In *Brain Mapping: Indications and Techniques*, editors Alfredo Quinones-Hinojosa, Kaisorn Chaichana, and Deependra Mahoto have assembled a superb cast of international authors who specialize in different aspects of brain mapping as it relates to brain tumor surgery.

The book begins with a discussion on brain anatomy and pathology, including the history of brain mapping, and a review of eloquent cortical regions and critical white matter tracts. The work then transitions to details about preoperative brain mapping adjuncts including functional MRI and tractography, PET and SPECT imaging, electroencephalograms, and electrocorticography. A detailed discussion of the necessary components for awake and asleep brain mapping follows, including insights into operating room equipment, anesthetic requirements, language mapping, motor mapping, subcortical mapping of critical white matter tracts, insular and visual cortices, epilepsy mapping, and brainstem mapping. Lastly, the work concludes with important chapters on postoperative management including physical therapy, promoting neuroplasticity, and radiation therapy following brainmapping surgery. Important to the practitioners who are involved with brain mapping surgery, this book focuses on the latest advancements in brain mapping as explained by recognized experts; the case examples are an excellent tool bringing out the nuances of the techniques highlighted. With the increased literature supporting brain mapping as a way of understanding and preserving neurological function, these techniques are ever more critical as a tool in the neurosurgeon's armamentarium.

The neurosurgical literature has been lacking a single source volume that encompasses the different options and approaches for various pre-, intra-, and postoperative mapping techniques to understand brain function. This book addresses these limitations by providing a comprehensive source of information that encompasses these different aspects of brain mapping techniques including advantages and disadvantages, bail out options, and considerations. By bringing together many perspectives on brain mapping into a single tome, the editors have created a tour de force overview of this important topic. I enjoyed this book, and I hope that health care providers who are involved in the perioperative planning and implementation of these techniques for patients with brain tumors will find it a valuable addition to their personal library as a must-read contribution to the neurosurgical literature.

Bob S. Carter, MD, PhD
William and Elizabeth Sweet Professor of Neurosurgery
Harvard Medical School
Chief of Neurosurgery
Massachusetts General Hospital
Boston, Massachusetts

Preface

The human brain has been a mystery for thousands of years. The brain was first described by the ancient Egyptians in 3000 BC in the Edwin Smith Papyrus, where detailed examination, diagnosis, treatment, and prognosis of 48 surgical cases involving the central nervous system.[1,2] Despite these early accounts, the brain was originally not considered a "special" organ.[3-5] Ancient Egyptians used the transnasal exenteration technique for removal of the brain through the nostril during their mummification process.[2,6] In the Western Hemisphere, the first evidence of trepanation on a living person as a neurosurgical procedure was performed in the Ancient Pre-Columbian Peruvian era dating back to 400 BC. Aristotle, in 335 BC, believed that the brain functioned as a cooling agent for the heart, and believed that thought came from the heart.[3-5] However, during this same time period, with observation, the functions of the brain were becoming more elucidated. Galen hypothesized that the brain was responsible for thought based on the consequences of people he observed with head injuries.[3-5] Hippocrates observed epilepsy cases and believed these events were due to disturbances in the brain, and that the brain was the seat of intelligence.[3-5] Plato, in 387 BC, believed that the brain was the center of mental processes; and Herophilus, in 300 BC, believed that the ventricles were the seat of human intelligence.[3-5]

Human cadaveric dissection led to improved knowledge of the brain. In the 1500s, Leonardo da Vinci produced wax casts of the human ventricles, Vesalius (1543) described the pineal gland, and Varolio (1573) described the brainstem.[3-5] In the 1600s, Thomas Willis described the vascular anatomy, cranial nerves, and the function of choroid plexus in producing cerebrospinal fluid.[3-5] Carl Wernicke in 1874 described different types of aphasias, and Sir Victor Horsley published the somatotopic map of the monkey motor cortex.[3-5] These advances led to intraoperative understanding of the human brain. In 1909, Harvey Cushing was the first to stimulate the human sensory cortex, and, the same year, Brodmann was able to describe 52 discrete cortical areas of the brain.[3-5] Walter Dandy used air to elucidate the ventricles in 1918. From their work with electrical stimulation in 1957, Penfield and Rasmussen provided illustrations of the motor and sensory homunculus.[3-5]

The history of electrical brain stimulation is equally interesting. In 1791, Luis Galvani discovered that the nerves and muscles were excitable when he applied electricity to spinal nerves and elicited muscle contractions in frogs.[7] Giovanni Aldini applied electrical currents to recently hanged and decapitated prisoners and erroneously thought he was stimulating the brain and spinal cord to induce movement, but it was concluded that he was actually directly stimulating the muscles.[7] Luigi Rolando and Pierre Flourens then used electrical stimulation to study brain localization of function. Rolando mistakenly concluded, based on stimulation, that the cerebellum was the source of limb movements.[7] Even though they were erroneous, they indirectly showed that the central nervous system was excitable.[7] The pioneering work of mapping the cortex with electrical stimulation was done in 1870s by Eduard Hitzig and Gustav Fritsch, where they stimulated the cortex of dogs and were able to obtain contralateral movement of the face and limbs.[7] They were also able to decipher that movement occurred in hindlimbs with more medial stimulation, while forelimb movement occurred with more lateral stimulation.[7] Based on this work, they were able to devise a somatotopic organization of the brain of dogs.[7] This led to David Ferrier's work in 1875 where he was able to map 29 different cortical functions in dogs and monkeys.[7]

The history of mapping the human brain, however, is more recent.[7] This is mainly due to centuries of the human brain being thought of as "no man's land" because of religious and medical ideologies, as well as the high morbidity and mortality associated with surgery in this area.[7] Sir Charles Scott Sherrington and Harvey Cushing extensively mapped the cortex of great apes in 1901, which led to studies in humans. Roberts Batholow stimulated the cortex from a patient with skull erosion down to the dura, and was able to induce contralateral limb movement.[7] Krause stimulated patients' brain and obtained the same localization as previously performed in animal experiments.[7] Wilder Penfield and colleagues at the Montreal Neurological Institute proved this more conclusively when they devised the motor and sensory homunculus.[7] At a similar time, Sir Victor Horsley and Robert Clarke were able to map the effects of stimulating deep-seated structures (i.e., limbic system, basal ganglia, thalamus) using a cartesian coordinate system.[7] In the 1940s, Lars Leksell developed stereotactic devices, which allowed for the study of lesioning, including the globus pallidus, basal ganglia, and other deep-seated areas.[7]

The use of electrical stimulation is now commonplace for a variety of both cortical and subcortical intracranial lesions.[8-10] In cortical areas, electrical stimulation is designed to identify motor and somatosensory cortices, language regions including Broca's and Wernicke's, as well as visual cortex, seizure foci, and cognitive function, among others.[8-10] In subcortical areas, electrical stimulation is designed to identify different white matter tracts including projection (i.e., corticospinal tract), commissural (i.e., corpus callosum), and association fibers (i.e., superior longitudinal fasciculus, arcuate fasciculus, inferior frontal occipital fasciculus, inferior longitudinal fasciculus), among others.[8-10] In meta-analyses, the use of electrical stimulation has been shown to improve extent of resection (gross total resection: 75% vs. 58%) and reduce neurological deficits (3.4% vs. 8.2%).[8] We have shown similar results with regional vs. general anesthesia for peri-Rolandic tumors in regards to achieving gross total resection (25.9% vs. 6.5%, p = 0.04) and decreased hospital stay (4.2 vs. 7.9 days, p = 0.049).[9] In addition, we have showed decreased cost, increased quality of life, and improved postoperative neurological function for patients who undergo awake surgery with brain mapping as compared to those under general anesthesia.[10]

The human brain is perhaps the most complex of organs. While it accounts for only 2% of the body's total weight, it demands at least 20% of the body's total energy.[11,12] Furthermore, the average brain only weighs three pounds, yet it is estimated to have roughly 86 billion neurons and glial cells that are in constant communication.[11,12] Through patch clamping techniques, it is well understood that neurons transmit information via action potentials that have been recorded to travel at an impressive 268 miles per hour.[13] The complexity of billions of neurons interacting to create over 100 trillion neural connections to define eloquent areas of the brain has made brain mapping a very appealing and challenging topic for neuroscientists and neurosurgeons alike.[14]

In brain tumor surgery, it is becoming well established that increasing extent of resection without developing a neurological deficit is associated with improved outcomes.[15–23] There have been several surgical developments to facilitate extent of resection including, but not limited to, intraoperative MRI, fluorescence-guided surgery, surgical navigation, and augmented reality.[24] In addition, there have been developments in imaging techniques to identify eloquent cortical areas and subcortical white matter tracts including functional MRI, diffusion tensor imaging, and magnetoencephalography, among others.[25] Despite these advances, the only way of obtaining real-time information about critical cortical and subcortical areas with high sensitivity and specificity is brain mapping.[26,27]

This book will serve as a comprehensive overview of the critical aspects of brain mapping from international experts. It will be divided into three sections. The first section will cover the preoperative aspects of brain mapping surgery. The second will feature aspects of brain mapping surgery. The third section will be on postoperative care after brain mapping surgery. In the first section, a review of the history of brain mapping will be given, as well as the anatomy of the eloquent cortical and subcortical regions. In addition, the various preoperative imaging techniques for identifying eloquent regions will be discussed including direct and indirect functional mapping, neurophysiology, and extra operative brain mapping. The second section will be devoted to what occurs in the operating room. It will describe anesthesia requirements, operating room setup, and awake and asleep brain mapping of the different cortical and subcortical regions. The last section will feature rehabilitation, neuroplasticity, and postoperative adjuvant therapy. We hope you enjoy this book as much as we enjoyed putting this book together with experts in the field in order to provide a comprehensive text for surgeons, residents, fellows, and other health providers interested in brain mapping and surgery in eloquent regions.

Alfredo Quinones-Hinojosa, MD
Kaisorn L. Chaichana, MD
Deependra Mahato, DO, MS

References

[1] Brandt-Rauf PW, Brandt-Rauf SI. History of occupational medicine: relevance of Imhotep and the Edwin Smith papyrus. Br J Ind Med 1987;44(1):68–70

[2] Santoro G, Wood MD, Merlo L, Anastasi GP, Tomasello F, Germanò A. The anatomic location of the soul from the heart, through the brain, to the whole body, and beyond: a journey through Western history, science, and philosophy. Neurosurgery 2009;65(4):633–643, discussion 643

[3] Frati P, Frati A, Salvati M, et al. Neuroanatomy and cadaver dissection in Italy: History, medicolegal issues, and neurosurgical perspectives. J Neurosurg 2006;105(5):789–796

[4] Moon K, Filis AK, Cohen AR. The birth and evolution of neuroscience through cadaveric dissection. Neurosurgery 2010;67(3):799–809, discussion 809–810

[5] Nanda A, Khan IS, Apuzzo ML. Renaissance Neurosurgery: Italy's Iconic Contributions. World Neurosurg 2016;87:647–655

[6] Fanous AA, Couldwell WT. Transnasal excerebration surgery in ancient Egypt. J Neurosurg 2012;116(4):743–748

[7] Sanai N, Berger MS. Surgical oncology for gliomas: the state of the art. Nat Rev Clin Oncol 2018;15(2):112–125

[8] De Witt Hamer PC, Robles SG, Zwinderman AH, Duffau H, Berger MS. Impact of intraoperative stimulation brain mapping on glioma surgery outcome: a meta-analysis. J Clin Oncol 2012;30(20):2559–2565

[9] Eseonu CI, Rincon-Torroella J, ReFaey K, et al. Awake Craniotomy vs Craniotomy Under General Anesthesia for Perirolandic Gliomas: Evaluating Perioperative Complications and Extent of Resection. Neurosurgery 2017;81(3):481–489

[10] Eseonu CI, Rincon-Torroella J, ReFaey K, Quiñones-Hinojosa A. The Cost of Brain Surgery: Awake vs Asleep Craniotomy for Perirolandic Region Tumors. Neurosurgery 2017;81(2):307–314

[11] Azevedo FA, Carvalho LR, Grinberg LT, et al. Equal numbers of neuronal and nonneuronal cells make the human brain an isometrically scaled-up primate brain. J Comp Neurol 2009;513(5):532–541

[12] Chang CY, Ke DS, Chen JY. Essential fatty acids and human brain. Acta Neurol Taiwan 2009;18(4):231–241

[13] Pettersen KH, Hagen E, Einevoll GT. Estimation of population firing rates and current source densities from laminar electrode recordings. J Comput Neurosci 2008;24(3):291–313

[14] Zimmer C. 100 trillion connections. Sci Am 2011;304(1):58–63

[15] Chaichana KL, Cabrera-Aldana EE, Jusue-Torres I, et al. When gross total resection of a glioblastoma is possible, how much resection should be achieved? World Neurosurg 2014;82(1-2):e257–e265

[16] Chaichana KL, Chaichana KK, Olivi A, et al. Surgical outcomes for older patients with glioblastoma multiforme: preoperative factors associated with decreased survival. Clinical article. J Neurosurg 2011;114(3):587–594

[17] Chaichana KL, Garzon-Muvdi T, Parker S, et al. Supratentorial glioblastoma multiforme: the role of surgical resection versus biopsy among older patients. Ann Surg Oncol 2011;18(1):239–245

[18] Chaichana KL, Jusue-Torres I, Navarro-Ramirez R, et al. Establishing percent resection and residual volume thresholds affecting survival and recurrence for patients with newly diagnosed intracranial glioblastoma. Neuro-oncol 2014;16(1):113–122

[19] Chaichana KL, Parker SL, Olivi A, Quiñones-Hinojosa A. Long-term seizure outcomes in adult patients undergoing primary resection of malignant brain astrocytomas. Clinical article. J Neurosurg 2009;111(2):282–292

[20] Chaichana KL, Zadnik P, Weingart JD, et al. Multiple resections for patients with glioblastoma: prolonging survival. . J Neurosurg 2013;118(4):812–820

[21] McGirt MJ, Chaichana KL, Attenello FJ, et al. Extent of surgical resection is independently associated with survival in patients with hemispheric infiltrating low-grade gliomas. Neurosurgery 2008;63(4):700–707, author reply 707–708

[22] McGirt MJ, Chaichana KL, Gathinji M, et al. Independent association of extent of resection with survival in patients with malignant brain astrocytoma. J Neurosurg 2009;110(1):156–162

[23] McGirt MJ, Mukherjee D, Chaichana KL, Than KD, Weingart JD, Quinones-Hinojosa A. Association of surgically acquired motor and language deficits on overall survival after resection of glioblastoma multiforme. Neurosurgery 2009;65(3):463–469, discussion 469–470

[24] Garzon-Muvdi T, Kut C, Li X, Chaichana KL. Intraoperative imaging techniques for glioma surgery. Future Oncol 2017;13(19):1731–1745

[25] Sternberg EJ, Lipton ML, Burns J. Utility of diffusion tensor imaging in evaluation of the peritumoral region in patients with primary and metastatic brain tumors. AJNR Am J Neuroradiol 2014;35(3):439–444

[26] Duffau H. Long-term outcomes after supratotal resection of diffuse low-grade gliomas: a consecutive series with 11-year follow-up. Acta Neurochir (Wien) 2016;158(1):51–58

[27] Duffau H, Mandonnet E. The "onco-functional balance" in surgery for diffuse low-grade glioma: integrating the extent of resection with quality of life. Acta Neurochir (Wien) 2013;155(6):951–957

Video Contents

Video 6.1 Video showing a high-density circular grid for neuro-intraoperative monitoring and afterdischarge detection during electrocortical stimulation

Video 9.1 Case Presentation 1: Left frontal/insular awake craniotomy with cortical and subcortical mapping and neuromonitoring using the circular grid

Video 9.2 Case Presentation 2: Left-sided awake craniotomy for temporal lobectomy and speech mapping

Video 10.1 Preoperative scalp block

Video 12.1 Awake motor mapping technique—An illustrative case video

Video 14.1 Awake monitoring of an anterior cingulate glioma surgery

Video 17.1 Intraoperative seizure mapping

Video 18.1 Asleep motor mapping

Contributors

Russell Addeo, PhD, ABPP-CN
Director
Behavioral Medicine
Brooks Rehabilitation
Jacksonville, Florida, USA

Rechdi Ahdab, MD, PhD
Associate Professor
Department of Neurology
Lebanese American University Medical Center, Rizk
  Hospital
Beirut, Lebanon

John P. Andrews, MD
Department of Neurological Surgery
University of California-San Francisco
San Francisco, California, USA

Juan A. Barcia, MD, PhD
Professor and Head
Department of Neurosurgery
Hospital Clínico San Carlos, Universidad Complutense de
  Madrid
Madrid, Spain

Perry Bechtle, DO
Chair, Division of Neurosurgical Anesthesiology
Department of Anesthesiology and Perioperative Medicine
Mayo Clinic
Jacksonville, Florida, USA

Mitchel S. Berger, MD, FACS, FAANS
Berthold and Belle N. Guggenhime Professor
Chairman, Department of Neurological Surgery
Director, Brain Tumor Center
University of California, San Francisco
San Francisco, California, USA

Elird Bojaxhi, MD
Assistant Professor
Department of Anesthesiology and Perioperative Medicine
Mayo Clinic
Jacksonville, Florida, USA

Antonio Cesar de Melo Mussi, MD, PhD
Staff Neurosurgeon
Department of Neurosurgery
Hospital Governador Celso Ramos
Florianopolis, SC, Brazil

Kaisorn L. Chaichana, MD
Consultant Neurosurgeon and Associate Professor of
  Neurosurgery
Department of Neurosurgery
Mayo Clinic
Jacksonville, Florida, USA

Sarah Chamberlin, MSOT, OTR/L
Occupational Therapist
Brain Injury Program
Brooks Rehabilitation Hospital
Jacksonville, Florida, USA

Edward F. Chang, MD
Professor
Department of Neurological Surgery
University of California, San Francisco
San Francisco, California, USA

Shao-Ching Chen, MD
Attending Physician
Division of General Neurosurgery, Neurological Institute
Taipei Veterans General Hospital
Taipei, Taiwan

D. Ceri Davies, PhD
Professor
Human Anatomy Unit
Department of Surgery and Cancer
Imperial College London
London, United Kingdom

Andrea J. Davis, MSN, RN, NE-BC, CRRN, CBIS
Certified Rehabilitation Specialist
Orange Park Inpatient Rehabilitation
Orange Park, Florida, USA
Adjunct Clinical Faculty
School of Nursing
Brooks College of Health
University of North Florida
Jacksonville, Florida, USA

Hugues Duffau, MD, PhD
Professor and Chairman
Department of Neurosurgery
University of Montpellier
Montpellier, France

Christine Edwards, MS
Deakin University PhD Candidate
Mayo Visiting Graduate Student
Deakin University School of Engineering
Mayo Clinic Graduate School of Biomedical Sciences
Rochester, Minnesota, USA

Kathleen H. Elverman, PhD
Aurora Neuroscience Innovation Institute
Aurora St. Luke's Medical Center
Milwaukee, Wisconsin, USA

Sanjeet S. Grewal, MD
Department of Neurologic Surgery
Mayo Clinic
Jacksonville, Florida, USA

Vivek Gupta, MD
Assistant Professor and Consultant Neuroradiologist
Department of Radiology
Mayo Clinic Florida
Jacksonville, Florida, USA

N. U. Farrukh Hameed, MBBS, MCh
Research Fellow, PhD Candidate
Department of Neurosurgery
Huashan Hospital
Fudan University
Shanghai, China

Tasneem F. Hasan, MD, MPH, CPH
Resident Physician
Department of Neurology
Ochsner Louisiana State University Health Sciences Center
Shreveport, Louisiana, USA

Shawn Hervey-Jumper, MD
Associate Professor
Department of Neurosurgery
University of California San Francisco
San Francisco, California, USA

Alison U. Ho, DO
Neurosurgery Resident
Department of Neurosurgery
Desert Regional Medical Center
Palm Springs, California, USA

George I. Jallo, MD
Director, Institute for Brain Protection Sciences
Professor of Neurosurgery, Pediatrics and Oncology
Department of Pediatric Neurosurgery
Johns Hopkins All Children's Hospital
St. Petersburg, Florida, USA

Emily L. Johnson, MD
Assistant Professor
Department of Neurology
Johns Hopkins School of Medicine
Baltimore, Maryland, USA

Matthew A. Kirkman, FRCS, MEd
Specialty Registrar in Neurosurgery
Victor Horsley Department of Neurosurgery
The National Hospital for Neurology and Neurosurgery
Queen Square
London, United Kingdom

Abbas Z. Kouzani, PhD
Professor
Department of Engineering
Deakin University
Geelong, Victoria, Australia

Kendall H. Lee, MD, PhD
Director, Neural Engineering Laboratories
Professor of Neurologic Surgery
Professor of Physiology
Department of Neurologic Surgery
Director, Mayo Clinic MD/PhD Program
Mayo Clinic
Rochester, Minnesota, USA

Deependra Mahato, DO, MS
Attending Neurosurgeon
Neurological Surgery Residency Program
Riverside University Health System
Moreno Valley, California, USA

Lina Marenco-Hillembrand, MD
Research Fellow
Department of Neurosurgery
Mayo Clinic
Jacksonville, Florida, USA

Erik H. Middlebrooks, MD
Associate Professor
Departments of Radiology and Neurosurgery
Mayo Clinic Florida
Jacksonville, Florida, USA

Jodi Morgan, MA CCC-SLP
Brooks Rehabilitation Aphasia Center Manager and Clinical
  Assistant Professor
Communication Science Disorder
Jacksonville University
Jacksonville, Florida, USA

Kenneth Ngo, MD
Medical Director, Brain Injury Program
Associate Medical Director, BRH
Brooks Rehabilitation
Jacksonville, Florida, USA

Kyle Noll, PhD
Assistant Professor
Department of Neuro-Oncology
The University of Texas M.D. Anderson Cancer Center
Houston, Texas, USA

Cristina Nombela, RPsy, PhD
Clinical Psychologist
Department of Neurosurgery
Hospital Clínico San Carlos, Universidad Complutense de
  Madrid
Madrid, Spain

Mohammad Hassan A. Noureldine, MD, MSc
Postdoctoral Research Fellow
Department of Neurosurgery
Johns Hopkins University School of Medicine
Institute for Brain Protection Sciences
Johns Hopkins All Children's Hospital
St. Petersburg, Florida, USA

Evandro de Oliveira, MD, PhD
Adjunct Professor of Neurological Surgery
Mayo Clinic
Jacksonville, Florida, USA

Courtney Pendleton, MD
Fellow
Department of Neurosurgery
Mayo Clinic
Rochester, Minnesota, USA

Wang Peng, MD
Resident
Department of Neurosurgery
Huashan Hospital, Fudan University
Shanghai, China

María Pérez-Garoz, RPsy, MSc
Neuropsychologist
Department of Neurosurgery
Hospital Clínico San Carlos, Universidad Complutense de
  Madrid
Madrid, Spain

Jennifer L. Peterson, MD
Associate Professor
Department of Radiation Oncology
Mayo Clinic
Jacksonville, Florida, USA

Karim ReFaey, MD
Postdoctoral Fellow
Department of Neurosurgery
Mayo Clinic
Jacksonville, Florida, USA

Eva K. Ritzl, MD, MBA, FRCP (Glasgow)
Associate Professor of Neurology
Director, Intraoperative Neuromonitoring
Director, Continuous-video-EEG Monitoring
Johns Hopkins University and Johns Hopkins Hospital
Baltimore, Maryland, USA

Erika Ross, PhD
Neuroscience Director
Department of Neuroscience
Cala Health
Burlingame, California, USA

Henry Ruiz-Garcia, MD
Post-Doctoral Research Fellow
Department of Radiation Oncology
Mayo Clinic
Jacksonville, Florida, USA

Vicent Quilis-Quesada, MD, PhD
Neurosurgeon
Department of Neurosurgery
University Clinic Hospital
Associate Professor of Neuroanatomy
Department of Human Anatomy and Embryology
Faculty of Medicine. University of Valencia
Valencia, Spain
Adjunct Assistant Professor of Neurosurgery
College of Medicine and Science
Mayo Clinic, USA

Alfredo Quinones-Hinojosa, MD
Chair and the William J. and Charles H. Mayo Professor
Department of Neurosurgery
Mayo Clinic
Jacksonville, Florida, USA

David S. Sabsevitz, PhD
Department of Psychology and Psychiatry, Department of
  Neurological Surgery
Mayo Clinic
Jacksonville, Florida, USA

George Samandouras, MD, FRCS
Consultant Neurosurgeon
Victor Horsley Department of Neurosurgery
The National Hospital for Neurology and Neurosurgery
University College London Hospitals NHS Trust
University College London
Institute of Neurology
Queen Square, London, United Kingdom

Nir Shimony, MD
Johns Hopkins University & Medicine
Institute of Brain Protection Sciences
Johns Hopkins All Children's hospital
St. Petersburg, Florida, USA
Assistant Professor
Department of Clinical Sciences - Neurosurgery and
  Neurology
Geisinger Commonwealth School of Medicine
Scranton, Pennsylvania, USA
Assistant Professor
Department of Neurosurgery and Department of Pediatrics
Lewis Katz School of Medicine, Temple University
Philadelphia, Pennsylvania, USA

Javed Siddiqi, HBSc, MD, DPhil (Oxon), FRCSC, FACS, FAANS
Professor & Chair, Department of Surgery, California
  University of Science & Medicine
Chief of Neurosurgery, Arrowhead Regional Medical Center
Colton, California, USA

Michael E. Sughrue, MD
Associate Professor
Department of Neurosurgery
Prince of Wales Private Hospital
Randwick, NSW, Australia

William O. Tatum, DO
Professor
Department of Neurology
Mayo Clinic
Jacksonville, Florida, USA

Daniel M. Trifiletti, MD
Assistant Professor
Department of Radiation Oncology
Department of Neurological Surgery
Mayo Clinic
Jacksonville, Florida, USA

Shashwat Tripathi
Department of Mathematics
University of Texas at Austin
Austin, Texas, USA

Prasanna G. Vibhute, MD
Consultant
Department of Radiology
Mayo Clinic
Jacksonville, Florida, USA

Jennifer Walworth, PT
Physical Therapist
Brain Injury Program
Brooks Rehabilitation Hospital
Jacksonville, Florida, USA

Jeffrey Wefel, PhD
Associate Professor
Department of Neuro-Oncology
The University of Texas M.D. Anderson Cancer Center
Houston, Texas, USA

Jinsong Wu, MD, PhD
Vice Director, Professor, Glioma Surgery Division,
  Department of Neurosurgery, Huashan Hospital,
  Fudan University
Director, Brain Function Laboratory, Neurosurgical Institute
  of Fudan University
Vice Director (Deputy), Huashan Brain Tumor Biobank,
  Neurosurgical Institute of Fudan University
Shanghai, China

Geng Xu, BS
Technician
Surgery Division, Neurosurgery Department
Huashan Hospital
Shanghai Medical College, Fudan University
Shanghai, China

Jie Zhang, MD, PhD
Glioma Doctor
Surgery Division, Neurosurgery Department
Huashan Hospital
Shanghai Medical College, Fudan University
Shanghai, China

Section I

Preoperative Brain Mapping Features

1 The Early History of Intraoperative Brain Mapping

Courtney Pendleton, Kaisorn L. Chaichana, and Alfredo Quinones-Hinojosa

Abstract

Intraoperative brain mapping has become a standard of care in neurosurgery, allowing more aggressive resection of intracranial lesions while preserving eloquent cortex. The development of brain mapping required centuries of work understanding neuroanatomic structures and functional networks, as well as technological developments in the understanding and harnessing of electricity. Combining multiple scientific disciplines allowed early neurosurgeons to introduce brain mapping to the operating room, forming the foundation for contemporary applications.

Keywords: neurosurgery, brain mapping, neural networks, microanatomic structure

1.1 Introduction

The practice of intraoperative brain mapping has become a standard of care across multiple subspecialties within neurosurgery.[1,2,3,4] It allows for safe delineation of eloquent cortex in awake and asleep patients intraoperatively and provides ways to monitor electrical function and networks in epilepsy patients in and out of the operating room. The multitude of devices available to the contemporary neurosurgeon for brain mapping, including bipolar and unipolar stimulation, and strip and grid electrodes, allow for a broadly stocked armamentarium.

Cartography relies on a general understanding of the environment in question, and brain mapping developed only after centuries of painstaking work elucidating the gross and microanatomic structures of the brain, the role of specialized cells in creating and maintaining neural networks, and the role of functional localization in organizing the brain into interlinked eloquent regions.[2]

1.2 Neuroanatomic Basis of Brain Mapping

At the heart of intraoperative neural mapping is the concept of functional localization, which relies on a thorough understanding of the micro- and macrostructure of the human brain. The work of Camille Golgi and Santiago Ramon y Cajal played a pivotal role in delineating individual neural cell characteristics and localizing specific cell types to certain anatomic regions.[5] Foster and Sherrington further expanded on this and coined the term "synapse" in describing how certain neurons communicate with one another.[6]

From the microscopic staining of individual neurons, neuroanatomists began to understand the functional implications of these specialized cell clusters, leading to descriptions of motor and sensory cortices, as well as deep white matter tracts. The presence of white matter tracts was described by Vesalius in his anatomic dissections, and further delineated by Willis, with some of the preeminent dissections done by Josef Klingler.[7] The functional implications of these tracts were elucidated with Cajal's studies on neural connections.[8] Clinical observations coupled with intraoperative and postmortem examination of the brain allowed surgeons and researchers to begin the process of functional localization. Paul Broca offered multiple lectures and publications describing the location of injury in patients with deficits in speech production, which have been recently revalidated using magnetic resonance imaging (MRI) of the particular patients' brains, although the involved area was found to extend beyond the bounds Broca noted in his studies.[9] Wernicke published the results of his case series of receptive aphasia,[10] localizing the sensory component of language function.

Fritsch and Hitzig were credited with the first use of intraoperative electrical stimulation of the cortex, using bipolar electrodes and galvanic current during canine motor mapping experiments.[11] The motor mapping was first used in the human brain a few years later.[1,12]

Hitzig's canine experiments led him to theorize that the motor cortex remained anterior to the central sulcus. However, experiments by Horsley and Ferrier demonstrated motor responses with stimulation of the postcentral gyrus, and the division of the cortex into motor and sensory regions was bitterly contested, with Sir Victor Horsley maintaining the motor–sensory cortex was intertwined along the central sulcus, and studies by Sherrington and Cushing demonstrating separate sensory and motor cortices divided by the central sulcus.[1,13] One of Sherrington's students, Alfred Campbell, combined information from the cytoarchitecture of the pre- and postcentral gyri with cortical stimulation results, and concluded that the high concentration of motor-associated Betz cells in the precentral region indicated the "motor center" resided solely in this region.[14] Horsley maintained that his experimental intraoperative mapping deviated from models based on chimpanzee mapping experiments, going so far as to deliver the Linacre Lecture in 1909, titled "The Function of the So-Called Motor Cortex."[15] This report described clinical observations in patients without intraoperative mapping, as well as intraoperative findings of a patient undergoing bipolar electrode stimulation for mapping, with subsequent resection of "motor" cortex resulting in combined sensorimotor deficit. These findings placed Horsley in direct opposition to the theories proposed by Sherrington and Cushing, with a narrow motor strip anterior to the central sulcus. This controversy was compounded further in that structures seen in chimpanzee models were notably absent in human brain studies. It was not until Penfield's later work delineating our contemporary notion of the homunculus, as well as the work of Woolsey regarding the associated supplemental cortices, that the boundaries of motor and sensory cortices were more fully understood.[16]

1.3 Development of Mechanisms for Mapping Techniques

Understanding of electricity in the natural world is a longstanding phenomenon. Its role in medical therapy was

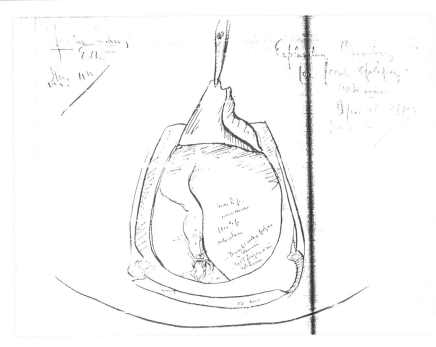

Fig. 1.1 Motor cortex in intraoperative mapping procedure. Labels from top to bottom: bottom lip, [illegible], upper lip, orbicularis, thumb and index fingers in extension, 3rd-5th fingers in extension.

described as early as ancient Rome, where shocks from stepping on electricity-generating fish were used to alleviate peripheral symptoms of gout.[17] From Benjamin Franklin's experiments with kites and keys, through the work of Volta, Ampere, Faraday, and Galvani, the understanding of how to produce, contain, and control electricity evolved over the 18th and 19th centuries. While Volta demonstrated the first device to produce large-scale electric current in 1800, it was Faraday's development of an electromagnetic induction coil in 1831 that laid the groundwork for generating electric currents on demand in the operating room.

Once introduced to the operating room, brain mapping and stimulation was accomplished with either faradic or galvanic current via rudimentary unipolar instruments. The split between faradic and galvanic current echoes the controversies brewing between Nikolai Tesla and Thomas Edison at the turn of the century. Faradic devices rely on high-frequency alternating currents, while galvanic devices employ lower frequency interrupted direct currents. In Penfield's experiments, faradic current was used to replicate seizure activity, while galvanic current was used for mapping of the sensorimotor cortex.

1.4 Review of Historical Applications

As in contemporary neurosurgery, the historical applications of brain mapping ran the gamut, and included resection of epileptogenic foci, sectioning of subcortical white matter tracts, and delineation of neoplasms to enable safe resection while sparing eloquent cortex.

Cortical mapping was utilized in epilepsy surgery in the late 19th century, with direct stimulation used to determine epileptogenic foci. Hadra's publication described the difficulty of epilepsy mapping given overlap and redundancy within functional

cortex, and emphasized that the role of mapping in these cases is not solely to locate the motor cortex associated with symptoms, but "to use the induced current … to find the spot from where an epileptic attack of the same nature the patient is accustomed to suffer from can be started."[18] In 1888, Keen described the use of cortical mapping to resect the "hand center" in a patient with intractable epilepsy by employing bipolar faradic stimulation of both cortex and subcortical white matter following his cortical resection.[19] Cushing spent time working with Sherrington, and brought his techniques for cortical mapping back to his practice in Baltimore. His intraoperative use of faradic stimulation demonstrated postcentral sensory cortex, and what he coined as the *narrow motor strip* within the precentral cortex (▶ Fig. 1.1, ▶ Fig. 1.2). Cushing reported his intraoperative sensory mapping in patients with epilepsy and used intraoperative cortical mapping in nearly 50 cases of epilepsy, tumor resection, and trauma with glial scarring or encephalomalacia.[1]

1.5 Looking Forward

Despite significant limitations in available technology, early neuroanatomists, neurologists, and neurosurgeons were able to advance our understanding of functional localization within the human brain, laying the groundwork for more advanced neuromonitoring and intraoperative mapping techniques. While brain mapping is currently considered standard of care in neuro-oncologic and functional surgery, a review of the history of the field demonstrates the tremendous advances in knowledge and technology that have been made since the early days of the special field of neurosurgery. The future of mapping is here and includes more precise preoperative functional imaging, which is then translated into the operating room where we are beginning to be more precise with our ability to identify areas of abnormal functional activity in patients with epilepsy

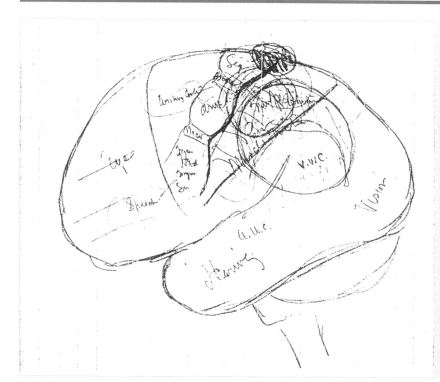

Fig. 1.2 Motor cortex mapping intraoperatively, with additional functional localization notations based on prior publications and Cushing's own intraoperative and laboratory-based observations. Motor areas from top to bottom: leg, arms, neck, face, head, tongue, and eye. Frontal lobe regions for eye movement and speech labeled, temporal region for hearing labeled, and occipital region for vision cortex labeled.

and/or tumors, among others.[20,21] Our ability to map the brain is allowing us to do more precise resections of lesions as well as understand plasticity and functions of the human brain so we can increase our capacity to regenerate following injury.

References

[1] Pendleton C, Zaidi HA, Chaichana KL, et al. Harvey Cushing's contributions to motor mapping: 1902–1912. Cortex. 2012; 48(1):7–14

[2] Eseonu CI, Rincon-Torroella J, ReFaey K, et al. Awake craniotomy vs craniotomy under general anesthesia for perirolandic gliomas: evaluating perioperative complications and extent of resection. Neurosurgery. 2017; 81(3):481–489

[3] Eseonu CI, Rincon-Torroella J, Lee YM, ReFaey K, Tripathi P, Quinones-Hinojosa A. Intraoperative seizures in awake craniotomy for perirolandic glioma resections that undergo cortical mapping. J Neurol Surg A Cent Eur Neurosurg. 2018; 79(3):239–246

[4] Quiñones-Hinojosa A, Lyon R, Du R, Lawton MT. Intraoperative motor mapping of the cerebral peduncle during resection of a midbrain cavernous malformation: technical case report. Neurosurgery. 2005; 56(2) Suppl:E439–, discussion E439

[5] Zamora-Berridi GJ, Pendleton C, Ruiz G, Cohen-Gadol AA, Quiñones-Hinojosa A. Santiago Ramón y Cajal and Harvey Cushing: two forefathers of neuroscience and neurosurgery. World Neurosurg. 2011; 76(5):466–476

[6] Foster M, Sherrington CS. A Textbook of Physiology. London: Macmillan; 1897

[7] Agrawal A, Kapfhamer JP, Kress A, et al. Josef Klingler's models of white matter tracts: influences on neuroanatomy, neurosurgery, and neuroimaging. Neurosurgery. 2011; 69(2):238–254

[8] Cajal S. The Croonian lecture: la fine structure des centres nerveux. Proc R Soc Lond. 1894; 55:444–468

[9] Dronkers NF, Plaisant O, Iba-Zizen MT, Cabanis EA. Paul Broca's historic cases: high resolution MR imaging of the brains of Leborgne and Lelong. Brain. 2007; 130(Pt 5):1432–1441

[10] Wernicke C. The aphasic symptom complex: a psychological study on an anatomical basis. Arch Neurol. 1970; 22(3):280–282

[11] Fritsch G, Hitzig E. Ueber die elektrische Erregbarkeit des Groshirns. Arch Anat Physiol Wissenschaftl Med. 1870; 37:300–332

[12] Bartholow R. Experimental investigations into the functions of the human brain. Am J Med Sci. 1874(67):305–315

[13] Grunbaum A, Sherrington CS. Observations on the physiology of the cerebral cortex of some of the higher apes. (Preliminary communication.). Proc R Soc Lond. 1901; 69:206–209

[14] Campbell AW. The localization of cerebral function. Cambridge University Press, 1905.Cushing H. A note upon the faradic stimulation of the postcentral gyrus in conscious patients. Brain. 1909; 32:44–53

[15] Horsley V. The function of the so-called motor area of the brain (Linacre lecture). BMJ. 1909; 11:125–132

[16] Woolsey CN, Settlage PH, Meyer DR, Sencer W, Pinto Hamuy T, Travis AM. Patterns of localization in precentral and "supplementary" motor areas and their relation to the concept of a premotor area. Res Publ Assoc Res Nerv Ment Dis. 1952; 30:238–264

[17] Gildenberg PL. Evolution of neuromodulation. Stereotact Funct Neurosurg. 2005; 83(2)(-)(3):71–79

[18] Hadra BE. VII. An improved method of brain localization in epilepsy. Ann Surg. 1894; 19(2):212–222

[19] Keen W. Three successful cases of cerebral surgery. Am J Med Sci. 1888; 96 (5):452–464

[20] Hua J, Miao X, Agarwal S, et al. Language mapping using T2-prepared BOLD functional MRI in the presence of large susceptibility artifacts - initial results in patients with brain tumor and epilepsy. Tomography. 2017; 3(2):105–113

[21] Feyissa AM, Worrell GA, Tatum WO, et al. High-frequency oscillations in awake patients undergoing brain tumor-related epilepsy surgery. Neurology. 2018; 90(13):e1119–e1125

2 Anatomy of Eloquent Cortical Brain Regions

Antonio Cesar de Melo Mussi and Evandro de Oliveira

Abstract

We review the anatomy of eloquent cortical brain regions. Eloquent cortical areas are areas of the cortex that if removed may result in loss of linguistic ability, motor function, or sensory perception. These areas commonly include the precentral gyrus (primary motor cortex), postcentral gyrus (primary sensory cortex), supplementary motor area (speech and motor function), the perisylvian area (language), medial occipital lobe (primary visual cortex), and medial temporal lobe (memory). The localization of function in certain anatomical cortical regions, such as Broca area, is variable among individuals and the surgeon depends upon cortical stimulation and cortical mapping to correlate function and anatomy with certainty. However, knowledge of the anatomy of the sulci and gyri of the brain is helpful in planning stimulation, tumor resection, understanding tumor extensions, and correlating the findings of the magnetic resonance imaging with the operative field. We review the anatomy of the sulci and gyri of the cerebrum and divide it into seven lobes: frontal, central (precentral, postcentral, and paracentral gyri), parietal, occipital, temporal, insular, and limbic.

Keywords: cortical anatomy, sulci and gyri, motor cortex, opercula, insula, frontal lobe, central lobe, parietal lobe, limbic lobe

2.1 Introduction

Eloquent cortical areas are areas of the cortex that if removed may result in loss of linguistic ability, motor function, or sensory perception. These areas commonly include the precentral gyrus (primary motor cortex), postcentral gyrus (primary sensory cortex), supplementary motor area (speech and motor function), perisylvian area (language), medial occipital lobe (primary visual cortex), and medial temporal lobe (memory). Eloquent cortical area will depend also on whether the area is in the dominant hemisphere, as in the case of speech areas. Although the whole cortex may be regarded as eloquent if we consider function, we use the term eloquent to distinguish specific areas of the brain that carry a higher risk of morbidity and disability in the postoperative period.

The localization of function and certain anatomical cortical regions, such as Broca area, is variable among individuals and the surgeon depends upon cortical stimulation and cortical mapping to correlate function and anatomy with certainty.[1] Localization of function cannot depend only on anatomical landmarks. However, knowledge of the anatomy of the sulci and gyri of the brain provides the surgeon with several key elements to plan procedures.[2,3,4,5] First, understanding the relation of the tumors with the sulci and gyri is helpful in planning the craniotomy for tumor resection.[2] Second, tumor location and extensions are often correlated with the anatomy of the gyri, as tumors are often located in a specific gyrus or lobe, and tumors are known to extend depending on the cytoarchitecture of the area where they originated.[4] Examples are tumors extending in

the limbic lobe and tumors commonly spreading from the opercula to the insula. Third, there is a relationship between brain structure and brain function that allows the surgeon to plan in advance which intraoperative monitoring may be necessary for specific brain regions.[1,6,7,8]

The cerebrum is commonly divided into five lobes: frontal, temporal, parietal, occipital, and insula. Yasargil[4] proposed a division into seven cerebral lobes: frontal, central (precentral, postcentral, and paracentral gyri), parietal, occipital, temporal, insular, and limbic. Yasargil's division was a surgical conception of the cerebrum, taking in consideration function and the embryological aspects of cortical organization. We follow Yasargil's division, since this separates the central lobe in a distinct lobe, highlighting its importance as the primary sensory–motor area. We discuss the anatomy of the opercula and the insula as we review the anatomy of the Sylvian fissure. We review the anatomy of the cortical arteries as they relate to the sulci and gyri.

Although there is great variation in the anatomy of the sulci and gyri among individuals, there is a common pattern in the organization of the sulci and gyri of the cerebrum that can be recognized and studied.[3,4,5] Only four sulci are consistently uninterrupted: the Sylvian fissure, the collateral sulcus, the callosal sulcus, and the parieto-occipital sulcus. The central sulcus and the calcarine sulcus are uninterrupted in 92% of the cases.[4,5] Because most of the sulci are interrupted, the anatomical boundaries of the gyri are not always clearly demarcated. Often, we consider a gyrus as areas of the brain consisting of several gyri, as in the case of the paracentral and medial frontal gyri. One gyrus may be continuous in another surface of the hemisphere: the inferior temporal gyrus (both lateral and basal surface of the temporal lobe) with the parahippocampal gyrus (both medial and basal surface of the temporal lobe).

2.2 Central Lobe

The central lobe is formed by the precentral and postcentral gyri on the lateral surface and by the paracentral lobule on the medial surface of the hemisphere.[3,4,8]

2.2.1 Lateral Surface

The central lobe on the lateral surface of the hemisphere includes the precentral and postcentral gyri, divided by the central sulcus (▸ Fig. 2.1). The central lobe is one of the most important eloquent area of the brain, as it corresponds to the primary motor (precentral gyrus) and sensory (postcentral gyrus) area of the cortex. The anterior and posterior limits of the central lobule are the precentral and postcentral sulci, respectively. The central sulcus originates at the medial hemisphere and runs on the lateral surface from a posterior to an anterior direction toward the Sylvian fissure (▸ Fig. 2.1). The central sulcus usually does not reach the Sylvian fissure and it is separated from the fissure by a continuation of the precentral gyrus with the postcentral gyrus, called subcentral gyrus.

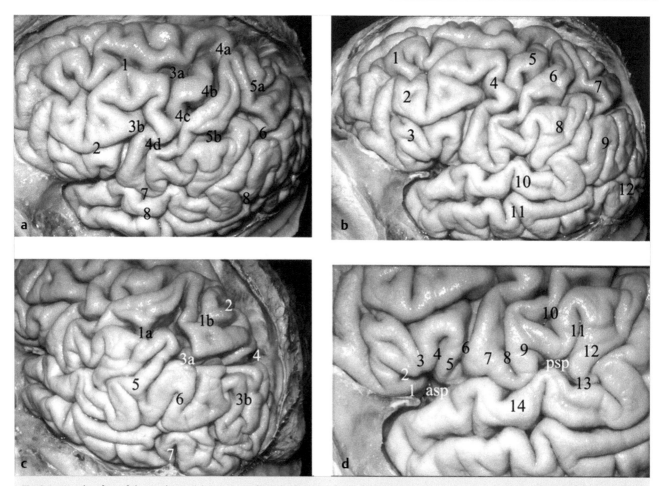

Fig. 2.1 Lateral surface of the cerebrum. **(a)** 1, Superior frontal sulcus. 2, Inferior frontal sulcus. 3a, Superior part of the precentral sulcus. 3b, Inferior part of the precentral sulcus. 4a, Superior curve of the central sulcus. 4b, Middle loop of the central sulcus. 4c, Inferior curve of the central sulcus. 4d, Inferior part of the central sulcus. 5a, Superior part of the postcentral sulcus. 5b, Inferior part of the postcentral sulcus. 6, Intraparietal sulcus. 7, Sylvian fissure. 8, Superior temporal sulcus. **(b)** 1, Superior frontal gyrus. 2, Middle frontal gyrus. 3, Inferior frontal gyrus. 4, Connection of the middle frontal gyrus with the precentral gyrus. 5, Precentral gyrus. 6, Postcentral gyrus. 7, Superior parietal lobule. 8, Supramarginal gyrus. 9, Angular gyrus. 10, Superior temporal gyrus. 11, Middle temporal gyrus. 12, Occipital lobe. **(c)** Inferior part of the postcentral sulcus. 1b, Superior part of the postcentral sulcus. 2, Superior end of the marginal ramus. 3a, Intraparietal sulcus. 3b, Intraoccipital sulcus. 4, Parieto-occipital sulcus. 5, Supramarginal gyrus around the posterior end of the Sylvian fissure. 6, Angular gyrus around the posterior end of the superior temporal sulcus. 7, Preoccipital notch. **(d)** 1, Pars orbitalis. 2, Horizontal ramus. 3, Pars triangularis. 4, Ascending ramus. 5, Pars opercularis. 6, Precentral sulcus. 7, Precentral gyrus. 8, Central sulcus. 9, Postcentral gyrus. 10, Postcentral sulcus. 11, Posterior ascending ramus of the Sylvian fissure. 12, Supramarginal gyrus. 13, Inferior descending ramus of the Sylvian fissure. 14, Superior temporal gyrus. Asp, anterior Sylvian point; psp, posterior Sylvian point.

Parallel to the central sulcus there are two interrupted sulci, one anterior (the precentral sulcus) and another posterior (the postcentral sulcus). The central sulcus is usually continuous and has a sinusoidal shape with three curves (▸ Fig. 2.2). The first curve is near the midline and here the sulcus has its convexity facing anteriorly. Then it curves again, making the middle genu, with its convexity facing posteriorly. Finally, the third curve has its convexity facing anteriorly. The precentral gyrus has the shape of an inverted Greek letter omega (υ) at the level of the second curve of the central sulcus, where the convexity of the sulcus is facing posteriorly (▸ Fig. 2.2). The omega on the precentral gyrus is where the motor representation of the hand is located.[6] The omega is easily seen on the CT or magnetic resonance imaging (MRI) scans because deeply inside the central sulcus there are two parallel sulci that run toward the base of the central sulcus on the superior and inferior aspects of the omega, giving its shape even in deeper cuts[6] (▸ Fig. 2.2a, b). The omega is also called the central knob. Another important anatomical relationship in this area is that the posterior part of the superior frontal sulcus ends at the level of the omega. After its third curve, the central sulcus continues inferiorly toward the Sylvian fissure in a sinusoidal line.[9,10,11] The part of the precentral gyrus in front of the last segment of the central sulcus is where the motor representation of the tongue is usually located.[9] Also, characteristic is the bifurcation of the superior end of the postcentral sulcus with the marginal ramus of the cingulate gyrus located between this bifurcation[10] (▸ Fig. 2.2).

2.2.2 Medial Surface

On the medial surface of the hemisphere the central lobule has a quadrangular shape and its gyri are called the paracentral

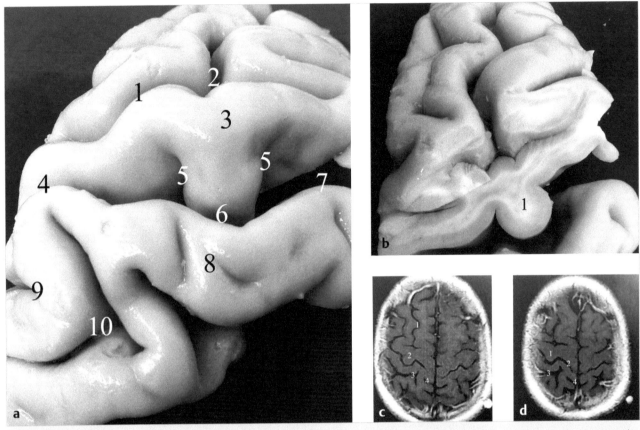

Fig. 2.2 Closer view of the area around the knob of the central sulcus. **(a)** 1, Precentral sulcus. 2, Posterior end of the superior frontal sulcus. 3, Knob of the precentral gyrus. 4, Superior curve of the central sulcus. 5, Longitudinal sulci forming the omega inside the second curve of the central sulcus. 6, Second loop of the central sulcus. 7, Third curve of the central sulcus. 8, Postcentral gyrus. 9, Superior parietal lobule. 10, Intraparietal sulcus. **(b)** 1, Omega (Ω) of the precentral gyrus. **(c)** 1, Superior frontal sulcus. 2, Knob of the precentral gyrus. 3, Superior end of the postcentral sulcus bifurcating around the marginal ramus. 4, Marginal ramus of the cingulate sulcus. **(d)** 1, Knob of the precentral gyrus. 2, Superior loop of the central sulcus. 3, Superior part of the postcentral sulcus. 4, Marginal ramus.

gyrus or lobule (▶ Fig. 2.3). This quadrangular shape is given by the limits of the paracentral gyrus: the cingulate sulcus inferiorly, the paracentral sulcus or ramus anteriorly, and the marginal ramus posteriorly. The paracentral sulcus has an upward direction and it is a sulcus that originates from the cingulate sulcus at the level of the middle of the corpus callosum. The marginal ramus is the posterior part of the cingulate sulcus as it curves upward at the level of the splenium of the corpus callosum. The most posterior part of the marginal ramus near the lateral surface is located at the level of the postcentral gyrus. The marginal ramus can be identified in the MRI in the middle of the bifurcation of the postcentral sulcus. The paracentral gyrus includes the continuation of the precentral and postcentral gyri on the medial surface. The supplementary motor area is an area that does not have clear boundaries, but it includes the paracentral gyrus anterior to the precentral gyrus and the posterior part of the superior frontal gyrus.[12] Stimulation in this area may cause complex postural movement, arrest of movement, or speech arrest. The supplementary area syndrome consists of reversible contralateral weakness and mutism following resection of the dominant supplementary motor area.[12]

2.3 Frontal Lobe

The frontal lobe includes the superior, middle, and inferior frontal gyri on the lateral surface; the orbital and rectus gyrus on the inferior surface; and the medial frontal gyrus on the medial surface of the hemisphere.

2.3.1 Lateral Surface

The frontal lobe on the lateral surface of the hemisphere is limited posteriorly by the precentral sulcus and inferiorly by the Sylvian fissure (▶ Fig. 2.1, ▶ Fig. 2.2, ▶ Fig. 2.3). The frontal lobe is divided by two longitudinal sulci, the superior and inferior frontal sulci, into three gyri, the superior, middle, and inferior frontal gyri. The superior and inferior sulci have an anterior to posterior direction and end at the precentral sulcus. The precentral sulcus is anterior and parallel to the central sulcus. The superior frontal sulcus has its posterior portion near the omega of the precentral gyrus. The superior frontal gyrus runs parallel to the midline, between the interhemispheric fissure and the superior frontal sulcus. The middle frontal gyrus is the most prominent of the frontal gyri, located between the superior

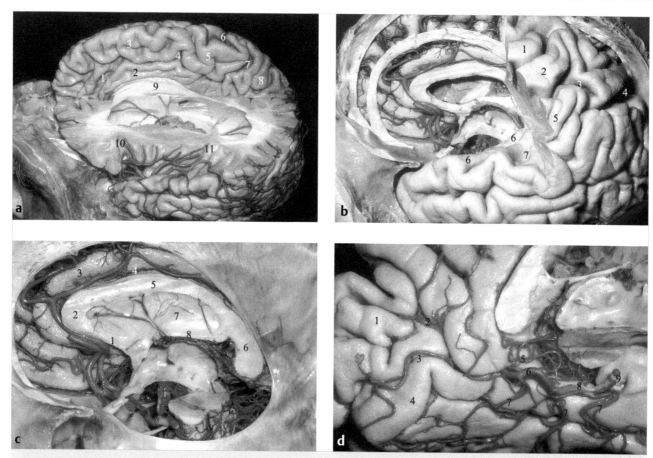

Fig. 2.3 Medial surface of the cerebrum. (a) 1, Cingulate sulcus. 2, Cingulate gyrus. 3, Medial frontal gyrus. 4, Paracentral sulcus. 5, Paracentral lobule. 6, Central sulcus. 7, Marginal ramus of the cingulate sulcus. 8, Precuneus. 9, Body of the corpus callosum. 10, Anterior limiting sulcus of the insula. 11, Heschl gyrus at the posterior part of the insula near the posterior limb of the internal capsule. (b) 1, Knob of the precentral gyrus. 2, Postcentral gyrus. 3, Intraparietal sulcus. 4, Parieto-occipital sulcus. 5, Supramarginal gyrus. 6, Heschl gyrus. 7, Temporal plane. (c) 1, Rostrum of the corpus callosum. 2, Genu of the corpus callosum. 3, Cingulate gyrus. 4, Callosal sulcus. 5, Body of the corpus callosum. 6, Splenium. 7, Septum pellucidum. 8, Fornix. (d) 1, Cuneus. 2, Parieto-occipital sulcus. 3, Calcarine sulcus. 4, Lingual gyrus. 5, Isthmus of the cingulate gyrus. 6, P3 segment of the PCA. 7, Inferior temporal branches of the PCA. 8, P2 P segment. 9, P2A segment at the level of the uncal sulcus.

frontal sulcus and the inferior frontal sulcus. There may be an intermediary sulcus inside the middle frontal gyrus that separates the middle frontal gyrus in two middle frontal gyri. The middle frontal gyrus is continuous with the precentral gyrus. This continuation interrupts the precentral sulcus in two portions, superior and inferior. The continuation of the middle frontal gyrus with the precentral gyrus is used as a landmark for reference in the MRI.[11] The inferior frontal gyrus is located between the inferior frontal sulcus and the Sylvian fissure. The horizontal and ascending rami of the Sylvian fissure give a characteristic shape to the inferior frontal gyrus, dividing it into three portions: pars orbitalis, pars triangularis, and pars opercularis. There may be a sulcus along the pars opercularis, the diagonal sulcus. When it is present, the diagonal sulcus is posterior and parallel to the ascending ramus. Broca speech area consists of pars triangularis and pars opercularis on the dominant hemisphere.[7]

2.3.2 Medial Surface

The frontal lobe in the medial aspect of the hemisphere extends from the paracentral sulcus posteriorly until the cingulate

sulcus inferiorly, forming the anterior surface of the hemisphere until the anterior cranial base. The frontal lobe on the medial aspect is called the medial frontal gyrus and it is a continuation of the superior frontal gyrus on the medial aspect of the hemisphere. Below and in front of the genu of the corpus callosum, the medial frontal gyrus has two small sulci on its surface: the superior and inferior rostral sulci.

2.3.3 Inferior Surface

The inferior surface of the frontal lobe lies over the orbit and has a concave shape to its surface (▶ Fig. 2.4). The inferior surface of the frontal lobe is divided by the olfactory sulcus into a small rectus gyrus medial to the sulcus and a larger area comprising the orbital gyri lateral to the sulcus. The rectus gyrus is continuous on the medial surface of the hemisphere with the medial frontal gyrus. The orbital sulcus is a complex sulcus, resembling the letter "H." This sulcus divides the orbital gyri in four parts: anterior, posterior, medial, and lateral orbital gyri. The lateral and posterior orbital gyri are continuous on the lateral surface with the pars orbitalis of the inferior frontal gyrus.

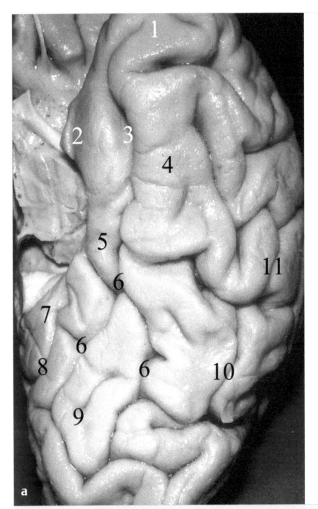 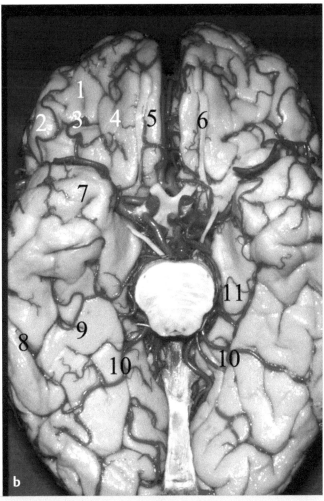

Fig. 2.4 Inferior view of the basal surface of the left temporal lobe. **(a)** 1, Temporal pole. 2, Uncus. 3, Rhinal sulcus continuous with the collateral sulcus. 4, Fusiform gyrus. 5, Parahippocampal gyrus. 6, Collateral sulcus and its bifurcation posteriorly. 7, Isthmus of the cingulate gyrus posterior to the splenium of the corpus callosum. 8, Anterior part of the calcarine sulcus. 9, Lingual gyrus. 10, Occipitotemporal sulcus. 11, Inferior temporal gyrus. **(b)** Inferior view of the basal surface of the frontal and temporal lobe. 1, Anterior orbital gyrus. 2, Lateral orbital gyrus. 3, Orbital sulcus. 4, Medial orbital gyrus. 5, Rectus gyrus. 6, Olfactory tract along the olfactory sulcus. 7, Temporal pole. 8, Occipitotemporal sulcus. 9, Fusiform gyrus. 10, Collateral sulcus. 11, Parahippocampal gyrus.

2.4 Parietal Lobe

The parietal lobe is formed by the superior and inferior parietal lobules on the lateral surface and by the precuneus on the medial side of the hemisphere.

2.4.1 Lateral Surface

The parietal lobe is limited on the lateral surface anteriorly by the postcentral sulcus (▶ Fig. 2.1c). The limit between the parietal lobe and the occipital lobe is an imaginary line, the lateral parietotemporal line. The lateral parietotemporal line runs from the parieto-occipital sulcus to the preoccipital notch. Another imaginary line divides the parietal lobe from the temporal lobe: temporo-occipital line. The temporo-occipital line runs from the end of the Sylvian fissure until it intersects the lateral parieto-occipital line in a right angle.

The postcentral sulcus runs posterior and parallel to the central sulcus. The postcentral sulcus is usually interrupted. The intraparietal sulcus runs posteriorly from the postcentral sulcus on the lateral surface of the parietal lobe in the direction of the occipital lobe. This configuration of the postcentral sulcus and intraparietal sulcus may be compared with a mirror image of the precentral and superior frontal sulcus, considering the central sulcus as the mirror in the middle.

The intraparietal sulcus divides the parietal lobe in two parietal lobules: superior and inferior parietal lobules (▶ Fig. 2.1c). The superior parietal lobule has a quadrangular configuration, limited by the postcentral, intraparietal and the parieto-occipital sulci. The inferior parietal lobule lies below the intraparietal sulcus and it is formed by the supramarginal gyrus and the angular gyrus. The supramarginal gyrus is the gyrus that turns around the posterior end of the Sylvian fissure. The angular gyrus is the gyrus that turns around the posterior end of the superior temporal sulcus.

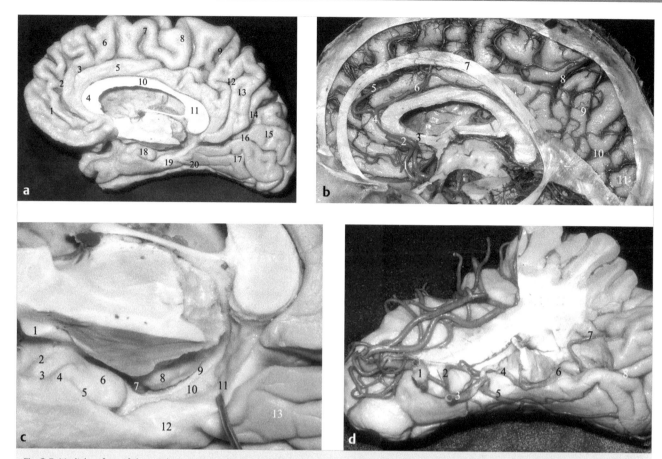

Fig. 2.5 Medial surface of the cerebrum. **(a)** 1, Inferior rostral sulcus. 2, Superior rostral sulcus. 3, Cingulate sulcus. 4, Genu of the corpus callosum. 5, Cingulate gyrus. 6, Medial frontal gyrus. 7, Paracentral sulcus. 8, Paracentral lobule. 9, Marginal ramus of the cingulate sulcus. 10, Body of the corpus callosum. 11, Splenium. 12, Subparietal sulcus. 13, Precuneus. 14, Parieto-occipital sulcus. 15, Cuneus. 16, Calcarine sulcus. 17, Lingual gyrus. 18, Uncus. 19, Parahippocampal gyrus. 20, Collateral sulcus. **(b)** 1, A2 segment of the ACA. 2, Beginning of A3 segment of the ACA. 3, Rostrum of the corpus callosum. 4, A3 segment of the ACA. 5, Pericallosal artery. 6, A4 or horizontal segment of the ACA. 7, Inferior edge of the falx. 8, Marginal ramus of the cingulate sulcus. 9, Precuneus. 10, Parieto-occipital sulcus. 11, Cuneus. **(c)** Closer view of the medial temporal lobe. 1, Optic tract. 2, Semilunar gyrus. 3, Semianular sulcus. 4, Ambient gyrus. 5, Uncal sulcus. 6, Posteromedial part of the uncus. 7, Inferior choroidal point. 8, Pulvinar of the thalamus. 9, Fimbria. 10, Dentate gyrus. 11, Subiculum. 12, Parahippocampal gyrus. 13, Lingual gyrus. **(d)** Medial temporal lobe and the PCA. 1, Carotid artery. 2, Anterior choroidal artery at the upper part of the uncus. 3, Posterior choroidal artery at the level of the uncal sulcus. 4, P2 P segment of the PCA above the subiculum. 5, Inferior temporal branch of the PCA. 6, P4 segment of the PCA inside the calcarine sulcus. 7 Parieto-occipital artery. 8, Calcarine sulcus.

2.4.2 Medial Surface

The parietal lobe on the medial surface of the hemisphere is called the precuneus (▶ Fig. 2.5). The precuneus is limited by the marginal ramus of the cingulate gyrus, the cingulate gyrus and the parieto-occipital sulcus. The precuneus is the continuation of the superior parietal lobule on the medial surface of the hemisphere. The precuneus has a complex sulcus on its surface: the subparietal sulcus. The subparietal sulcus is a complex sulcus and its inferior part is like the posterior continuation of the cingulate sulcus.

2.5 Temporal Lobe

The temporal lobe is formed by the superior, middle and inferior temporal gyri on the lateral surface and by the inferior temporal gyrus, the fusiform gyrus and the parahippocampal on the inferior surface, the temporal pole and the uncus on its anterior surface and by the parahippocampal gyrus and the uncus on its medial surface[13,14] (▶ Fig. 2.4, ▶ Fig. 2.5). The uncus and the parahippocampal gyrus are considered as part of the limbic lobe.

2.5.1 Lateral Surface

The lateral surface of the temporal lobe has the superior, middle and inferior temporal gyri. These gyri are separated by the superior and inferior temporal sulci. Both the temporal gyri and sulci have an antero-posterior direction. The inferior temporal gyrus is part both of the lateral and inferior surface of the temporal lobe. The superior, middle and inferior gyri converge on the anterior surface of the temporal lobe to form the temporal pole.

2.5.2 Inferior Surface

The limit between the inferior surface of the temporal lobe and the inferior surface of the occipital lobe is given by an imaginary line: the inferior parietotemporal line. The inferior parietotemporal line begins in the junction of the parieto-occipital sulcus with the calcarine sulcus and it runs until the preoccipital notch. The inferior surface of the temporal lobe is divided into three gyri: inferior temporal gyrus, fusiform gyrus, and parahippocampal gyrus (▶ Fig. 2.4). The inferior temporal gyrus is separated from the fusiform gyrus by the occipitotemporal sulcus. The occipitotemporal sulcus is usually discontinuous and has a curved shape, with the convexity facing laterally. The collateral sulcus originates below the calcarine sulcus. The collateral sulcus runs from lateral to medial, then posterior to anterior, and then medial to lateral. The shapes of the collateral sulcus and the occipitotemporal sulcus give a fusiform configuration to the fusiform gyrus between them. The fusiform gyrus is also called the lateral occipitotemporal gyrus and the lingual gyrus is also called the medial occipitotemporal gyrus. The inferior temporal and the fusiform gyri converge to also form the temporal pole. The posterior part of the collateral sulcus is usually divided into two branches.

The temporal pole is separated from the uncus by the rhinal sulcus. The rhinal sulcus is often continuous with the collateral sulcus.

2.6 Sylvian Fissure and Insula
2.6.1 Sylvian Fissure

The Sylvian fissure has a superficial and a deep part.[15] The superficial part of the Sylvian fissure has a stem parallel to the sphenoid bone and three rami on the lateral surface of the cerebrum. The stem of the Sylvian fissure divides in three rami at the anterior Sylvian point: horizontal ramus, ascending ramus, and posterior ramus (▶ Fig. 2.1d, ▶ Fig. 2.6). The anterior Sylvian point is easily recognized as it is located in a widening of the fissure just below pars triangularis. The anterior Sylvian point is an important landmark because it is located at the level of the apex of the insula and near the anterior limiting sulcus of the insula. The horizontal and ascending rami are small compared with the posterior ramus. The horizontal and ascending rami divide the inferior frontal gyrus in three parts: pars orbitalis, pars triangularis, and pars opercularis. Pars orbitalis has a characteristic bulging shape easily seen in the most anterior portion of the frontal operculum. Pars orbitalis is continuous with the lateral orbital gyrus on the basal surface of the frontal lobe. Pars triangularis can be recognized by its triangular shape that is

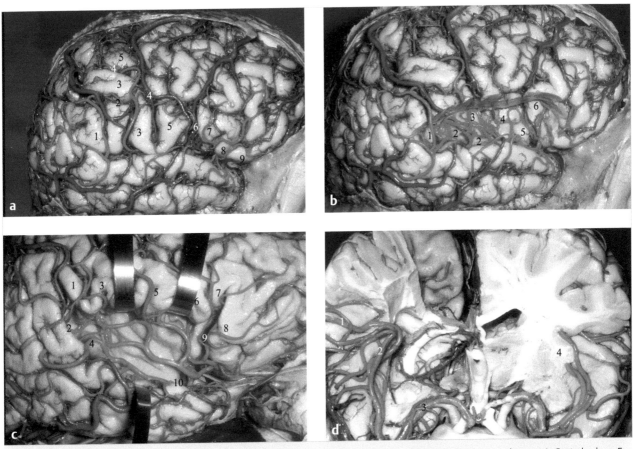

Fig. 2.6 Lateral surface: Sylvian fissure and the opercula. **(a)** 1, Supramarginal gyrus. 2, Postcentral sulcus. 3, Postcentral gyrus. 4, Central sulcus. 5, Precentral gyrus. 6, Precentral sulcus. 7, Pars opercularis. 8, Pars triangularis. 9, Pars orbitalis. **(b)** Removal of the frontal and parietal opercula. 1, Temporal plane. 2, Heschl gyrus. 3, Long gyrus of the insula. 4, Short gyri of the insula. 5, Apex of the insula. 6, Anterior part of the insula near the level of the inferior frontal sulcus. **(c)** Retraction of the frontal and parietal opercula. 1, Supramarginal gyrus. 2, Temporal plane. 3, Postcentral gyrus. 4, Heschl gyrus. 5, Precentral gyrus. 6, Pars opercularis. 7, Pars triangularis. 8, Pars orbitalis. 9, Anterior limiting sulcus of the insula. 10, Limen of the insula. **(d)** Anterior view of the Sylvian fissure after a coronal cut along the frontal lobe on the left side. 1, M3 at the level of the temporal plane. 2, M2 segment of the MCA. 3, M1 segment. 4, Insula.

defined by the direction of the horizontal ramus anteriorly and the ascending ramus posteriorly. The pars opercularis is continuous with the precentral gyrus posteriorly.

The posterior ramus forms most of the Sylvian fissure on the lateral surface of the hemisphere. The posterior ramus has one small subcentral ramus below the precentral gyrus and another below the postcentral gyrus. The posterior end of the posterior ramus divides at the posterior Sylvian point into a posterior ascending ramus and a posterior descending ramus. In summary, the gyri above the Sylvian fissure from anterior to posterior are pars orbitalis, pars triangularis, pars opercularis, precentral gyrus, postcentral gyrus, and supramarginal gyrus. The gyrus located below the Sylvian fissure is the superior temporal gyrus. The superior temporal gyrus extends inside the Sylvian fissure. If we remove the frontal and parietal opercula, we see that the superior temporal gyrus has a characteristic shape (▶ Fig. 2.7). Lateral to the insula, the superior temporal gyrus has a concave surface. Posterior to the insula, the superior temporal gyrus has a flat surface, making it much more difficult to open the fissure at this level. The concave superior surface is called the polar plane (▶ Fig. 2.7a, d). The flat surface is formed

by the anterior transverse temporal gyrus (Heschl gyrus) and the temporal plane. The temporal plane consists of two posterior transverse gyri. There is a correspondence between the frontoparietal and the temporal opercula (▶ Fig. 2.6). The temporal plane is located just below the marginal gyrus. Heschl gyrus lies below the postcentral gyrus. The polar plane is below the precentral and the inferior frontal gyrus (pars opercularis, triangularis, and orbitalis). The deep part of the Sylvian fissure also has a horizontal segment and a lateral segment. The deep lateral segment of the Sylvian fissure is called the operculoinsular segment.

2.6.2 Insula

The insula is a triangular shaped area clearly separated from the hemisphere by three sulci: the anterior, superior, and inferior circular or limiting sulci of the insula[15,16] (▶ Fig. 2.6, ▶ Fig. 2.7). The insula has a smaller anterior part and a larger lateral part. The anterior part of the insula is a small area facing anteriorly and hidden by pars orbitalis. The lateral side of the insula has a convex shape and its most lateral part is the apex

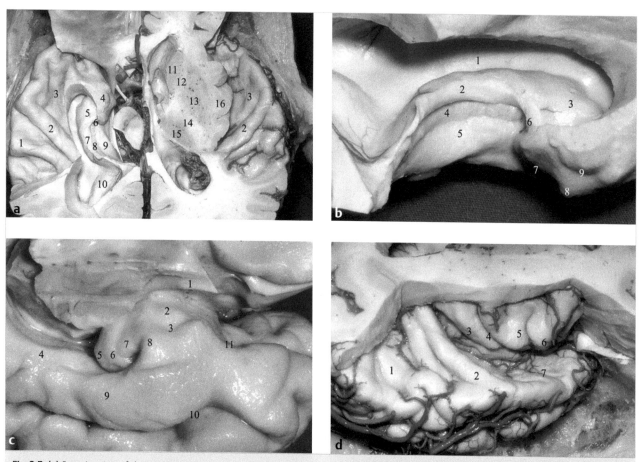

Fig. 2.7 (a) Superior view of the superior temporal gyrus. 1, Temporal plane. 2, Heschl gyrus. 3, Polar plane. 4, Uncus. 5, Head of the hippocampus. 6, Inferior choroidal point. 7, Fimbria. 8, Dentate gyrus. 9, Subiculum. 10, Calcar avis. 11, Head of the caudate nucleus. 12, Anterior limb of the internal capsule. 13, Lentiform nucleus. 14, Posterior limb of the internal capsule. 15, Thalamus. 16, Insula. (b) Medial temporal lobe with exposure of the temporal horn. 1, Collateral eminence. 2, Fimbria. 3, Head of the hippocampus. 4, Dentate gyrus. 5, Subiculum. 6, Inferior choroidal point. 7, Uncal sulcus. 8, Ambient gyrus. 9, Semianular sulcus. (c) Closer view of uncus. 1, Optic tract. 2, Semilunar gyrus. 3, Semianular sulcus. 4, Subiculum. 5, Intralimbic gyrus. 6, Band of Giacomini. 7, Uncinate gyrus. 8, Ambient gyrus. 9, Parahippocampal gyrus. 10, Rhinal sulcus. 11, Impression of the rhinal sulcus. (d) Insula and superior temporal gyrus. 1, Temporal plane. 2, Heschl gyrus. 3, Long gyrus of the insula. 4, Central sulcus of the insula. 5, Short gyri of the insula. 6, Apex of the insula. 7, Polar plane.

of the insula. The insula is divided into anterior and posterior parts by the central sulcus of the insula. The central sulcus of the insula has a similar orientation and position with the central sulcus of the cerebral hemisphere. The central sulcus of the insula is the sulcus on the surface of the insula that goes until near the limen of the insula. The anterior part of the insula is formed by four or five small gyri that converge to the insular pole. The most lateral projection of the anterior part of the insula is called the apex of the insula. The apex of the insula is located at the level of the anterior Sylvian point. The posterior part of the insula is formed by two long parallel gyri. The posterior part of the insula is smaller than the anterior part. The insula may be considered as the lateral wall of the insular block or the central core of the brain.[17] Deeper to the insula are the claustrum, putamen, globus pallidum, internal capsule, caudate nucleus, and thalamus. The most anterior portion of the insula is related to the anterior limb of the internal capsule and the most posterior part of the insula is related to posterior limb.

2.7 Limbic Lobe

The limbic lobe forms a **C**-shaped ring around the corpus callosum. This ring is limited by a discontinuous sulcus composed succes-

sively by the cingulate, subparietal, calcarine, collateral, and rhinal sulcus (▶ Fig. 2.5). The cortical part of the limbic lobe includes the uncus, the parahippocampal gyrus, the isthmus of the cingulate gyrus, the cingulate gyrus, and the subcallosal area.[4,14]

2.7.1 Medial Surface of the Hemisphere

The limbic lobe occupies part of the medial surface of the hemisphere (▶ Fig. 2.6, ▶ Fig. 2.7, ▶ Fig. 2.8). The medial surface of the hemisphere is composed of three layers: corpus callosum, cingulate gyrus, and the medial aspect of the frontal, central, parietal, temporal, and occipital lobes (▶ Fig. 2.5a). The cingulate gyrus is continuous on the medial side of the temporal lobe with the parahippocampal gyrus. The corpus callosum is divided into four parts: rostrum, genu, body, and splenium (▶ Fig. 2.3c). The corpus callosum is separated from the cingulate gyrus by a continuous sulcus, the callosal sulcus. The cingulate sulcus is the upper limit of the cingulate gyrus. The cingulate sulcus originates below the rostrum of the corpus callosum and ends as the marginal ramus. There are two small sulci below the rostrum of the corpus: the anterior and posterior parolfactory sulci. The area between the anterior and posterior parolfactory sulci is the subcallosal area. The small

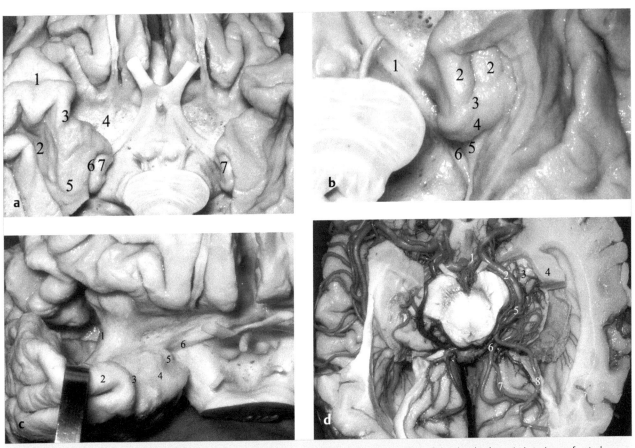

Fig. 2.8 Inferior surface of the temporal lobe. **(a)** 1, Temporal pole. 2, Rhinal sulcus. 3, Impression of the rhinal sulcus. 4, Anterior perforated substance. 5, Parahippocampal gyrus. 6, Uncal sulcus. 7, Uncus. **(b)** Closer view of the uncus after resection of the parahippocampal gyrus below the uncal sulcus. 1, Optic tract. 2, Uncinate gyrus. 3, Band of Giacomini. 4, Intralimbic gyrus. 5, Fimbria. 6, Inferior choroidal point. **(c)** Anterior view of the uncus and the horizontal part of the Sylvian fissure. 1, Limen insulae. 2, Temporal pole. 3, Impression of the rhinal sulcus. 4, Anterior part of the uncus. 5, Semianular sulcus. 6, Optic tract. **(d)** PCA and inferior surface of the temporal lobe after opening the temporal horn. 1, P1 segment of the PCA. 2, P2A segment of the PCA. 3, Posterior part of the uncus (extraventricular part of the head of the hippocampus). 4, Head of the hippocampus (intraventricular part). 5, P2 P segment of the PCA. 6, P3 segment. 7, Calcarine branch inside the calcarine sulcus. 8, Posterior inferior temporal branch of the PCA.

area between the posterior parolfactory sulcus and the lamina terminalis is the paraterminal gyrus. The cingulate sulcus gives rise to small sulci that have a radiating pattern upward. One of these sulci, on the middle of the corpus callosum, is the paracentral sulcus. The subparietal sulcus is present on the surface of the precuneus. The subparietal sulcus is like the continuation of the cingulate sulcus after the marginal ramus. It separates the posterior part of the cingulate gyrus from the precuneus. Posterior to the splenium of the corpus callosum and above the anterior part of the calcarine sulcus, the cingulate gyrus becomes thinner. This segment of the cingulate gyrus is the isthmus of the cingulate gyrus. The isthmus is separated from the lingual gyrus by the anterior part of the calcarine sulcus. The isthmus of the cingulate gyrus continues as the parahippocampal gyrus on the medial temporal lobe.

2.7.2 Medial Temporal Lobe

The medial temporal lobe is formed by the uncus, the parahippocampal gyrus, the dentate gyrus, and the fimbria[13,14] (► Fig. 2.2, ► Fig. 2.5, ► Fig. 2.7, ► Fig. 2.8). When seen from above, the parahippocampal gyrus has a flat surface, called the subiculum. It is important to remember that the structure lying just above the subiculum is the pulvinar of the thalamus (► Fig. 2.5c, d). When seen from medially, the medial surface of the temporal lobe posterior to the uncus is formed by the fimbria above, the dentate gyrus in the middle, and the parahippocampal gyrus below (► Fig. 2.5c, ► Fig. 2.7). The fimbria is separated from the dentate gyrus by the fimbriodentate sulcus. The dentate gyrus is separated from the subiculum by the hippocampal sulcus.

The uncus is the anterior portion of the parahippocampal gyrus (► Fig. 2.5, ► Fig. 2.6, ► Fig. 2.7). The uncus is formed by a posterior reflection of the anterior portion of the parahippocampal gyrus. This creates a sulcus, the uncal sulcus, on the anterior portion of the parahippocampal gyrus. From a surgical perspective, the uncus may be divided into an anterior part related to the amygdala, a medial part located above the uncal sulcus, and an inferior part consisting of the part of the parahippocampal gyrus below the uncal sulcus. The anterior part of the uncus is separated from the temporal pole by the impression of the rhinal sulcus. The impression of the rhinal sulcus is either the continuation of the rhinal sulcus on the anterior surface of the temporal lobe or is just a depression separating the temporal pole laterally from the uncus medially. The anterior portion of the uncus has a small depression: the semianular sulcus.[14] The small semilunar gyrus is located just above the semianular sulcus. The area of the uncus surrounding the anterior end of the uncal sulcus is called the ambient gyrus of the uncus. The ambient gyrus is the most medial aspect of the uncus. The portion of the uncus above the uncal sulcus is divided into three gyri from anterior to posterior: uncinate gyrus, band of Giacomini, and intralimbic gyrus.[13,14] These three gyri constitute the extraventricular portion of the head of the hippocampus. The head of the hippocampus has a ventricular and extraventricular portion (► Fig. 2.8d). The ventricular portion is the one seen when opening the temporal horn. The ventricular portion of the head of the hippocampus has small digitations that resemble the paw of a lion, the so-called pes hippocampi.

The hippocampus and the collateral eminence form the floor of the temporal horn. The collateral eminence is the superior projection of the collateral sulcus. The hippocampus has a head, body, and tail. Both the head and tail of the hippocampus are curved medially, whereas the body has an anterior to posterior direction. Posterior to the head of the hippocampus is the inferior choroidal point, the most inferior part of the choroidal fissure. The choroidal fissure is a virtual space between the fornix on one side and the thalamus on the other side. At the level of the temporal horn, the choroidal fissure is located between the fimbria of the fornix and the thalamus. The fimbria of the fornix begins posteriorly to the head of the hippocampus and runs posteriorly on the superior and medial aspect of the hippocampus.

The choroidal fissure is a very important anatomical landmark. The structures below the choroidal fissure (hippocampus, subiculum, and parahippocampal gyrus) may be removed in a medial temporal resection. But above the choroidal fissure is the thalamus. If we look at the roof of the temporal horn from below, we see that there is no clear demarcation between the thalamus and the roof of the temporal horn. Resection of the roof of the temporal horn medial to the level of the choroidal fissure will damage the thalamus. Anterior to the anterior choroidal point, there is no more choroidal fissure. Anterior to this point, if resection of the uncus is needed, we may use the optic tract as a landmark. The optic tract is at the upper limit of the uncus (► Fig. 2.5c, ► Fig. 2.7c, ► Fig. 2.8c). Resection above the optic tract damages the basal ganglia. The optic tract may be followed in a subpial resection of the uncus.

2.8 Occipital Lobe

The occipital lobe has a lateral, inferior, and medial surface.

2.8.1 Lateral Surface

The intraparietal sulcus continues in the occipital lobe toward the occipital pole. After it passes the level of the parieto-occipital sulcus into the occipital lobe, the intraparietal sulcus is called the intraoccipital sulcus[18] (► Fig. 2.1c). The two other consistent sulci on the lateral surface of the occipital lobe are the lateral occipital sulcus and the transverse occipital sulcus. The lateral occipital sulcus is like the continuation of the superior temporal sulcus into the occipital lobe. The transverse occipital sulcus is the sulcus that originates near the midline posterior to the parieto-occipital sulcus and usually transverses the intraoccipital sulcus. The lateral surface of the occipital lobe is commonly divided into three gyri: superior, middle, and inferior occipital gyri. The superior occipital gyrus is between the interhemispheric fissure and the intraoccipital sulcus. The middle occipital gyrus is between the intraoccipital sulcus and the lateral occipital sulcus, and the inferior occipital gyrus is the one below the lateral occipital sulcus. The three gyri converge to form the occipital pole. The superior occipital gyrus is continuous on the medial surface with the cuneus and the inferior occipital gyrus is continuous on the basal surface with the lingual gyrus.

2.8.2 Medial and Basal Surface

The cuneus and the lingual gyrus form the medial and basal surface of the occipital lobe. The cuneus is on the medial surface of the hemisphere and it is limited by the calcarine sulcus and the parieto-occipital sulcus (▶ Fig. 2.5a). The calcarine sulcus is a continuous deep sulcus. The calcarine sulcus extends laterally near the atrium and the occipital horn. The most lateral extension of the calcarine sulcus forms the calcar avis on the medial side of the atrium, just below the bulb of the corpus callosum (▶ Fig. 2.7a, ▶ Fig. 2.8d). The calcarine sulcus has a characteristic shape, with its convexity facing upward. The parieto-occipital sulcus is also a continuous sulcus and it separates the calcarine sulcus in an anterior and a posterior segment. The primary visual cortex occupies the upper and lower lips of the posterior part of the calcarine sulcus, including its depths and extending to parts of the cuneus and lingual gyrus. The lingual gyrus lies both on the medial and basal surface of the occipital lobe. The lingual gyrus is located below the calcarine sulcus and medial to the posterior end of the collateral sulcus. As the collateral sulcus is usually divided into its most posterior part, the medial division of the collateral sulcus may be inside the lingual gyrus. The lingual gyrus is the posterior continuation of the parahippocampal gyrus.

2.9 Arteries

The main arteries related to the sulci and gyri are the carotid artery, the anterior choroidal artery (AChA), the anterior cerebral artery (ACA), the middle cerebral artery (MCA), and the posterior cerebral artery (PCA). The arteries are reviewed in their relation to the sulci and gyri.[19]

2.9.1 Carotid Artery and Anterior Choroidal Artery

The carotid bifurcation lies on the anterior aspect of the uncus (▶ Fig. 2.6d). The AChA arises from the carotid artery and courses below the optic tract to reach the superior and medial side of the uncus (▶ Fig. 2.5d, ▶ Fig. 2.6d). It continues through the inferior choroidal point to irrigate the choroidal plexus of the temporal horn.

2.9.2 Anterior Cerebral Artery

The ACA arises from the carotid bifurcation and runs medially above the optic tract and chiasm to supply most of the medial surface of the frontal and parietal lobes (▶ Fig. 2.5b). It is divided into five segments. A1 runs from the carotid bifurcation until the anterior communicating artery (ACoA). A2 runs from the ACoA to the rostrum of the corpus callosum. A3 is the segment of the ACA that goes around the genu of the corpus callosum. A4 and A5 form the horizontal segment, separated by convention by the coronal suture. The horizontal segment runs above the corpus callosum. The main branch of the ACA that runs along the cingulate sulcus is the callosomarginal artery. The segments of the ACA distal to the ACoA is also called the pericallosal artery.

2.9.3 Middle Cerebral Artery

The MCA supplies the lateral surface of the hemispheres, the insula, the lateral aspect of the inferior surface, and the superior medial surface of the cerebrum (▶ Fig. 2.5). It also gives rise to important perforating branches to the anterior perforated substance. And it arises from the carotid bifurcation below the anterior perforated substance. It runs laterally parallel to the sphenoid wing. At the limen of the insula, it turns laterally to run inside the operculoinsular compartment of the Sylvian fissure. The course of the MCA is shaped by the configuration of the insula and the opercula. At the superior limiting sulcus of the insula, the MCA undergoes sharp turns to run along the cleft between the opercula. At the level of the temporal plane, the MCA has a straight course that can be identified in the angiogram. The MCA is divided into four segments: M1, M2, M3, and M4. M1 runs from the carotid bifurcation to the arterial curve at the limen insulae. The bifurcation of the MCA usually lies in the M1 segment. M2 runs from the limen insulae to the limiting sulcus of the insula. It is the segment closely related to the insula. M3 is the opercular segment, where the artery courses between the frontoparietal opercula and the temporal operculum. M4 is the cortical segment.

2.9.4 Posterior Cerebral Artery

The PCA arises from the rostral end of the basilar artery. It encircles the midbrain and supplies the medial surface of the occipital lobe and the medial and basal surfaces of the temporal lobe (▶ Fig. 2.5d, ▶ Fig. 2.8d). And it also has branches that irrigate the thalamus, midbrain, lateral and third ventricular walls, and choroid plexus. The PCA may be divided into four segments: P1, P2, P3, and P4. The P1 segment arises at the basilar artery and ends at the junction with the posterior communicating artery (PCoA). P2 segment is from the PCoA to posterior part of the midbrain. P2 is divided at the posterior margin of the cerebral peduncle in P2A and P2P. P2A is located between the medial part of the uncus and the midbrain. The PCA runs near the uncal sulcus. P2P is the segment related to the subiculum. The hippocampal arteries arise from the PCA to irrigate the uncus and the hippocampus. The P2A and P2P give rise to the inferior temporal arteries (anterior, middle, and posterior temporal arteries) that irrigate the medial and basal surfaces of the temporal lobe. The P3 segment begins at the posterior part of the midbrain and ends inside the calcarine sulcus. P3 is a short cisternal segment, and it can easily be identified in the angiogram because the PCAs approach each other near the midline just posterior to the colliculi. P4 is the cortical segment and it includes the calcarine and parieto-occipital arteries.

References

[1] Ojemann G, Ojemann J, Lettich E, Berger M. Cortical language localization in left, dominant hemisphere. An electrical stimulation mapping investigation in 117 patients. J Neurosurg. 1989; 71(3):316–326

[2] Ribas GC, Yasuda A, Ribas EC, Nishikuni K, Rodrigues AJ, Jr. Surgical anatomy of microsurgical key points. Neurosurgery. 2006; 59(4) Suppl 2:ONS117–ONS211

[3] Ribas GC. The cerebral sulci and gyri. Neurosurg Focus. 2010; 28(2):E2

[4] Yasargil MG. Microneurosurgery IVB. New York, NY: Thieme; 1996

[5] Ono M, Kubik S, Abernathey CD. Atlas of Cerebral Sulci. Stuttgart: Thieme, 1990

[6] Yousry TA, Schmid UD, Alkadhi H, et al. Localization of the motor hand area to a knob on the precentral gyrus. A new landmark. Brain. 1997; 120(Pt 1): 141–157

[7] Dronkers NF, Plaisant O, Iba-Zizen MT, Cabanis EA. Paul Broca's historic cases: high resolution MR imaging of the brains of Leborgne and Lelong. Brain. 2007; 130(Pt 5):1432–1441

[8] Frigeri T, Paglioli E, de Oliveira E, Rhoton AL, Jr. Microsurgical anatomy of the central lobe. J Neurosurg. 2015; 122(3):483–498

[9] Fesl G, Moriggl B, Schmid UD, Naidich TP, Herholz K, Yousry TA. Inferior central sulcus: variations of anatomy and function on the example of the motor tongue area. Neuroimage. 2003; 20(1):601–610

[10] Naidich TP, Blum JT, Firestone MI. The parasagittal line: an anatomic landmark for axial imaging. AJNR Am J Neuroradiol. 2001; 22(5):885–895

[11] Naidich TP, Valavanis AG, Kubik S. Anatomic relationships along the low-middle convexity: Part I–Normal specimens and magnetic resonance imaging. Neurosurgery. 1995; 36(3):517–532

[12] Rostomily RC, Berger MS, Ojemann GA, Lettich E. Postoperative deficits and functional recovery following removal of tumors involving the dominant hemisphere supplementary motor area. J Neurosurg. 1991; 75(1):62–68

[13] Wen HT, Rhoton AL, Jr, de Oliveira E, et al. Microsurgical anatomy of the temporal lobe: Part 1: Mesial temporal lobe anatomy and its vascular relationships as applied to amygdalohippocampectomy. Neurosurgery. 1999; 45(3): 549–591, discussion 591–592

[14] Duvernoy HM. The Human Hippocampus: Functional Anatomy, Vascularization and Serial Sections with MRI. Berlin: Springer; 1998

[15] Wen HT, Rhoton AL, Jr, de Oliveira E, Castro LHM, Figueiredo EG, Teixeira MJ. Microsurgical anatomy of the temporal lobe: Part 2–Sylvian fissure region and its clinical application. Neurosurgery. 2009; 65(6) Suppl:1–35, discussion 36

[16] Türe U, Yaşargil DCH, Al-Mefty O, Yaşargil MG. Topographic anatomy of the insular region. J Neurosurg. 1999; 90(4):720–733

[17] Ribas EC, Yagmurlu K, de Oliveira E, Ribas GC, Rhoton AL, Jr. Microsurgical anatomy of the central core of the brain. J Neurosurg. 2017; 22:1–18

[18] Alves RV, Ribas GC, Párraga RG, de Oliveira E. The occipital lobe convexity sulci and gyri. J Neurosurg. 2012; 116(5):1014–1023

[19] Rhoton AL, Jr. The supratentorial arteries. Neurosurgery. 2002; 51(4) Suppl: S53–S120

3 Anatomy of Eloquent White Matter Tracts

Vicent Quilis-Quesada and Shao-Ching Chen

Abstract

Lesions in eloquent areas represent a great challenge for neurosurgeons due to its surgical complexity. While the "eloquent area" is a concept that is more frequently linked to cortical regions alone, the role of deep fiber tracts in the proper functioning of the brain is often underestimated. At the same time, neurosurgical procedures ordinarily require passage through one or multiple fiber tracts to reach the target in intrinsic brain lesions. Ignorance of the functioning fiber bundles and accidental injury may result in postoperative neurological deficits. Hence, the stereoscopic structures of the brain, better than a pure cortical conception, should be taken into account when considering the "eloquence" of the brain. In this chapter, we will introduce the most relevant eloquent white matter tracts and their relationship with surgical approaches. The detailed knowledge of the three-dimensional brain anatomy is the key to avoid impairing brain functions during surgery.

Keywords: white matter tract, fiber dissection, eloquent area, three-dimensional anatomy, surgical approach

3.1 Introduction

The white matter is made up of bundles of myelinated axons, known as fiber tracts. White matter tracts carry nerve impulses between neurons that resided in gray matter, acting as relays and coordinating communications between different brain areas. Any damage to the white matter tracts may result in impairments of certain brain function.

As axons of neurons, fiber tracts are generally not regarded as "eloquent areas" of the brain. Eloquent brain regions are defined as being essential for carrying out readily identifiable neurological functions, including the sensorimotor, verbal, acoustic, and visual cortex; the thalamus and hypothalamus; the internal capsule; and the brainstem.[1,2] If the fiber bundles do not function properly, neurological deficits will present regardless if eloquent cortical areas remain intact. Hence the idea of "eloquent areas" should be expanded to include deep structures rather than a purely cortical concept. And for the same reason, detailed knowledge of the white matter tracts is of paramount importance while dealing with intrinsic lesions in the brain[3] (▶ Fig. 3.1).

3.2 General Aspects

White matter tracts in the brain are categorized into association, commissural, and projection fibers. Short association fibers, also known as U-fibers, lie immediately beneath the gray matter, and connect adjacent gyri, whereas long association fibers connect the more widely separated gyri in the same hemisphere. The main long association fibers are the uncinate fasciculus (UF), the cingulum, the superior longitudinal fasciculus (SLF), the inferior longitudinal fasciculus (ILF), the arcuate fasciculus (AF), the occipitofrontal fasciculus, and the fornix.

Commissural fibers, which are axons connecting the two hemispheres of the brain, include the corpus callosum, the anterior commissure, the posterior commissure, and the hippocampal commissure. Projection fibers consist of efferent and afferent fibers connecting the cerebral cortex with the brainstem and the spinal cord. The main efferent projection fibers are the corticospinal tracts and the corticopontine fibers, while the principal afferent projection fibers are the optic and acoustic radiations as well as fibers arising from thalamus and reaching different cortical areas through thalamic peduncles.[4]

3.3 Relationship of Fiber Tracts and Operative Approaches

3.3.1 Lateral Surface

Among white matter tracts, association fibers are most vulnerable to neurosurgical procedures. In the lateral aspect of the hemisphere, after removing the cortex and the short association U-fibers, three main fiber systems are shown. The SLF/AF system is the longest association fiber system at the lateral surface, connecting the frontal, temporal, parietal, and occipital lobes. In the frontal and temporal region, anteriorly, the UF originated from the frontal lobe displays a **C**-shape configuration and reaches the temporal pole. In contrast, the occipitofrontal fasciculus courses posteriorly to join the sagittal stratum and terminates in the temporal and occipital cortex (▶ Fig. 3.2).

In the dominant side, the occipitofrontal fasciculus is considered to be related with language function, while the UF is linked to memory, language, and social–emotional processing.[5] As the SLF/AF system connects the more extensive area of the cerebrum, it is suggested to be related to motor regulation, language, memory, and cognitive functions. Thus, when carrying out operative approaches to deep lesions in the frontal lobe, surgeons should be aware of possible motor or language deficits if the fiber tracts are damaged, especially in the dominant hemisphere. In the meanwhile, surgeons should pay more attention to the psychiatric and neurological illness related to the UF, which is frequently severed during the transsylvian approach to the temporal horn.

In the temporal lobe, the SLF/AF system connects the auditory area to the frontal lobe. As a result, it is considered to be involved in the language pathway. Deep to the occipitofrontal fasciculus and the fibers of the anterior commissure, a projection fiber system named as optic radiation forms the roof of the temporal horn. It carries the visual signal from the lateral geniculate body toward the striate cortex in the occipital lobe. Thus, the language and visual pathways may be at risk during surgical approaches to the temporal lobe. On the other hand, surgeons could also consider the feasibility of different plans, for instance, the transsylvian approach or the supracerebellar transtentorial approach to access the temporal horn, rather than the transsulcal approach, to avoid visual defect postoperatively.

In the frontoparietal region, the pyramidal tract and the thalamocortical pathway correlate to the precentral and the

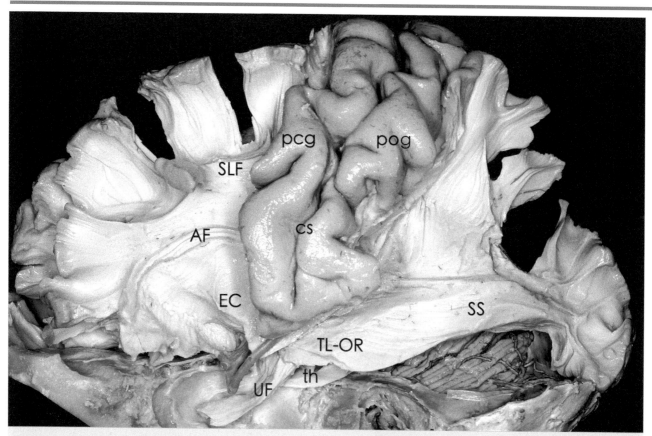

Fig. 3.1 The spatial relationship between some eloquent fiber tracts and cortical areas. AF, arcuate fasciculus; cs, central sulcus; EC, extreme capsule; pcg, precentral gyrus; pog, postcentral gyrus; SLF, superior longitudinal fasciculus; SS, sagittal stratum; th, temporal horn; TL-OR, temporal loop of the optic radiation; UF, uncinate fasciculus.

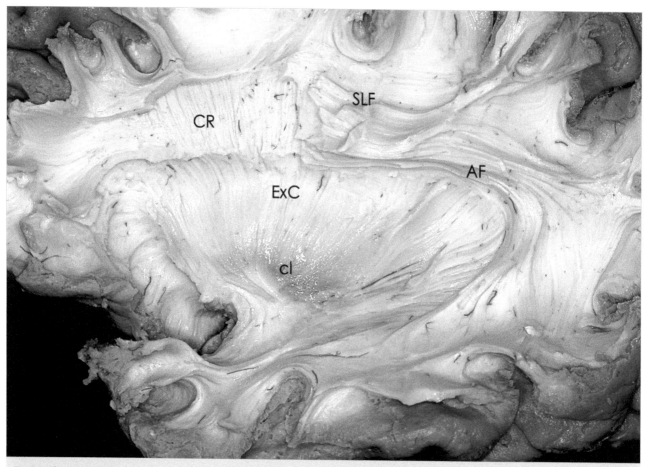

Fig. 3.2 The SLF and the AF. AF, arcuate fasciculus; cl, claustrum; CR, corona radiata; ExC, external capsule; SLF, superior longitudinal fasciculus.

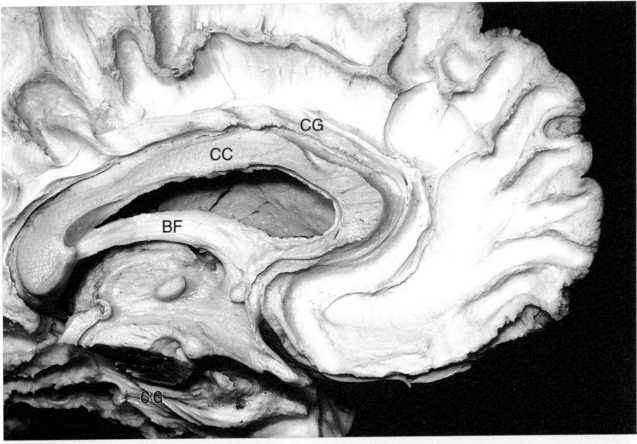

Fig. 3.3 The cingulum, a **C**-shape fiber tract, is the longest association fiber system in the medial side. CG, cingulum; CC, corpus callosum; BF, body of fornix.

postcentral gyrus, respectively. These are two of the most eloquent projection fiber systems, transmitting motor and sensory signals to and from the spinal cord. However, postoperatively, motor weakness may present despite the intactness of the corticospinal tract if the supplementary motor area (SMA) is disrupted. The SLF is believed to play a role in coordinating the motor area and the SMA. Damage to the SLF in this region may also result in motor weakness.

Meanwhile, the motor and sensory pathways could also be injured in another segment, that is, the internal capsule. In the insular lobe, surgical interventions may cause damage to the internal capsule due to either direct interruption or vascular insults. On the other hand, although the extreme and the external capsule are proposed as long association fiber pathways related to the language circuit (since they connect the Wernicke area and the Broca area), the verbal deficit is not significant when they are severed.

3.3.2 Medial Surface

In the medial surface, the cingulum is the longest association fiber system as well as the main fiber tracts of the limbic lobe, connecting not only the cingulate gyrus and the parahippocampal gyrus, but also the neighboring frontal, parietal, occipital, and temporal lobe. The function of the anterior section of the cingulum is linked to emotion, while the posterior part is more related to cognitive function. Therefore, surgical disruption of the anterior cingulum, known as cingulotomy, is proposed to treat depression and obsessive–compulsive disorder as psychosurgery. Deep brain stimulation in this region is also an option to neuromodulate and treat all these psychiatric disorders (▶ Fig. 3.3).

The corpus callosum, formed by the strongest commissural fibers called callosal fibers, can also be best inspected at the medial aspect of the cerebrum. It is the broadest, thickest, and largest fiber tract in the human brain, extensively radiating to various parts of different lobes, thus interconnecting each hemisphere. Hence, a corpus callosotomy can be performed to treat patients with refractory epilepsy produced by unilateral epileptogenic foci. In addition, parts of the corpus callosum are frequently opened in order to gain access to the ventricles while dealing with intraventricular pathologies. A well-known adverse effect of callosotomy is the "disconnection syndrome." Language impairments and memory deficits are also reported, but most complications are transient.[6]

3.3.3 Basal Surface

The ILF is the major association fiber pathway in the basal surface. It connects the temporal–occipital region of the brain to the anterior temporal area. With its extensive anatomic connections, this white matter bundle seems to involve a relatively

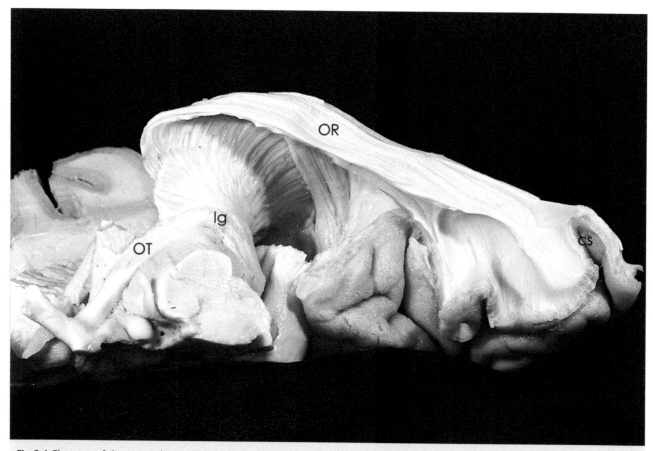

Fig. 3.4 The route of the optic radiation. lg, lateral geniculate body; OR, optic radiation; OT, optic tract.

vast array of brain functions, but mainly relates to visually guided decisions and behaviors. Consequently, disruption of the ILF may associate with neuropsychological impairments of visual cognition, for example, the visual agnosia, prosopagnosia, and alexia.[7] The ILF is frequently in danger while performing the subtemporal approach or the supracerebellar transtentorial approach toward the basal temporal surface.

3.4 Most Relevant Eloquent Fiber Tracts

3.4.1 Optic Radiation

In the mid-19th century, Gratiolet described a fiber system that came from the optic tract and traveled to the posterior part of the cerebral cortex, terminating in a particular part of the brain (striate cortex). His observation was the first confirmation of a specific sensory pathway linked to a defined cortical area and was also the beginning of discoveries of the cerebral functional map. At the beginning of the 20th century, Meyer gave the first detailed configuration of the optic radiation, and it was popularized by Cushing's illustration later known as the "Meyer loop" because of its peculiar temporal detour.[8]

Optic radiation refers to axons of neurons in the lateral geniculate body that finally reach the visual cortex (Brodmann area 17). This projection fiber system passes under the lentiform

nucleus and makes an initial anterior detour anteriorly before going posteriorly to join the sagittal stratum, forming a loop in the anterior temporal region. Dissecting from the basal surface, after removing the ependymal layer of the temporal horn and tapetal fibers, the "temporal loop" or "Meyer loop" can be exposed (▶ Fig. 3.4).

When the optic radiation is severed, the patient may present with contralateral superior quadrantanopsia of both visual fields. Besides, recent reports propose that rather than only individual optic radiation fibers, the temporal loop is composed of various projection fibers that travel through the sublenticular internal capsule.[9,10] As a result, for any surgeons planning to conduct a surgical approach toward the temporal horn or around the temporo-occipital region, the three-dimensional relationship between the lesion and optic radiation should always be taken into consideration.

3.4.2 Fornix

The discovery of fornix can trace back to the 1st century when Galen described it as a "vault" or an "arch." Thomas Willis changed this term with an equivalent word in Latin expression—Fornix. For more than a thousand years, as its name indicated, fornix was considered as a supportive structure to sustain the lateral and third ventricles. It was not until 1820—when Treviranus noted the connection between the olfactory nerve, hippocampus, and fornix, and drew a remarkable

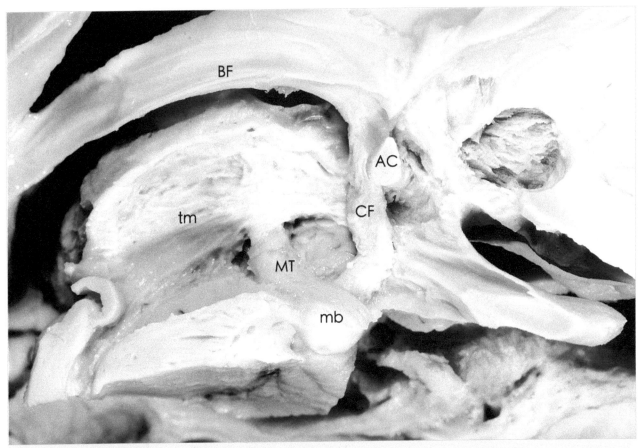

Fig. 3.5 Subdivisions of the fornix. AC, anterior commissure; BF, body of fornix; CF, column of fornix; mb, mammillary body; MT, mammillothalamic tract; tm, thalamus.

conclusion that these structures may be involved in a higher mental function, perhaps that of memory—that the role of fornix started to link to the modern concept.[11]

The fornix is a **C**-shape nerve bundle that acts as the primary efferent fibers of the hippocampus, a structure that is involved in memory formation and recall. It is part of the limbic system, and it terminates in the mammillary body. The fornix is divided into the fimbria, crura, commissure, body, and columns. Most parts of the fornix are long (▶ Fig. 3.5, ▶ Fig. 3.6).

The fornix has a close relationship with the lateral ventricle, third ventricle, and thalamus. For approaches toward these areas, the relationship between the lesion and each part of the fornix should be thoroughly evaluated before carrying any procedure. As the major efferent fibers of the hippocampi, damage to the fornix may result in transient or permanent amnesia.[12,13]

3.5 Internal Capsule and Corona Radiata

In the 17th century, Vieussens described the white matter of the centrum ovale and was the first to demonstrate that these connections were composed of projection fibers coming from the cortical gray matter to the spinal cord. At the beginning of the 19th century, Reil coined the term "corona radiata" to describe the radiation fibers in Vieussens' centrum and empha-

sized the relationship between these fibers, the internal capsule, and the cerebral peduncles. Corona radiata fibers are the most prominent projection fibers transmitting information to and from the cerebral cortex. They continue with the cerebral peduncle via the internal capsule, then keep traveling downward through the brainstem and spinal cord.

The internal capsule is bordered by the lentiform nucleus laterally as well as the caudate nucleus and thalamus medially. It is divided into five parts—the anterior limb, genu, posterior limb, sublenticular part, and retrolenticular part. While the sublenticular internal capsule covers the auditory radiations and the retrolenticular internal capsule carries the optic radiations, the posterior limb of the internal capsule is passed by two of the most eloquent fiber bundles—the pyramidal tract and the thalamocortical somatosensory tract (▶ Fig. 3.7, ▶ Fig. 3.8).

The pyramidal tract was composed of the corticobulbar and corticospinal tract. They are efferent fibers of the upper motor neurons that originate from not only the primary motor area (Brodmann area 4) at the precentral gyrus, but also the premotor and somatosensory cortex.[14,15] The corticobulbar tract terminates at the brainstem and carries impulses to the cranial nerves, whereas the spinothalamic tract conducts impulses to the spinal cord for the voluntary movement after making a decussation in the medulla oblongata. On the other hand, thalamocortical somatosensory fibers originate from the

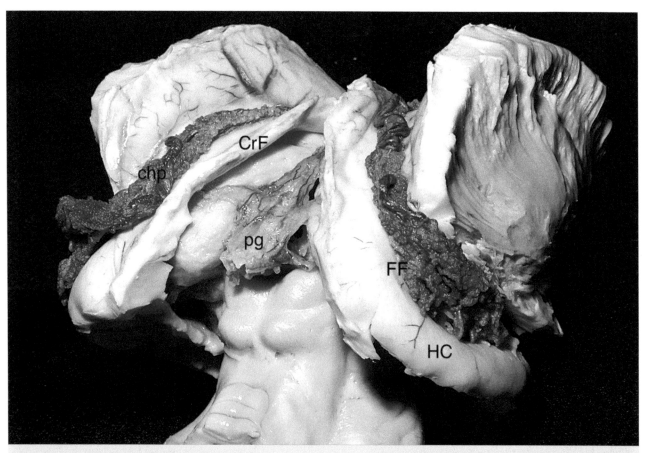

Fig. 3.6 Subdivisions of the fornix (continued with ▶ Fig. 3.3). chp, choroid plexus; CrF, crura of fornix; FF, fimbria fornix; HC, hippocampus; pg, pineal gland.

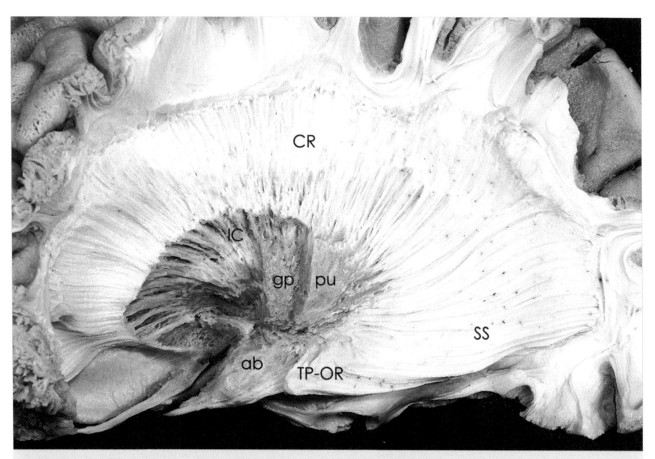

Fig. 3.7 The course of the corona radiata, the internal capsule, and the temporal loop in the lateral surface. ab, amygdaloid body; CR, corona radiata; IC, internal capsule; gp, globus pallidus; pu, putamen; TP-OR, temporal loop of optic radiation; SS, sagittal stratum.

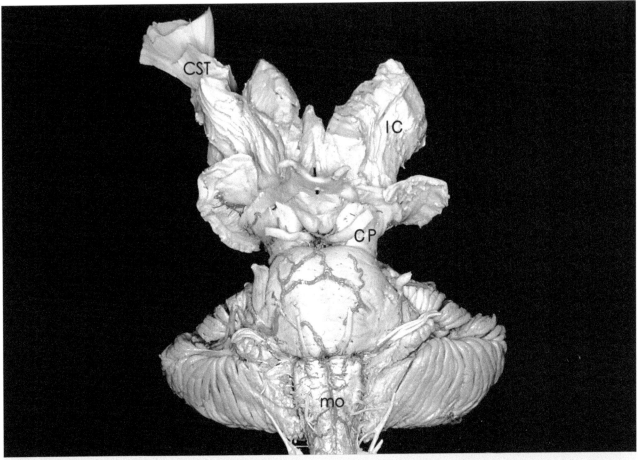

Fig. 3.8 The course of the pyramidal tract in the coronal view. CP, cerebral peduncle; CST, corticospinal tract; IC, internal capsule; mo, medulla oblongata.

ventroposterior nucleus of the thalamus and project to the first and second somatic sensory areas of the cortex in the postcentral gyrus. The somatosensory radiation accounts for transferring the sensory information including touch, pain, and nociception.[16,17]

When the connections of the pyramidal tract are disrupted, the patient may present with hemiplegia on the corresponding side of the body. Frequently, the fiber tracts are not damaged by direct transaction, but by vascular insults. The lenticulostriate arteries and the posterior perforating arteries supply the internal capsule. These small vessels are particularly vulnerable to surgical manipulations. Consequently, infarctions resulted from vascular events may also cause hemiparesis to the patient.

3.5.1 Superior Longitudinal Fasciculus and Arcuate Fasciculus

The SLF and AF have been considered synonymous in the human for centuries. At the beginning of the 19th century, Reil was the first to describe the SLF/AF system and Burdach later provided a more comprehensive description. Subsequently, Dejerine acknowledged Burdach's observation and designated the pathway as the arcuate fasciculus of Burdach, using this term interchangeably with SLF or fasciculus arcuatus. Not until

recent years, when the technique of in vivo diffusion tensor imaging (DTI) progressed, the subcomponents of the SLF were depicted by magnetic resonance image.[18,19] Although the accurate subdivisions of SLF are challenging to be shown by classic gross fiber dissection methods, many attempts have been performed.[20,21]

In the lateral surface of the cerebrum, the SLF is shown after removal of the cortex and adjacent U-fibers of the frontal, temporal, and parietal opercula, as well as the middle and inferior frontal gyri, superior and middle temporal gyri, and the inferior parietal lobule. This fasciculus is a deep long association fiber system, traveling variable distances and reaching different destinations in the frontal, temporal, parietal, and occipital lobe. It originates from the temporal lobe and runs posteriorly superiorly into the occipital lobe, then circles around the Sylvian fissure through the parietal lobe and eventually reaches the frontal lobe. At a deeper level, the SLF/AF system surrounds the outer edges of the insula (▸ Fig. 3.2).

The AF is a subcomponent of the SLF, known as the long segment. Common understanding has been that the AF originates from the superior and middle temporal gyri and terminates at the frontal operculum, connecting the Wernicke area and the Broca area as a major language processing bundle.[22,23] Nevertheless, as the techniques of DTI and fiber dissection improved, the connectivity of the AF has been depicted to correspond to more cortical areas. Instead of being a language processing bundle per se, ongoing discussions propose that the AF may play a role in the motor sequencing necessary to utter word components or spatial attributes of acoustic stimuli and auditory processing.[19,24,25,26]

While the exact function of AF is still subject to debate, the SLF is understood to connect more divergent functions as it connects many different cortical areas. It is suggested that the SLF is involved in regulating motor behavior as it connects the premotor and motor areas in the frontal lobe. Meanwhile, spatial recognition, language, working memory, and even cognitive function are also proposed to be related to the SLF while it connects the parietal lobe to other extensive cortical regions.[27,28,29] Any damage to the SLF/AF system, therefore, may lead to neurological deficits in the aforementioned features.

3.6 Conclusion

Generally, "eloquent area" is a concept used by neurologist and neurosurgeons for areas of cortex that—if removed—may result in paralysis, linguistic disability, or loss of sensory processing. However, cortical areas alone cannot carry out any of the tasks that our brain is meant to do. The white matter tracts pass messages between different cortical regions, and their connectivity makes it possible for the central nervous system to function properly. Inadvertent injury to the fiber tracts in the cerebrum may cause more serious or irreversible neurological deficits than damage to the cortical area.[30] Therefore, when planning any surgical approach, surgeons should consider more relevant the three-dimensional anatomical knowledge of the brain including the deep "eloquent fiber tracts" rather than a pure cortical conception. Furthermore, the thorough four-dimensional knowledge of the fiber bundles, that is, the topographic three-dimensional anatomical relationship plus the functions it carries out through their connection, cannot be overemphasized before any preprocedural planning.

Also, we should keep in mind that the central nervous system is a harmonic organic system and it works as a whole. The brain can function properly if and only if both the cortical areas and the subcortical fiber tracts operate appropriately. Regardless of how subtle or significant the function of each specific fiber bundle is, whenever we interrupt the continuity of any white matter tract, we disrupt the integrity of the brain.

References

[1] Chang EF, Clark A, Smith JS, et al. Functional mapping-guided resection of low-grade gliomas in eloquent areas of the brain: improvement of long-term survival. Clinical article. J Neurosurg. 2011; 114(3):566–573

[2] Spetzler RF, Martin NA. A proposed grading system for arteriovenous malformations. J Neurosurg. 1986; 65(4):476–483

[3] Berger MS, Hadjipanayis CG. Surgery of intrinsic cerebral tumors. Neurosurgery. 2007; 61(1) Suppl:279–304, discussion 304–305

[4] Schmahmann J, Pandya D. Fiber Pathways of the Brain. New York: Oxford; 2006

[5] Von Der Heide RJ, Skipper LM, Klobusicky E, Olson IR. Dissecting the uncinate fasciculus: disorders, controversies and a hypothesis. Brain. 2013; 136(Pt 6): 1692–1707

[6] Stigsdotter-Broman L, Olsson I, Flink R, Rydenhag B, Malmgren K. Long-term follow-up after callosotomy–a prospective, population based, observational study. Epilepsia. 2014; 55(2):316–321

[7] Herbet G, Zemmoura I, Duffau H. Functional anatomy of the inferior longitudinal fasciculus: from historical reports to current hypotheses. Front Neuroanat. 2018; 12(77):77

[8] Catani M, Jones DK, Donato R, Ffytche DH. Occipito-temporal connections in the human brain. Brain. 2003; 126(Pt 9):2093–2107

[9] Goga C, Türe U. The anatomy of Meyer's loop revisited: changing the anatomical paradigm of the temporal loop based on evidence from fiber microdissection. J Neurosurg. 2015; 122(6):1253–1262

[10] Güngör A, Baydin S, Middlebrooks EH, Tanriover N, Isler C, Rhoton AL, Jr. The white matter tracts of the cerebrum in ventricular surgery and hydrocephalus. J Neurosurg. 2017; 126(3):945–971

[11] Meyer A. Historical Aspects of Cerebral Anatomy. Oxford, England: Oxford University Press; 1971

[12] Hodges JR, Carpenter K. Anterograde amnesia with fornix damage following removal of IIIrd ventricle colloid cyst. J Neurol Neurosurg Psychiatry. 1991; 54(7):633–638

[13] Apuzzo MLJ, Chikovani OK, Gott PS, et al. Transcallosal, interfornicial approaches for lesions affecting the third ventricle: surgical considerations and consequences. Neurosurgery. 1982; 10(5):547–554

[14] Martino AML, Strick PL. Corticospinal projections originate from the arcuate premotor area. Brain Res. 1987; 404(1–2):307–312

[15] Schulz R, Park E, Lee J, et al. Interactions between the corticospinal tract and premotor-motor pathways for residual motor output after stroke. Stroke. 2017; 48(10):2805–2811

[16] Ploner M, Schmitz F, Freund HJ, Schnitzler A. Parallel activation of primary and secondary somatosensory cortices in human pain processing. J Neurophysiol. 1999; 81(6):3100–3104

[17] Padberg J, Cerkevich C, Engle J, et al. Thalamocortical connections of parietal somatosensory cortical fields in macaque monkeys are highly divergent and convergent. Cereb Cortex. 2009; 19(9):2038–2064

[18] Catani M, Howard RJ, Pajevic S, Jones DK. Virtual in vivo interactive dissection of white matter fasciculi in the human brain. Neuroimage. 2002; 17(1):77–94

[19] Makris N, Kennedy DN, McInerney S, et al. Segmentation of subcomponents within the superior longitudinal fascicle in humans: a quantitative, in vivo, DT-MRI study. Cereb Cortex. 2005; 15(6):854–869

[20] Martino J, De Witt Hamer PC, Berger MS, et al. Analysis of the subcomponents and cortical terminations of the perisylvian superior longitudinal fasciculus: a fiber dissection and DTI tractography study. Brain Struct Funct. 2013; 218 (1):105–121

[21] Yagmurlu K, Vlasak AL, Rhoton AL, Jr. Three-dimensional topographic fiber tract anatomy of the cerebrum. Neurosurgery. 2015; 11 Suppl 2:274–305, discussion 305

[22] Catani M, Jones DK, ffytche DH. Perisylvian language networks of the human brain. Ann Neurol. 2005; 57(1):8–16

[23] Rilling JK, Glasser MF, Preuss TM, et al. The evolution of the arcuate fasciculus revealed with comparative DTI. Nat Neurosci. 2008; 11(4):426–428

[24] Bernal B, Ardila A. The role of the arcuate fasciculus in conduction aphasia. Brain. 2009; 132(Pt 9):2309–2316

[25] Parker GJ, Luzzi S, Alexander DC, Wheeler-Kingshott CA, Ciccarelli O, Lambon Ralph MA. Lateralization of ventral and dorsal auditory-language pathways in the human brain. Neuroimage. 2005; 24(3):656–666

[26] Rauschecker JP. An expanded role for the dorsal auditory pathway in sensorimotor control and integration. Hear Res. 2011; 271(1–2):16–25

[27] Shinoura N, Suzuki Y, Yamada R, Tabei Y, Saito K, Yagi K. Damage to the right superior longitudinal fasciculus in the inferior parietal lobe plays a role in spatial neglect. Neuropsychologia. 2009; 47(12):2600–2603

[28] Dick AS, Tremblay P. Beyond the arcuate fasciculus: consensus and controversy in the connectional anatomy of language. Brain. 2012; 135(Pt 12): 3529–3550

[29] Vestergaard M, Madsen KS, Baaré WF, et al. White matter microstructure in superior longitudinal fasciculus associated with spatial working memory performance in children. J Cogn Neurosci. 2011; 23(9):2135–2146

[30] Duffau H. The "frontal syndrome" revisited: lessons from electrostimulation mapping studies. Cortex. 2012; 48(1):120–131

4 Direct Functional Mapping Using Radiographic Methods (fMRI and DTI)

Erik H. Middlebrooks, Vivek Gupta, and Prasanna G. Vibhute

Abstract

Methods for noninvasively mapping neuronal activity (e.g., functional magnetic resonance imaging) and white matter connections (e.g., diffusion tensor imaging) have rapidly evolved. These techniques have greatly enhanced our understanding of normal brain function and anatomy. Their use in surgical planning has also had a positive impact on patient outcomes, operative times, and survival; however, these techniques remain subject to several potential pitfalls and limitations. In this chapter, we discuss the basics of these imaging methods and explore their current limitations.

Keywords: functional MRI, diffusion tensor imaging, connectomics, brain mapping, surgical planning

4.1 Functional MRI

The principles underlying the use of magnetic resonance imaging (MRI) to detect intrinsic changes in blood oxygenation related to neuronal activity were first reported in humans in 1991 by Belliveau et al[1] using dynamic susceptibility contrast and followed by the first human report of blood oxygen level dependent (BOLD) imaging in 1992 by Ogawa et al.[2] These early studies highlighted the potential of dynamic MRI in assessing brain activity. Since then, substantial progress has been made in functional neuroimaging, and BOLD imaging has become a standard tool used in understanding brain function in vivo.

4.1.1 Principles

The signal change detected in BOLD functional MRI (fMRI) results from a change in relative concentrations of oxy- and deoxyhemoglobin. At the onset of neuronal activity, local vasodilation that exceeds the increased energy demand results in an effective increase in oxyhemoglobin and a resultant small, 1 to 5%, change in MRI intensity. The physiologic effects are not instantaneous. The time dependency of these effects is modeled by the hemodynamic response function (HRF).[3] In the normal adult brain, oxyhemoglobin change peaks approximately 6 seconds after the onset of neuronal activity and does not return to baseline until nearly 16 seconds after the initial neuronal onset (► Fig. 4.1). While the exact timing varies slightly across brain regions and subjects, this "double-gamma" function generally applies. Unfortunately, in the setting of brain pathology, this model may be inaccurate, or the HRF may not exist at all. This breakdown of a normal blood flow response to neuronal activity is termed "neurovascular uncoupling" (NVU) and is a major limitation of current clinical fMRI applications.[4]

4.1.2 Task-Based Functional Magnetic Resonance Imaging

Currently, task-based fMRI is the most commonly applied method of performing functional imaging in the clinical setting. In task-based fMRI, the subject performs various tasks in the MRI scanner intended to elicit a specific brain function (e.g., tapping fingers to elicit hand motor activation). A block task design is most widely utilized and consists of short blocks of the active task (e.g., finger tapping) alternating with a control task (e.g., rest). Since BOLD signal is typically modeled as a linear time-invariant (LTI) system, rapid repetition of the task will scale the measured signal proportionally (e.g., back-to-back finger taps will produce twice the BOLD signal change as a single finger tap); however, the rate of signal rise and decay reaches a steady state at approximately 16 seconds. Therefore, individual blocks in task-based fMRI are typically short, on the order of 20 to 30 seconds. The block design remains a mainstay of clinical practice as it results in a maximum functional signal-to-noise ratio and the most robust activation given this summation of individual HRFs. The most common method of analysis of task-based fMRI is the general linear model (GLM) in which the

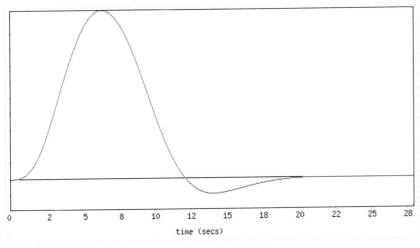

Fig. 4.1 Hemodynamic response function illustrating the expected MRI signal change over time in response to a single neural stimulus.

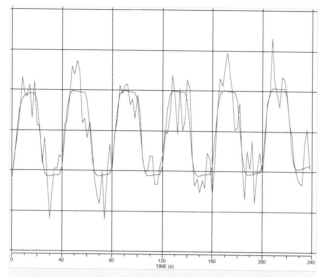

Fig. 4.2 Typical task-based fMRI time course showing the change in signal over time (red curve) and the expected time course in blue, obtained by convolution of the hemodynamic response function and the block design (on–off cycles of 20 seconds each × 6 cycles).

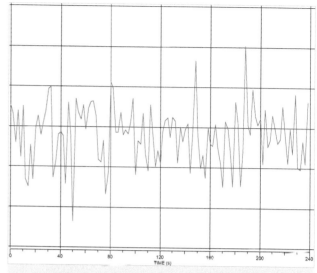

Fig. 4.3 Typical time course for resting-state fMRI. As opposed to task-based design, the expected time course is not known. Rather, a spontaneous oscillation of signal is present that represents a combination of neuronal resting activity and numerous sources of noise and unwanted signal.

expected variation in BOLD signal over time is predictable by a convolution of the block design (on and off block pattern) and the hemodynamic response curve (▶ Fig. 4.2).

4.1.3 Resting-State Functional Magnetic Resonance Imaging

In recent years, resting-state fMRI (rs-fMRI) has grown rapidly in popularity. Slow (< 0.1 Hz) spontaneous oscillations in BOLD signal had been initially considered noise in fMRI until these were first suggested to have a neural origin in a landmark study by Biswal et al in 1995.[5] In this study, Biswal et al were able to show that these seemingly erratic BOLD signal fluctuations in the motor cortex at rest were in close synchrony with the contralateral motor cortex.[5] Since this original paper, numerous resting brain networks have been shown including those in memory, language, executive function, and attention.

As opposed to task-based fMRI, no tasks are performed by the patient while in the scanner. Due to the absence of a task, the analysis of rs-fMRI data presents several major challenges. Recall that in the block design task-based fMRI, the expected BOLD signal change related to the task is already known by the convolution of the block design and the HRF allowing straightforward application of a GLM. In rs-fMRI, spontaneous BOLD signal changes are measured, and there is no preconceived knowledge of the expected time course of signal change (▶ Fig. 4.3). Thus, analysis of rs-fMRI requires a different mathematical approach.[6] Two of the most common approaches are seed-based analysis (SBA) and independent component analysis (ICA). SBA relies on choosing a reference region in the brain for which the BOLD signal time course can be extracted and used as the basis for a GLM in the remainder of the brain to find areas of similar spontaneous signal change. This is nicely illustrated by the original experiment of Biswal et al where the time

course for one motor cortex is used as a model for eliciting the remainder of the motor network.[5] SBA, therefore, relies on an a priori assumption about the network of interest. The SBA approach is often able to be applied to preoperative planning when a normal network seed is readily identified, such as the anatomic reliability of the normal contralateral motor cortex, but it can be problematic when such reliability is absent. For instance, given the lateralization of language networks and variance of functional anatomy relative to anatomical landmarks, choosing an appropriate seed point can be challenging. The ICA approach uses no a priori assumption, but rather decomposes the time course throughout the whole brain into multiple component maps that explain the variance in the data. It is important to note that much of the variance in the time course is explained by phenomena of no interest, such as the cardiac and respiratory cycle, motion, and thermal noise. Therefore, each component identified must then be categorized as a potential brain network versus a signal of no interest. ICA has been shown as potentially reliable for use in preoperative identification of brain networks; however, questions remain to be answered including the ideal number of components and the ideal way of identifying relevant component maps.[6]

Although seemingly easier to perform than task-based fMRI, rs-fMRI presents several additional challenges. First, the true origin of these resting BOLD signal fluctuations is not known. Recent evidence does support a neural origin; however, the lack of understanding of their origin means limited insight into the effects of brain pathology. Second, NVU has also been demonstrated in rs-fMRI, but the relationship of NVU with resting BOLD fluctuations is not entirely clear.[7] Last, in task-based fMRI, the extended experimental blocks of 20 to 30 seconds allow increased ability to remove sources of higher frequency noise (such as cardiac and respiratory signal) with the simple application on a bandpass filter. Unfortunately, the BOLD signal change of interest in rs-fMRI lies in the same frequency range as do these sources of noise and unwanted signal. Therefore, separation of true signal from background is more challenging in rs-fMRI. In summary, rs-fMRI provides a unique method of identifying brain networks and is likely applicable to a greater number of patients (including pediatric patients, patients with cognitive impairment, etc.); however, many unique challenges of rs-fMRI have prevented its widespread use in presurgical planning, to date.

4.1.4 Functional Magnetic Resonance Imaging in Surgical Planning

Some of the earliest studies assessing preoperative fMRI focused on sensorimotor mapping and were able to show a high correlation between intraoperative stimulation and task-based fMRI.[8,9,10] Studies also compared fMRI and the intracarotid sodium amobarbital (Wada) test for lateralizing language function, again showing a high agreement rate.[11,12] These studies, among others, were able to establish the reproducibility and reliability of fMRI as a clinical tool. In the subsequent years, several key studies were able to ascertain the clinical benefit of presurgical fMRI including a reduction in preoperative resources, such as avoidance of Wada testing, a change in operative planning in approximately half of patients, and reduction in operative time.[13,14,15] These studies, among others, ultimately led to the establishment of a Current Procedural Terminology (**CPT**) code for fMRI in January 2007, followed by the introduction of several Food and Drug Administration (FDA)-approved fMRI software platforms. To date, preoperative planning remains the only FDA approved use of clinical fMRI.

Due to the rapid adoption of fMRI into clinical practice, randomized clinical trials have been challenging to produce, and a majority of data is retrospective. Nevertheless, the addition of preoperative fMRI has been shown to reduce postoperative complications with a significant increase in extent of resection, postoperative KPS, and increased median survival, reducing the risk of death by nearly 50%.[16] Additionally, fMRI has proven to be significantly more accurate in localizing motor function in the setting of distorted anatomy when compared to expert review of structural imaging.[17] When assessing for the hand motor cortex in a tumor-affected hemisphere, structural imaging only allowed identification in 86% of subjects compared to 99% with fMRI.[17]

While motor mapping with fMRI has proven quite reliable, such high correlation with language mapping has proven challenging. Numerous factors contribute to the inconsistencies in language mapping. Most importantly, there is substantial variability in the protocols utilized across centers, and outdated anatomical models of language are also commonly encountered. Often, paradigms utilized for language mapping are unsatisfactory due to poor design, such as the use of rest as a control task, and poor linguistic control. Along these lines, the traditional use of the outdated dichotomous "receptive" and "expressive" model of language and the monikers of Wernicke and Broca areas have led to further confusion. Reliance on such outdated models of language function also leads to the inappropriate assessment of language tasks during awake mapping and often an erroneous assumption of a lack of correlation with fMRI results.[18] Despite these shortcomings, a recent meta-analysis of language mapping with fMRI showed a sensitivity of 67% and specificity of 55% for language fMRI.[19] As expected, this meta-analysis confirmed the significant effect on sensitivity and specificity due to language tasks, statistical thresholds, and imaging times.[19]

In summary, preoperative assessment of sensorimotor localization with fMRI has repeatedly been shown as highly reproducible with high correlation to intraoperative mapping. Language mapping has shown much higher variability that is likely confounded by inconsistent terminology, fMRI tasks, as well as similar variability in intraoperative testing. The use of fMRI in preoperative mapping has been shown to offer several benefits including altering surgical plans, reduced operative times, reduced complication rates, and increased tumor resection. Importantly, fMRI serves as a useful adjunct (▶ Fig. 4.4) but is not a substitute for meticulous intraoperative mapping.

4.2 Diffusion Tensor Imaging

Although cortical landmarks can often provide some inference of cortical function in the setting of brain tumors, the vector of displacement of critical white matter tracts is often more challenging. The emergence of white matter fiber tracking via MRI has proven to be a useful tool for preoperative subcortical mapping. The most commonly utilized method in the clinical setting remains the diffusion tensor imaging (DTI) model.

4.2.1 Principles

Diffusion-weighted imaging (DWI) is a commonly utilized technique in MRI that allows the quantification of microscopic water diffusion in vivo. Historically, DWI is widely used in routine brain MRI for detection and characterization of various brain pathologies, most notably playing a pivotal role in the assessment of stroke. Traditional DWI largely focuses on the general diffusibility of water in any direction; however, by applying directionally oriented magnetic field gradients in multiple directions, one can also quantify the preferential direction and magnitude of water diffusion in tissue. By quantifying the diffusion of water in a minimum of six different diffusion directions, a vector can be defined and is the basis of the tensor model (DTI). By modeling this tensor across the entire brain, white matter fiber bundles can be modeled by examining the relationship of any voxel of tissue with its neighbors (▶ Fig. 4.5).

Several important limitations of DTI are noteworthy. Most importantly, the modeling of a single vector per voxel of tissue is inherently flawed due to the presence of crossing fibers in a large portion of the white matter.[20] For example, if two fiber tracts cross at 90 degrees in a voxel, a single vector will result in an erroneous model of the fiber geometry such that the vector is oriented at 45 degrees between the true orientation of the two perpendicular fiber bundles. DTI also relies on a model-based approach with an assumption regarding the amount of water within the tissue that is bound by the cell membrane. Such model-based approaches typically fail to correctly model fiber anatomy in the presence of edema or tumor infiltration, which is a major shortcoming in the setting of planning tumor resection.[20] Despite these major limitations, DTI has remained commonplace in the clinical setting due to the lengthy acquisitions and complex modeling necessary in more modern approaches. Recent advances in diffusion imaging, notably

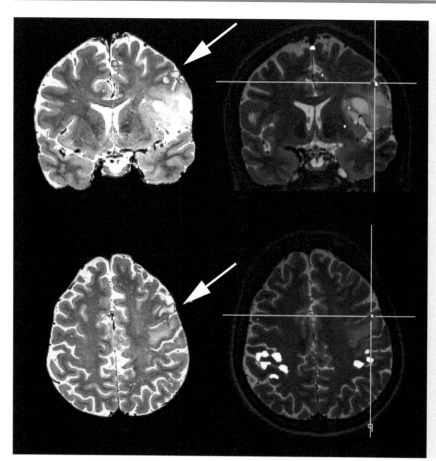

Fig. 4.4 Preoperative language fMRI using a sentence completion task shows activation in the left frontoparietal operculum (arrow) corresponding to the pars opercularis and ventral premotor cortex. Intraoperative navigation showing an area of speech arrest (green crosshairs) elicited by cortical stimulation.

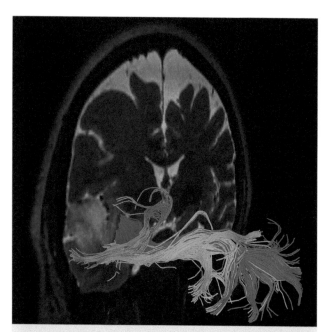

Fig. 4.5 Preoperative DTI highlights the displacement of the middle longitudinal fasciculus (orange), inferior longitudinal fasciculus (green), and inferior fronto-occipital fasciculus (blue) relative to a temporal lobe glioma.

simultaneous multislice (SMS) image acceleration, have resulted in the potential clinical feasibility of better model-free approaches like diffusion spectrum imaging (DSI) and q-ball imaging that are less prone to the aforementioned limitations.[20]

To summarize, DTI is a widely utilized noninvasive method of modeling white matter fiber tracts in the brain (▶ Fig. 4.6). While a major clinical benefit still exists using the DTI model, there are important limitations, such as modeling of crossing fibers and tracking in the setting of brain edema and tumor infiltration. Newer methods of fiber tracking are likely to supplant the clinical use of the DTI model in the near future; however, these methods present their own challenges (e.g., imaging time, computation resources, and sophisticated mathematical modeling).

4.2.2 Clinical Outcomes

Correlation between DTI and subcortical mapping has been shown to have high sensitivity (>90%) for both motor and language tracts.[21] Unlike fMRI, prospective studies have been performed to assess the effect of DTI on patient outcomes. In a prospective, randomized study of 238 patients, Wu et al found a significant reduction in postoperative motor deficits in the DTI group (32.8% of patients in the control group versus 15.3% of patients with DTI).[22] There was also a significantly higher Karnofsky Performance Scale score in patients with DTI (86 ±

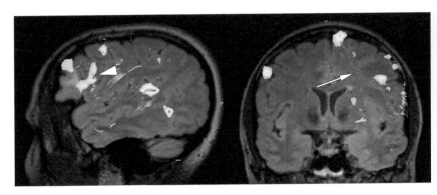

Fig. 4.6 Combined preoperative DTI and language fMRI using a sentence completion task in the sagittal (left) and coronal (right) planes. Opercular activation (arrowhead) corresponding to the combined pars opercularis and ventral premotor cortex is shown along the posterior margin of the tumor. The relationship of the frontal aslant tract (arrow) is also shown as it traverses from the pre-supplementary motor area to the frontal operculum.

20 vs. 74 ± 28 in the control group), as well as a survival benefit in high-grade gliomas (21.2 months median vs. 14.0 months in the control group).[22] The addition of DTI alone resulted in a 43.0% reduction in the risk of death.[22]

4.3 Conclusion

Despite several known limitations, fMRI and DTI have both proven to be valuable additions to the preoperative assessment of brain tumors and epilepsy. An understanding of the limitations and benefits of high-quality fMRI and DTI will assist with maximizing their efficacy and safety in clinical practice. The rapid advancement of technologies behind these tools, as well as an improved understanding of their performance in the abnormal brain, will only further enhance their utility in clinical medicine. Neither tool is a substitute for careful intraoperative mapping but allows improved preoperative planning, shorter operative times, and a benefit in functional outcomes and overall survival.

References

[1] Belliveau JW, Kennedy DN, Jr, McKinstry RC, et al. Functional mapping of the human visual cortex by magnetic resonance imaging. Science. 1991; 254 (5032):716–719

[2] Ogawa S, Tank DW, Menon R, et al. Intrinsic signal changes accompanying sensory stimulation: functional brain mapping with magnetic resonance imaging. Proc Natl Acad Sci U S A. 1992; 89(13):5951–5955

[3] Buxton RB, Uludağ K, Dubowitz DJ, Liu TT. Modeling the hemodynamic response to brain activation. Neuroimage. 2004; 23 Suppl 1:S220–S233

[4] Ulmer JL, Krouwer HG, Mueller WM, Ugurel MS, Kocak M, Mark LP. Pseudo-reorganization of language cortical function at fMR imaging: a consequence of tumor-induced neurovascular uncoupling. AJNR Am J Neuroradiol. 2003; 24(2):213–217

[5] Biswal B, Yetkin FZ, Haughton VM, Hyde JS. Functional connectivity in the motor cortex of resting human brain using echo-planar MRI. Magn Reson Med. 1995; 34(4):537–541

[6] Rosazza C, Zacà D, Bruzzone MG. Pre-surgical brain mapping: to rest or not to rest? Front Neurol. 2018; 9:520

[7] Agarwal S, Sair HI, Yahyavi-Firouz-Abadi N, Airan R, Pillai JJ. Neurovascular uncoupling in resting state fMRI demonstrated in patients with primary brain gliomas. J Magn Reson Imaging. 2016; 43(3):620–626

[8] Yetkin FZ, Mueller WM, Morris GL, et al. Functional MR activation correlated with intraoperative cortical mapping. AJNR Am J Neuroradiol. 1997; 18(7): 1311–1315

[9] Roux FE, Boulanouar K, Ranjeva JP, et al. Usefulness of motor functional MRI correlated to cortical mapping in Rolandic low-grade astrocytomas. Acta Neurochir (Wien). 1999; 141(1):71–79

[10] Hirsch J, Ruge MI, Kim KH, et al. An integrated functional magnetic resonance imaging procedure for preoperative mapping of cortical areas associated with tactile, motor, language, and visual functions. Neurosurgery. 2000; 47(3): 711–721, discussion 721–722

[11] Binder JR, Swanson SJ, Hammeke TA, et al. Determination of language dominance using functional MRI: a comparison with the Wada test. Neurology. 1996; 46(4):978–984

[12] Bahn MM, Lin W, Silbergeld DL, et al. Localization of language cortices by functional MR imaging compared with intracarotid amobarbital hemispheric sedation. AJR Am J Roentgenol. 1997; 169(2):575–579

[13] Petrella JR, Shah LM, Harris KM, et al. Preoperative functional MR imaging localization of language and motor areas: effect on therapeutic decision making in patients with potentially resectable brain tumors. Radiology. 2006; 240 (3):793–802

[14] Medina LS, Bernal B, Dunoyer C, et al. Seizure disorders: functional MR imaging for diagnostic evaluation and surgical treatment–prospective study. Radiology. 2005; 236(1):247–253

[15] Roessler K, Donat M, Lanzenberger R, et al. Evaluation of preoperative high magnetic field motor functional MRI (3 Tesla) in glioma patients by navigated electrocortical stimulation and postoperative outcome. J Neurol Neurosurg Psychiatry. 2005; 76(8):1152–1157

[16] Sang S, Wanggou S, Wang Z, et al. Clinical long-term follow-up evaluation of functional neuronavigation in adult cerebral gliomas. World Neurosurg. 2018; 119:e262–e271

[17] Wengenroth M, Blatow M, Guenther J, Akbar M, Tronnier VM, Stippich C. Diagnostic benefits of presurgical fMRI in patients with brain tumours in the primary sensorimotor cortex. Eur Radiol. 2011; 21(7):1517–1525

[18] Middlebrooks EH, Yagmurlu K, Szaflarski JP, Rahman M, Bozkurt B. A contemporary framework of language processing in the human brain in the context of preoperative and intraoperative language mapping. Neuroradiology. 2017

[19] Weng HH, Noll KR, Johnson JM, et al. Accuracy of presurgical functional MR imaging for language mapping of brain tumors: a systematic review and meta-analysis. Radiology. 2018; 286(2):512–523

[20] Wedeen VJ, Wang RP, Schmahmann JD, et al. Diffusion spectrum magnetic resonance imaging (DSI) tractography of crossing fibers. Neuroimage. 2008; 41(4):1267–1277

[21] Bello L, Gambini A, Castellano A, et al. Motor and language DTI fiber tracking combined with intraoperative subcortical mapping for surgical removal of gliomas. Neuroimage. 2008; 39(1):369–382

[22] Wu JS, Zhou LF, Tang WJ, et al. Clinical evaluation and follow-up outcome of diffusion tensor imaging-based functional neuronavigation: a prospective, controlled study in patients with gliomas involving pyramidal tracts. Neurosurgery. 2007; 61(5):935–948, discussion 948–949

5 Indirect Functional Mapping Using Radiographic Methods

Vivek Gupta, Erik H. Middlebrooks, and Prasanna G. Vibhute

Abstract

The anatomy of human brain demonstrates remarkable consistency of functional organization and serves as valuable adjunct to direct functional mapping with functional magnetic resonance imaging and diffusion tensor imaging. Identification of key anatomic landmarks provides reliable information about the topographic relationship of the lesions with functional regions and facilitates safe surgical resection. In this chapter, we provide an overview and a practical template for identification of the surgically relevant brain functional anatomy on cross-sectional images.

Keywords: MRI, functional neuroanatomy, somatotopy, brain mapping, surgical planning

5.1 Introduction

The human brain is structured on the basis of regional functional specialization and integration of these regions into task-defined networks. Regions of cortex and subcortical nuclei behave as functional modules, each with a distinct cytoarchitecture. All perceptual, executive, and motor functions recruit a subset of these functional modules into a network determined by the specific needs of the task. Thus, operations of these cortical functional "modules" are best viewed as serial or parallel subprocesses required for task execution. The white matter tracts serve as pathways of information flow across these modules.

Indirect, lesion-based data have been instrumental in defining the overall functional neuroanatomic organization of the brain. One of the highlights of brain organization is the remarkable consistency of regional functional specialization across human subjects and, to a slightly lesser extent, all primates. For example, the primary hand motor cortex can be reliably localized by identifying the "knob" or inverted "omega" in the precentral gyrus (pre-CG), and phonological information processing in posterior half of the superior temporal sulcus (STS). This chapter focuses on anatomic neuroimaging-based localization of sensorimotor and language regions, which are two of the most critical functions neurosurgeons aim to preserve. Surgical interventions in or adjacent to these "eloquent" brain regions carry higher risk of postoperative neurological deficits that majorly impact quality of life. Although there have been major advances in our ability to map brain function including widespread application of blood oxygen level dependent (BOLD) functional magnetic resonance imaging (fMRI), sound understanding of functional neuroanatomy remains critical in surgical decision-making. Interpretation and meaningful reporting of clinical fMRI cannot be performed without the knowledge of appropriate anatomic landmarks.

5.2 Primary Sensorimotor (Pericentral, Perirolandic, S1M1) and Supplementary Motor Cortex

Resections in this region involve risk of permanent motor and sensory deficits that seriously limit everyday function. Primary sensorimotor cortex has a consistent morphology that is readily and reliably identified by imaging landmarks (▶ Fig. 5.1, ▶ Fig. 5.2, ▶ Fig. 5.3, ▶ Fig. 5.4, ▶ Fig. 5.5). Fortunately, visualization of these landmarks is subject to little variation despite changes in scan orientation.

Several anatomic imaging landmarks and morphologic appearances can be used to reliably identify the primary sensorimotor cortex. In their practice, the authors begin by identifying in the axial images the superior frontal sulcus (SFS) located immediately paramedian to the anterior interhemispheric fissure. The SFS ends posteriorly by joining the precentral sulcus (pre-CS), which runs immediately anterior and parallel to the central sulcus (CS). The latter separates the anterior pre-CG from posterior postcentral gyrus (post-CG). CS is then confirmed by tracing it medially toward the interhemispheric fissure where it curves slightly posteriorly and ends in 94 to 96% of cases by pointing at the horizontal bracket formed by pars marginalis (pars "bracket" sign; ▶ Fig. 5.1a, ▶ Fig. 5.3).[1,2,3] Pars marginalis or the marginal ramus is a superior directed branch of the cingulate sulcus on the interhemispheric surface that terminates by curving over the apex of the cerebral convexity immediately posterior to the CS (▶ Fig. 5.1a, c). A highly reliable and readily applicable landmark along the CS is the precentral "knob," an inverted omega (℧) or less commonly a horizontal epsilon (ω) shape protuberance from the posterior face of pre-CG. This is located on the pre-CG, immediately lateral to the parasagittal plane passing through the SFS and is a site for hand motor area (▶ Fig. 5.1a, ▶ Fig. 5.2).[1] On the parasagittal image passing through the plane of insula, the precentral knob corresponds to the "precental hook" that snugly fits into a concavity of hand sensory region of the post-CG (▶ Fig. 5.1b, ▶ Fig. 5.5b).[1] Finally, the anteroposterior thickness of the pre-CG is always greater than that of the post-CG.[3] Together, the above features are highly reliable in confirming the location of the primary sensorimotor cortex.

Even when the regional anatomy is effaced and distorted by tumor mass effect and edema, the above methodology is invariably successful in identifying the CS (▶ Fig. 5.3, ▶ Fig. 5.4, ▶ Fig. 5.5). In the presence of subcortical vasogenic edema in the perirolandic region, a twofold difference in cortical thickness between the anterior and posterior banks of the CS uniquely identifies the CS on T2-weighted images despite the marked distortion of sulcal anatomy (▶ Fig. 5.4).[4,5] The face sensorimotor cortex can be fairly reliably localized about 2 cm inferolateral to the hand knob along the CS. Similarly, the primary sensorimotor localization of foot corresponds to the posterior paracentral lobule (PCL), located on the medial surface of the cerebrum, immediately anterior to the pars marginalis (▶ Fig. 5.2). Thus, the somatotopy of the primary sensorimotor cortex is laid out from lateral to medial. Compared to the precentral knob, which is highly specific for the hand motor region, anatomic approaches have limited accuracy for localization of the remaining primary sensorimotor homunculus. Despite excellent landmarks for identification of the S1M1, the anatomic approach for its localization can be rarely limited by occasional anatomic variants, extreme

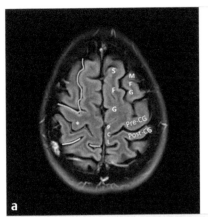
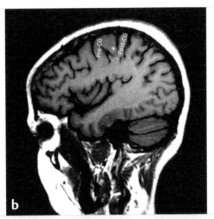
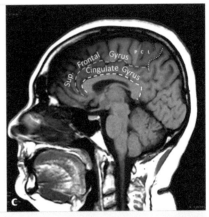

Fig. 5.1 Normal anatomy—sensorimotor region. (**a**) Axial plane: Step 1—Superior frontal sulcus (SFS—*blue line*) is identified as the parasagittal sulcus parallel to the interhemispheric fissure. Step 2—The SFS when traced posteriorly terminates into the precentral sulcus (pre-CS—*orange line*). Step 3—Immediately posterior to the pre-CS is the precentral gyrus (pre-CG), which in turn is separated from the postcentral gyrus (post-CG) by the central sulcus (CS—*red line*). Step 4—The CS is verified by (i) identifying the hand motor "knob" (•) on the posterior face of the pre-CG, which lies just lateral to the parasagittal line passing through the SFS; (ii) confirming that the medial end of the CS dips into the horizontal bracket formed by pars marginalis (PM—*green line*), known as the pars "bracket sign"; (iii) that the pre-CG is always thicker than the post-CG; and (iv) the cortical thickness of the anterior bank of the CS is thicker than the posterior bank of CS (best seen in the presence of vasogenic edema, see ▶ Fig. 5.4b). Note that the paracentral lobule (PCL) is contained between the SFG anteriorly and PM posteriorly. (**b**) Parasagittal plane passing through the plane of insula: the hand motor region can be readily identified on this image as a "hook" (•) that snuggly fits into a concavity of hand sensory region of the post-CG (*open arrow*). (**c**) Midsagittal plane: the medial surface of the cerebral hemisphere is made up of alternating arrangement of curvilinear sulci and gyri that are concentric to the corpus callosum. From inside out these are pericallosal sulcus (*broken white line*), cingulate gyrus, cingulate (a.k.a. callosomarginal) sulcus (*broken green line*), and superior (a.k.a. medial) frontal gyrus. Pars marginalis or marginal ramus (*dotted green*) is a branch of the cingulate sulcus that curves away toward the convexity and forms the posterior limit of the PCL. The CS (*dotted red*) dives over the medial margin of the cerebral convexity, notches the PCL, and is surrounded by primary S1M1 representation of the foot (*shaded red*). Immediately anteriorly is the SMA, occupying the frontal portion of the PCL and adjacent posterior one-third portion of the SFG (*shaded yellow*). Anterior to the SMA is pre-SMA within the mid one-third of the SFG (*shaded blue*).

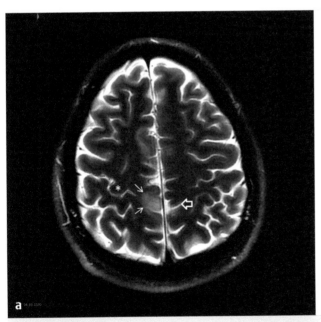
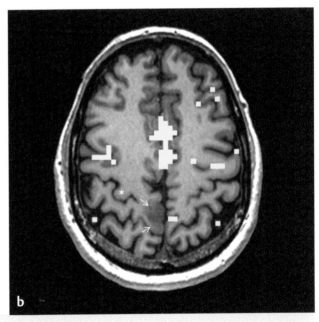

Fig. 5.2 Pathology—Primary sensorimotor foot region low-grade glioma (paracentral lobule [PCL]). (**a**) Axial T2-weighted image of a 42-year-old man presenting with insidious onset of left foot clumsiness reveals a low-grade glioma involving the right PCL (*small arrows*). The standard steps described in the normal anatomy (see legend of ▶ Fig. 5.1) were followed for localization of this tumor. The SFS was first sought on more superior axial views (not shown) and used to identify the pre-CS and CS. The CS (*broken red line*) was reconfirmed by presence of the precentral "knob" (*asterisk*). The lesion is located at the medial end of the CS, and therefore, involves the PCL. Note the effacement of right PM by the tumor in comparison to the contralateral left PM (*empty arrow*). PM was distinguished from the immediate posterior similar looking sulcus, by tracing the connection of the PM to the CS on the medial hemispheric surface on the orthogonal sagittal section (not shown). (**b**) BOLD fMRI activation map of simultaneous foot motor task shows deceptive absence of activation in the right PCM on bilateral foot motor task, even though the patient was able to move his left foot. Large areas of activation in the interhemispheric fissure anterior to the lesion represent SMA and pre-SMA. Activation overlying the pre-CS represents frontal eye fields.

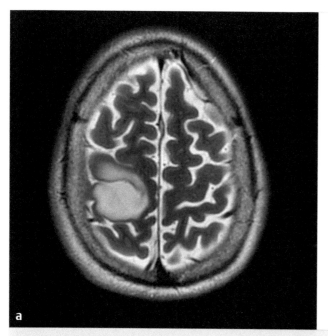
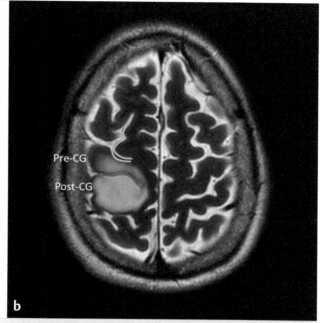

Fig. 5.3 Pathology—Primary sensorimotor hand region glioma. (**a, b**) Axial T2-weighted image at the level of ventricles reveals a perirolandic hyperintense T2 glioma, primarily expanding the post-CG. Although the regional anatomy is distorted with anterior displacement and complete effacement of the CS (*red*), the mass can be correctly localized by first identifying the SFS (*blue*) and following it posteriorly to the pre-CS (*orange*). Also, despite distortion by the mass effect, note the maintained relationship of PM (*green*) with medial end of CS (pars "bracket" sign). The effacement of pre-CG hand "knob" due to mass effect limits its use for localization.

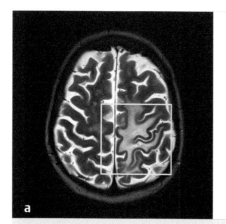
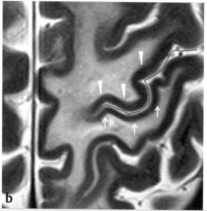
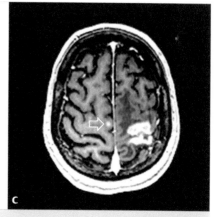

Fig. 5.4 Pathology—Primary sensorimotor region metastasis. (**a**) Axial T2-weighted image of a 65-year-old woman suffering from metastatic lung cancer shows extensive vasogenic edema involving the left frontoparietal junction. (**b**) Observation of twofold difference in cortical thickness between the anterior (*arrowheads*) and posterior (*arrows*) banks helps reliably identify the CS. Although normally seen, this finding becomes self-evident in presence of vasogenic edema, particularly on the axial T2-weighted sequence. This imaging pearl is elegantly revealed on the magnified boxed region of the axial T2-weighted image. Note the fulfilment of the pars "bracket" sign (*green*) and the greater thickness of the pre-CG compared to the post-CG lends additional evidence for accurate localization of the CS. (**c**) Axial T1-weighted postcontrast image immediately above the level of T2-image shows an irregular heterogeneously enhancing lesion straddling the left CS as the cause for this edema. An additional tiny enhancing juxta-cortical metastasis is seen within the right PCL (*open arrow*).

pathological distortions of anatomy, and functional reorganization induced by lesions.

The supplementary motor area (SMA) is located on the medial surface of the cerebral hemisphere in the anterior PCL and posterior end of the medial (superior) frontal gyrus (▶ Fig. 5.1c). On the axial plane, as the name implies, the PCL can be easily identified as a lobule at the medial end of the CS, located between the pars marginalis posteriorly and superior frontal gyrus (SFG) anteriorly (▶ Fig. 5.1a, c, ▶ Fig. 5.2). The somatotopy in SMA is from anterior to posterior: the SMA for lower extremity lies immediately anterior to the corresponding M1; the two are often inseparable on BOLD fMRI. Immediately anterior to the SMA lies the pre-SMA with a similarly oriented, albeit, coarser somatotopy. Pre-SMA appears to be involved in

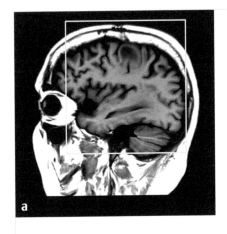
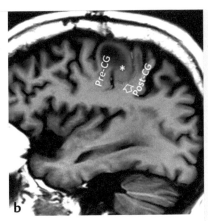
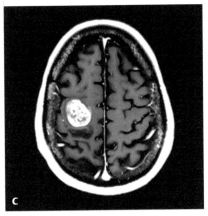
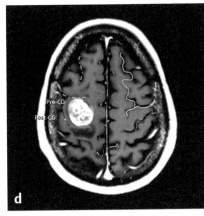

Fig. 5.5 Pathology—Primary sensorimotor hand region metastasis. (**a**) Noncontrast sagittal T1-weighted image: a metastasis localizing to the hand motor region of the pre-CG and seen as an expanded precentral "hook" (compare with normal anatomy in ▶ Fig. 5.1). This is better seen in the labeled magnified portion of the boxed region (**b**). (**c**) Postcontrast axial T1-weighted image: on axial image, accurate localization of the lesion is possible by orderly front to back identification of the SFS, pre-CS, and CS. Although effaced and posteriorly displaced, the CS continues to maintain its relationship with pars "bracket," which also is posteriorly displaced (*green*). For comparison, the right-sided sulci are outlined by broken lines and the normal left-sided sulci are outlined by solid lines with similar color scheme (**d**).

procedural aspects of cognitive processing, including higher order speech processing.[6]

5.3 Language and Speech Regions

Frontotemporal surgical approaches and resections are heavily governed by the relationship of the lesion with the language network (▶ Fig. 5.6, ▶ Fig. 5.7, ▶ Fig. 5.8, ▶ Fig. 5.9). This is particularly crucial when the lesion is located in dominant hemisphere. Although safe surgery is significantly facilitated by preoperative fMRI mapping of language function in relation to the lesion, the activation patterns are task dependent, delineating subsets of the language network. Therefore, good knowledge of the temporal lobe functional anatomy is imperative, particularly when intraoperative electrocorticography is considered. We will now review imaging anatomy of the language network.

The transverse temporal gyrus, also known as the gyrus of Heschl (HG) is the seat of the primary auditory cortex (▶ Fig. 5.6). In axial plane through the massa intermedia, the HG extends outwards anterolaterally from the posterior end of insula (▶ Fig. 5.6d). In the sagittal plane just lateral to the plane of insula, this is easily identified as a protuberance between the posterior insula and superior temporal gyrus (STG; ▶ Fig. 5.6a, b). On the coronal plane, the protuberance of the HG is seen at the depth of the posterior end of Sylvian fissure on the superior temporal surface (▶ Fig. 5.6c).[7] The HG processes simple acoustic stimuli such as sound burst and pure tones. Even though HG

is typically larger and longer on the left side, the correlation of its size with language dominance is debatable.[8] The size of triangular superior temporal surface, between the HG and posterior end of the Sylvian fissure, known as "planum temporale," however, appears to be positively correlated with the hemispheric language dominance.[9] The planum temporale, involved in language processing, is separated anteriorly from the HG by Heschl sulcus.

The initial cortical processing of speech takes place along the HG. The information then projects to the posterior half of the STS for phonological processing and representation (▶ Fig. 5.7). From here, language processing appears to split along two distinct streams, the ventral conceptual semantic network and the dorsal articulatory pathway (▶ Fig. 5.8).[10] The dorsal stream, comprising the traditionally described strongly left dominant language network, posteriorly includes the parietotemporal junction (posterior end of the STG, planum temporale, angular gyrus [AG] and supramarginal gyrus [SMG]) that functions as the sensorimotor interface and falls into the traditionally described Wernicke region. This region projects anteriorly via arcuate and superior longitudinal fasciculi onto the inferior frontal gyrus (IFG) and more superiorly onto the dorsolateral prefrontal cortex in the middle frontal gyrus immediately in front of the pre-CS.[11] The posterior planum temporale activation is highly correlated with inferior frontal motor language regions even in subvocal speech. Hence, the importance of this region in the left hemisphere not only in language comprehension but also in speech production tasks cannot be overemphasized.

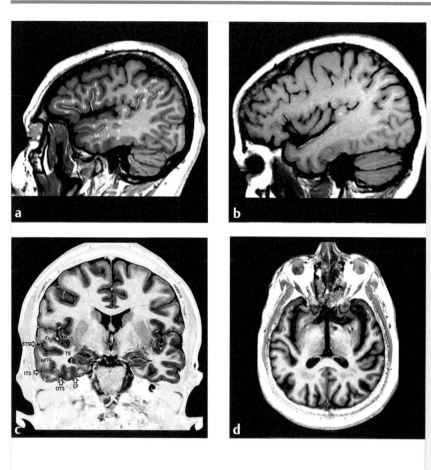

Fig. 5.6 Normal anatomy—Language. (**a**) Sagittal T1-weighted image through the operculum. The frontoparietal operculum above and the temporal operculum below border the Sylvian fissure and cover the insula. Note on the **M**-shaped configuration of the inferior frontal gyrus (IFG) created by the anterior horizontal (*blue*) and anterior vertical rami (*yellow*) of the Sylvian fissure, segmenting the IFG into pars orbitalis (or), pars triangularis (tr), and pars opercularis (op). The posterior ascending ramus (*orange*) of the Sylvian fissure is capped by the supramarginal gyrus (SMG). Posterior to the SMG is angular gyrus (AG) capping the upswing of the superior temporal sulcus (*dotted white line*). (**b**) Sagittal T1-weighted image through the plane of insula: Posteriorly within the Sylvian fissure, the Heschl gyrus (HG) is seen as an omega-shaped protuberance arising from the superior temporal surface. The HG divides the superior temporal surface into the anterior and posterior portions, known as planum polare (*dotted white*) and planum temporale (*dotted red*), respectively. (**c**) Coronal inversion recovery image: Note the superior (STG), middle (MTG), and inferior (ITG) temporal gyri, and the fusiform (FG) and parahippocampal (PHG) gyri fanning out from the temporal stem (TS) on the coronal image (**c**). Separating these gyri are the superior (STS) and inferior (ITS) temporal sulci, occipitotemporal sulcus (OTS), and collateral fissure or sulcus (CF), respectively. (**d**) Axial inversion recovery image: HG is seen extending outward anterolaterally from the posterior end of insula. In order to optimize visualization of the HG, axial images were reconstructed along the superior temporal plane. Note that the white matter of HG blends with that of STG laterally.

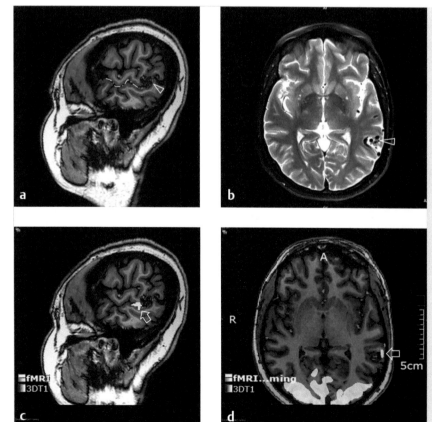

Fig. 5.7 Pathology—Superior temporal sulcus (STS) phonological processing and representation region arteriovenous malformation. (**a**) Axial T2 and (**b**) sagittal T1-weighted images reveal an incidental small arteriovenous malformation (*arrowheads*) centered within the posterior third of the left STS (*broken white line*). (**c**) Sagittal and (**d**) axial language task-based BOLD fMRI obtained as part of preoperative workup confirms left hemispheric language dominance with activation (*open arrows*) seen along the anterior margin of the arteriovenous malformation (AVM) with the STS. Lack of robust activation is likely due to neurovascular uncoupling from regional hemodynamic abnormalities caused by the AVM. In the dominant hemisphere, the posterior end of the STG, the planum temporale, AG, and SMG constitute posterior part of the dorsal language stream, also described as Wernicke region.

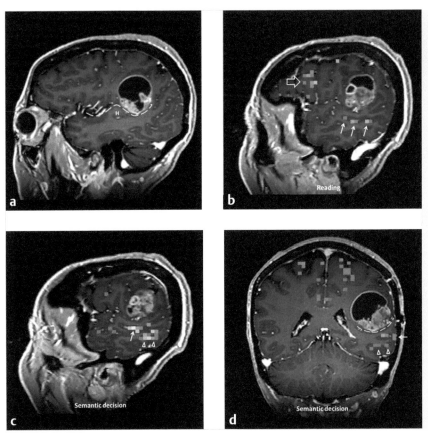

Fig. 5.8 Pathology—Dorsal language stream supramarginal gyrus (SMG) anaplastic glioma. (a) Sagittal T1-weighted MRI: anaplastic astrocytoma in the SMG at the posterior end of the Sylvian fissure. Despite the distorted anatomy, the tumor can be localized to the SMG (dorsal language stream) on the basis of its relationship to the Heschl gyrus (HG) and inferiorly displaced posterior end of the Sylvian fissure (*yellow line*). (b) Sagittal reading task fMRI: superior temporal sulcus (STS; *arrows*) and pars opercularis activation (*open arrow*, dorsal stream) is seen. (c) Sagittal and (d) coronal semantic decision task fMRI: additional activation surrounding the anterior STS and posterior ITS (*arrowheads*, ventral stream) can be seen. The lesion is again noted to abut the inferiorly displaced Sylvian fissure (*yellow line*).

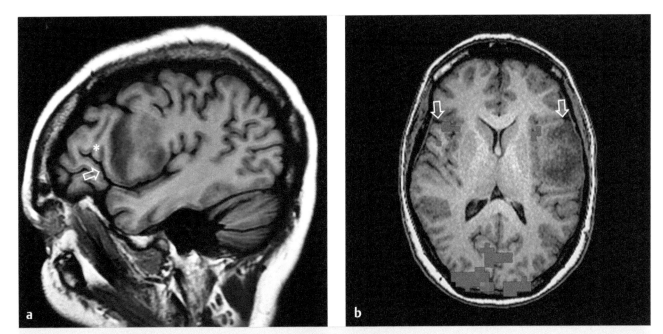

Fig. 5.9 Pathology—Dorsal language stream pars opercularis grade 2 oligodendroglioma. (a) Sagittal T1-weighted MRI: grade 2 oligodendroglioma. The location of the lesion in the pars opercularis is apparent by anterior displacement of the anterior ascending ramus (*arrow*) of the Sylvian fissure and intact pars triangularis (*asterisk*) immediately anterior to the mass. (b) A reading comprehension task fMRI reveals bilateral pars opercularis and anterior insular cortical activation.

35

The more recently understood ventral stream is bilaterally represented and is weakly left hemispheric dominant. This stream includes the posterior middle and inferior temporal gyri (MTG, ITG) that appear to serve as lexical interface between phonological and semantic order processing, and anterior MTG and ITG that serve as parts of combinatorial or syntactical network (▶ Fig. 5.8a, d).[12] This network projects onto ventrolateral prefrontal cortex (pars orbitalis and adjacent pars triangularis) via the inferior fronto-occipital fasciculus in the extreme capsule.[11]

Three horizontal gyri, the STG, MTG, and ITG separated by the STG and inferior temporal sulcus (ITS), form the lateral surface of the temporal lobe. The STG and MTG posteriorly merge into the parietal lobe. The ITG continues onto the inferior surface of the temporal lobe and is posteriorly separated from the inferior occipital gyrus by the preoccipital notch. The ITG is medially separated from the fusiform gyrus (FG) by occipitotemporal sulcus (OTS). While the collateral fissure or sulcus (CF) separates the FG from the medial parahippocampal gyrus (PHG). The posterior vertically oriented extension of the STS, also known as the angular sulcus, terminates in the AG, whereas the posterior ascending ramus of the Sylvian fissure is superiorly capped by the SMG (▶ Fig. 5.6).

The IFG, forming the ventrolateral prefrontal cortex, is classically considered to be the seat of the motor organization in the articulatory network, including silent (inner) speech. The triangular shaped IFG forms the inferolateral boundary of the frontal lobe posteriorly separated from the STG by the Sylvian fissure. The IFG is divided anteroposteriorly into the pars orbitalis (BA 47), pars triangularis (BA 45), and pars opercularis (BA 44) by the anterior horizontal and anterior ascending rami of the Sylvian fissure. These divisions are easily identified on sagittal MR sections by the characteristic "**M**" shape (▶ Fig. 5.6a).[13] The classic Broca area includes the pars opercularis and adjacent posterior pars triangularis and is connected to the Wernicke region by the arcuate fasciculus (AF), forming the dorsal stream.

The insula is covered by the frontoparietal operculum (pars opercularis, subcentral gyrus, and post-CG) superiorly and the temporal operculum (STG and HG) inferiorly and is separated from these by the Sylvian fissure (▶ Fig. 5.6). The insula is divided into anterior and posterior lobule by an obliquely coursing CS. The lesions of the left anterior lobule are known to cause speech apraxia.[14] It now appears that the anterior lobule of the left insula may be responsible for the motor speech function ascribed to IFG by Broca.[15] This is supported by frequent BOLD activation of the anterior insula on fMRI studies of language and speech (▶ Fig. 5.9b).

5.4 Conclusion

The human brain demonstrates a remarkably consistent anatomy that serves as the basis for functional organization. Despite individual variations, all methods of brain functional mapping, including fMRI and electrocorticography, begin with anatomy. In this chapter, we have described the anatomic features of the regions involved in sensorimotor and language functions and the algorithmic approach for their identification on routine clinical imaging.

References

[1] Yousry TA, Schmid UD, Alkadhi H, et al. Localization of the motor hand area to a knob on the precentral gyrus. A new landmark. Brain. 1997; 120(Pt 1): 141–157

[2] Naidich TP, Brightbill T. C. The pars marginalis: Part 1. A "bracket" sign for the central sulcus in axial plane CT and MRI. Inter J Neuroradiol. 1996a; 1:3–19

[3] Naidich TP. BTC. Systems for localizing fronto-parietal gyri and sulci on axial CT and MRI. Int J Neuroradiol. 1996b; 2:313–338

[4] Meyer JR, Roychowdhury S, Russell EJ, Callahan C, Gitelman D, Mesulam MM. Location of the central sulcus via cortical thickness of the precentral and postcentral gyri on MR. AJNR Am J Neuroradiol. 1996; 17(9):1699–1706

[5] Biega TJ, Lonser RR, Butman JA. Differential cortical thickness across the central sulcus: a method for identifying the central sulcus in the presence of mass effect and vasogenic edema. AJNR Am J Neuroradiol. 2006; 27(7):1450–1453

[6] Hertrich I, Dietrich S, Ackermann H. The role of the supplementary motor area for speech and language processing. Neurosci Biobehav Rev. 2016; 68: 602–610

[7] Yousry TA, Fesl G, Buttner A. Heschl's gyrus: anatomic description and methods of identification on magnetic resonance imaging. Int J Neuroradiol. 1997a; 3:2–12

[8] Warrier C, Wong P, Penhune V, et al. Relating structure to function: Heschl's gyrus and acoustic processing. J Neurosci. 2009; 29(1):61–69

[9] Foundas AL, Leonard CM, Gilmore R, Fennell E, Heilman KM. Planum temporale asymmetry and language dominance. Neuropsychologia. 1994; 32(10): 1225–1231

[10] Hickok G, Poeppel D. Dorsal and ventral streams: a framework for understanding aspects of the functional anatomy of language. Cognition. 2004; 92 (1–2):67–99

[11] Saur D, Kreher BW, Schnell S, et al. Ventral and dorsal pathways for language. Proc Natl Acad Sci U S A. 2008; 105(46):18035–18040

[12] Hickok G, Poeppel D. The cortical organization of speech processing. Nat Rev Neurosci. 2007; 8(5):393–402

[13] Naidich TP, Valavanis AG, Kubik S. Anatomic relationships along the low-middle convexity: Part I—Normal specimens and magnetic resonance imaging. Neurosurgery. 1995; 36(3):517–532

[14] Dronkers NF. A new brain region for coordinating speech articulation. Nature. 1996; 384(6605):159–161

[15] Price CJ. The anatomy of language: contributions from functional neuroimaging. J Anat. 2000; 197(Pt 3):335–359

6 Neurophysiology of Identifying Eloquent Regions

Tasneem F. Hasan and William O. Tatum

Abstract

Neurophysiological monitoring is a useful technique during functional brain mapping (FBM) with and without an identifiable brain lesion. It helps preserve functional integrity of tissue and optimal surgical resection leading to improved postoperative neurosurgical outcome. Examples of noninvasive FBM techniques include scalp electroencephalography, evoked potentials, magnetoencephalography, and transcranial magnetic stimulation. However, these techniques may be limited by their inability to precisely map the brain due to temporal or spatial constraints. Direct electrical stimulation has been the gold standard for FBM and demonstrates utility as a therapeutic tool for aiding resections in, near, or overlying regions of brain imparting eloquent function. Furthermore, a focus on preserving cortical function during FBM has led to additional insight in meticulously evaluating subcortical functional regions to avoid injury to the subcortical structures that lead to neurological deficits. Integrating multiple FBM techniques improves the precision of preserving eloquent brain regions. New noninvasive techniques advance hope of achieving greater safety profiles, better tolerability, and shorter procedure times to precisely outline the structural–functional relationships of an individual's brain anatomy, to optimize targeted resections and improve long-term functional outcomes.

Keywords: neurophysiology, eloquent, brain, epilepsy, seizures, direct electrocortical stimulation, neurostimulation, functional mapping

6.1 Introduction

Resection of brain tumors and other lesions adjacent to eloquent regions constitutes a principal challenge in neurosurgery. Because maximal gross total resection of abnormal tissue is desirable without introducing a postoperative neurological deficit, working knowledge of the brain's functional topography in and around the lesion is critical. Functional brain mapping (FBM) is routinely accomplished through the integration of various techniques. Noninvasive means to localize structural pathology center on high-resolution brain magnetic resonance imaging (MRI) with an epilepsy protocol. Functional procedures such as electroencephalography (EEG) and magnetoencephalography (MEG) identify physiological integrity of the neuron, tractography reflects function of the axons, functional MRI (fMRI) identifies vascular function, MR spectroscopy analyzes neurochemistry, positron emission tomography (PET) reflects metabolism, single photo emission computed tomography (SPECT) identifies regional blood flow, and Wada testing reflects neuropsychological function.

The human brain is segmented into *eloquent* and clinically *silent* regions. Eloquent cortex are areas responsible for essential function in daily life. If removed or injured, a loss of sensory function, paralysis, visual loss, or deficits in language may result. Indispensable regions where irreversible postoperative deficits can occur include primary motor cortex, primary sensory cortex, primary visual area, and anterior and posterior language areas. Other areas where deficits following surgery by virtue of network connectivity may occur but may not be long lasting include operable areas in the primary somatosensory and motor areas, primary auditory cortex, secondary sensory cortex, and basal temporal language area.[1] By contrast, resection of clinically silent areas of brain results in no discernible consequences of function.

Knowledge of the functional capability for brain that is surrounding a lesion is indicated for the resection adjacent to eloquent cortex (▶ Table 6.1, ▶ Fig. 6.1). This may include surgical resection of a seizure focus, brain tumor, or vascular lesion to cite a few common examples. FBM informs the operating surgeon to determine a safe balance between the extent of resection versus minimizing postoperative neurological deficits from injury to eloquent regions. FBM has evolved from within the boundaries of the operating room to the epilepsy monitoring unit (EMU). Intraoperative FBM may be performed for tumors and immediately prior to surgical resection but has limitations

Table 6.1 Primary and association cortex

Primary cortex	Association cortex

Motor
• Primary area involved (M1)
• Brodmann area 4
• Located in the frontal lobe, along the precentral gyrus
• Controls execution of motor function
	Motor
	• Secondary motor cortices
	  ○ Posterior parietal cortex—transforms visual information into motor commands
	  ○ Premotor cortex—integrates sensory input to guide movement; controls proximal and truncal musculature
	  ○ Supplementary motor area—planning and coordination of complex motor movement

Sensory
• Somatosensory cortex
  ○ Located in the parietal lobe, postcentral gyrus
  ○ Brodmann areas 1, 2, 3
  ○ Processes somatic sensation detected through touch, proprioception, nociception, and temperature
• Visual cortex
  ○ Located in the occipital lobe, on either side of the calcarine sulcus
  ○ Brodmann area 17
  ○ Informs about simple contours, boundaries, color, lighting, and location
• Auditory cortex
  ○ Located in the temporal lobe, posterior–superior aspect
  ○ Brodmann area 22 (simple pure tones)
	Sensory
	• Somatosensory cortex
	  ○ Assists in the ability to recognize objects by touch
	• Visual cortex
	  ○ Located superior and inferior to the primary visual cortex
	  ○ Brodmann area 18—Secondary cortex
	  ○ Brodmann area 19—Association cortex
	  ○ Combines information received from the primary area to help recognize complex objects (faces, animals)
	• Auditory cortex
	  ○ Located inferior and posterior to the primary cortex
	  ○ Assists in recognition of sound and identifies complex sound patterns (speech sounds)

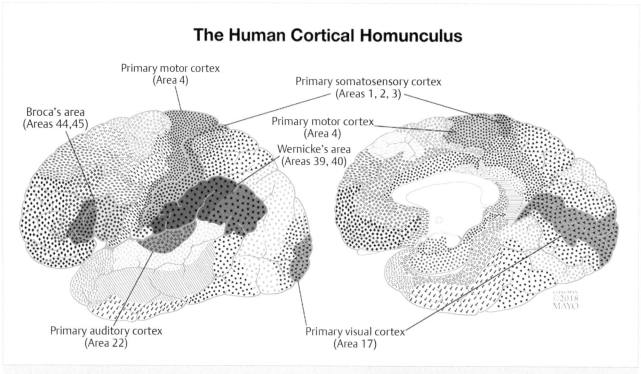

The Human Cortical Homunculus

Broca's area
(Areas 44,45)

Primary motor cortex
(Area 4)

Primary somatosensory cortex
(Areas 1, 2, 3)

Primary motor cortex
(Area 4)

Wernicke's area
(Areas 39, 40)

Primary auditory cortex
(Area 22)

Primary visual cortex
(Area 17)

Fig. 6.1 Homunculus. (Mayo Foundation for Medical Education and Research. Used with permission, all rights reserved.)

in the practical use of this procedure. By contrast, preoperative epilepsy surgery evaluation is typically performed within the EMU using intracranial electrodes (e.g., subdural, depth, and stereotactic), where the seizure focus is first delineated using noninvasive EEG electrodes. Following placement of intracranial electrodes, elective direct electrical stimulation (DES) of selected electrodes is utilized to identify and map the eloquent regions of brain surrounding the seizure focus. Development of novel FBM noninvasive techniques (e.g., fMRI, transcranial magnetic stimulation [TMS], passive electrocorticography [ECoG], spectral analysis of high gamma activity [HGA], and artificial intelligence/deep brain machine learning) is emerging given their potential to replace conventional methods using DES.[2] However, DES has remained pivotal to FBM as the *gold standard* for cortical and subcortical FBM since its recognition by Penfield and colleagues.[1,3,4,5] Of note, the Bonini paradox[6] illustrates the dichotomous nature of outlining territories involved in FBM—simpler maps are less accurate though more useful representations of the territory. Techniques used attempt to optimize the balance between accuracy and practicality when contemplating the most suitable technique for FBM.

The goals for this chapter are to provide the reader with an understanding of the variations in clinical neurophysiological techniques to identify crucial neuroanatomic sites serving as eloquent regions. FBM and different neurophysiologic techniques utilizing extra- and intracranial mapping are available to guide better patient outcomes in the hands of an experienced neurosurgical team.

6.2 Indications for Functional Brain Mapping

6.2.1 Epilepsy

Epilepsy surgery aimed at the resection of an epileptogenic foci was an initial area to use clinical neurophysiological techniques in FBM. Resective epilepsy surgery is a standard of care in patients with drug-resistant focal epilepsy and has shown to significantly improve long-term, seizure-free outcomes.[7] Often, areas of epileptogenesis may involve the eloquent cortex and mapping of cortical function is critical during presurgical planning (▶ Fig. 6.2). FBM has been utilized in the resection of perirolandic and dominant neocortical temporal lobe epilepsy. Remarkably, FBM during epilepsy surgery is distinct from resection of tumors such that FBM is primarily aimed at localizing the epileptogenic zone first, followed by mapping functional areas. Further, epilepsy surgery evaluations commonly occur outside the operating room and within the EMU using scalp video EEG monitoring. When noninvasive techniques fail to localize the seizure onset zone, intracranial electrodes are placed in the operating room and patients are then transferred to the EMU for seizure monitoring with video EEG. Subdural grids (▶ Fig. 6.3) may be used during intraoperative or extraoperative recording of intracranial EEG to localize the seizure onset zone and map large cortical areas for eloquent brain function.[8] Stereo-EEG monitoring is increasing and as a result electrical stimulation mapping has shown utility as a unique

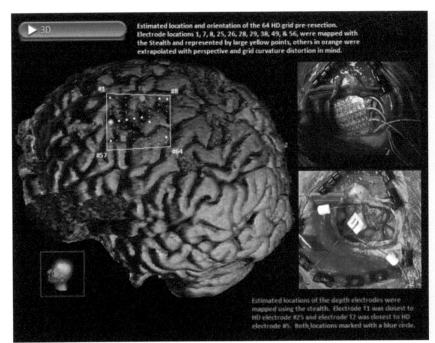

Fig. 6.2 Color brain map preresection with grid placement and active areas designated by *dots* (left) and intraoperative photos (right).

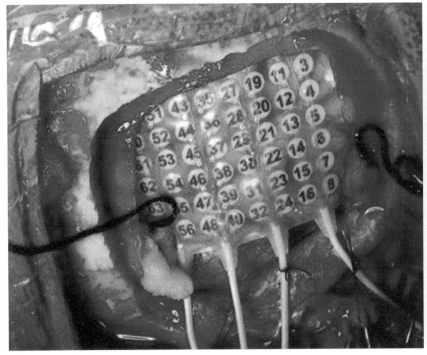

Fig. 6.3 Subdural grid recording 64-channel high-density intraoperative electrocorticography performed for assessment of epileptiform discharges and high-frequency oscillations (HFOs).

methodology associated with special advantages, disadvantages, and potential safety concerns relative to parameters that are used.[9] EEG technologist and specialized nurses are also present if a seizure were to occur and are responsible for fixing electrode dislodgement after a seizure event, monitor for cerebrospinal fluid leakage or bleeding, and rebandage the head to limit spread of infection.[10] After localizing the seizure focus, intracranial electrodes can then be used to map eloquent regions using DES extraoperatively after several habitual seizures have been recorded to characterize an individual's epilepsy syndrome for surgical resection or ablation of the epileptogenic

zone.[11] When intracranial monitoring (phase II) is required due to discordant information obtained on noninvasive evaluation,[12] DES is typically performed after localizing the seizure onset zone.

6.2.2 Brain Tumors

Primary brain tumors arise directly from the brain parenchyma, while secondary lesions are metastatic from another source. Low-grade gliomas often have a slow clinical course and balancing degree of resection with postoperative functional

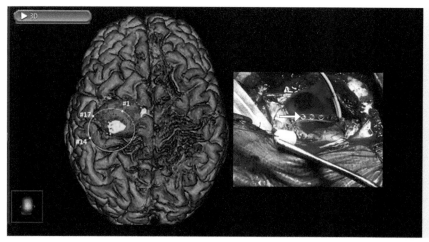

Fig. 6.4 Brain map (left) with tumor bed and surrounding contacts on a high-density grid (numbers) identifying placement for detection of epileptiform activity. An intraoperative image following resection (right). Note the electrode array for recording postresection electrocorticography (*arrow*).

neurological deficits is essential when tumors occur near or within eloquent brain regions. Low-grade gliomas have been found to contain functional tissue, and therefore, outcome may vary by extent of resection.[13] Postoperative outcome may be severely compromised when blindly resecting infiltrating gliomas without guidance.[14] FBM defines eloquent boundaries to improve surgical outcomes in glioma patients (▶ Fig. 6.4). In a meta-analysis of 90 reports on resective surgery for supratentorial infiltrative glioma with or without intraoperative DES, late severe neurological deficits were observed in only 3.4% of DES-resected patients, while 8.2% of the non–DES-resected patients demonstrated deficits.[15] Additionally, gross total resection was achieved in a greater number of patients undergoing DES for FBM despite patients having tumor in eloquent regions.[15] As a result, the authors recommend FBM as a standard of care in resecting brain tumors.

Brain metastases are the most frequent intracranial tumors and due to the overall poor prognosis, they should have surgical management individualized when they occur in close proximity or involve eloquent regions of the brain.[16,17] Palliative surgery seeks to optimize functional capacity without worsening the existing capacity or introducing new neurological deficits. Thus, localizing the eloquent cortices through a combination of intraoperative mapping techniques with neurophysiological monitoring has been recommended.[18,19] In a study of 33 patients with perirolandic metastases, DES was shown to improve surgical planning and resection, as well as spare the eloquent regions by precisely outlining the functional cortical and subcortical structures.[19] Gross total resection of the metastases was achieved in 31 patients (93.9%), and at 6 months follow up, 88.9% had a Karnofsky Performance Scale score greater than 80% and a mean survival time of 24.4 months.[19]

6.2.3 Other Brain Lesions

FBM has expanded to include the resection of any brain lesions at risk for postoperative neurological deficits from injury to the eloquent region. These lesions include vascular lesions, abscesses, granulomas, and trauma in addition to others. Resecting the complex interconnecting arteries and veins of arteriovenous malformations (AVMs) located within eloquent cortex is challenging and prognosis is often poor after surgical

resection.[20] Due to brain plasticity, reorganization of functional areas may commonly shift from their anticipated location during embryonic development of AVMs.[21] Functional imaging studies have been used to identify surgical landmarks during the preoperative management of cavernous malformation resection.[4] Neurophysiological procedures such as MEG have also demonstrated success in localizing the central sulcus as a reference point when AVMs are located near the motor cortex.[22]

FBM techniques may extend beyond just the preoperative planning phase. For example, in a patient with phantom limb pain, fMRI was used to guide the placement of a chronic motor cortex stimulator.[23] PET imaging has been used to visualize brain metabolic activity in an experimental model of heat allodynia.[24] Further, there are various neurostimulation techniques that have been used to restore functional integrity (e.g., epilepsy, Parkinson disease, chronic pain, and obsessive–compulsive disorder) and include deep brain stimulation (DBS), motor cortex stimulation (MCS), responsive neurostimulation (RNS), spinal cord stimulation (SCS), and vagus nerve stimulation (VNS). Further, neurostimulation has also been described as a technique for neural repair of motor function, cognition/memory, and vision.[25,26,27] Remarkably, functional mapping of the occipital cortex may assist with the development of a prosthesis for the blind using a brain–computer interface, and thus, stimulation of the primary visual cortex using intracortical stimulation may have a role in the treatment of cortical blindness.[28]

6.3 Clinical Neurophysiology Techniques

6.3.1 Electroencephalography

EEG records and monitors spontaneous electrical activity of the brain, and can be performed noninvasively by placing scalp electrodes, or invasively, through intracranial electrodes (▶ Fig. 6.5). EEG measures voltage oscillations from ionic current within the neurons and can be of great utility in the diagnosis of neurological conditions but is especially suited for detecting epileptiform abnormalities and seizures, disorders involving the level of consciousness (stupor and coma), stages of sleep, depth of anesthesia, and when confirming death.

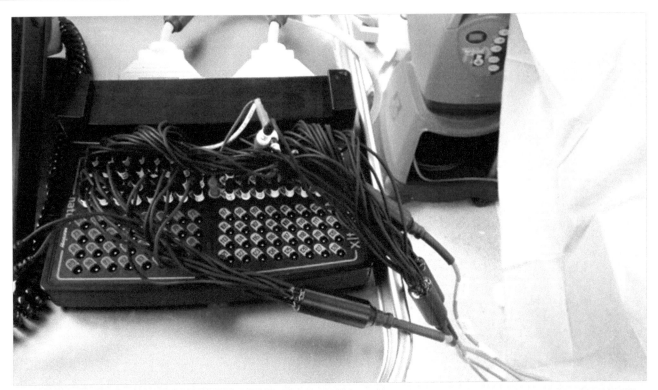

Fig. 6.5 Color coordinated jack box (left) directing electrical activity delivered by the neurostimulator (right) to the brain back to the EEG machine for recording and real-time visualization of electrocorticography by the neurophysiologist.

Intracranial EEG or ECoG has been used for studying electrophysiological correlates to functional brain activation (► Fig. 6.6). By contrast to standard scalp EEG recordings, ECoG produces waveforms that are approximately 10 times greater in amplitude, provides higher resolution and spatial information, and has better sensitivity and improved signal-to-noise ratio (high-frequency EEG activity) due to the adjacent proximity of the electrodes to the cortical surface. ECoG is particularly helpful in identifying potentially epileptogenic tissue in patients with drug-resistant focal epilepsy and has been widely used during motor and language mapping, in the pediatric population, and within the EMU setting.[29,30,31]

ECoG has also been used to study event-related dynamics of brain oscillations over a wide range of frequencies and within the somatosensory/motor systems, language networks, and visual and auditory systems.[2] Previously, noninvasive techniques have demonstrated event-related desynchronization/synchronization (ERD/ERS) within lower frequencies, and this observation has extended the use of ECoG in determining event-related responses within much higher gamma frequencies.[9,32] Changes in the broadband gamma range (> 60 Hz) are of clinical relevance and high-frequency oscillations, including gamma (30–80 Hz), ripples (80–250 Hz), and fast ripples (250–500 Hz), have been observed in various functional brain systems and can be recorded with equipment capable of high sampling rates (► Fig. 6.7).[33] The temporal and spatial localization of high gamma oscillations on passive ECoG are specific to unique activation of functional brain areas that are generated by large populations of neurons produced by a single task.[34]

ECoG offers similar precision when compared to DES, but has a greater safety profile, better patient tolerance, and a shorter procedure time.[35] Studies comparing results of sensorimotor mapping from ECoG to those of DES report sensitivities between 0.43 and 1.0 and specificities of 0.72 to 0.94.[36,37,38] Using ECoG and DES together has several benefits; it reflects the level of wakefulness by monitoring background activity, assesses the effects of anesthesia, verifies the integrity of DES by identifying stimulation-induced artifact, and obtains a recording with after-discharges resulting from overstimulation. Delineating after-discharges helps ascertain that electrographic seizures are not missed or result in provoked seizures due to repetitive stimulation.[39] A study evaluating extraoperative and intraoperative ECoG, DES, and fMRI during mapping of expressive language function reported that integration of multiple functional mapping techniques improved precision of functional localization of the eloquent language cortex.[35] In this study, extraoperative ECoG and DES were both found to be effective in outlining critical functional areas, which was later confirmed using intraoperative high-resolution ECoG. Nonetheless, limitations to ECoG exist. Brain mapping using ECoG either requires a staged procedure or be performed during an awake craniotomy (AC). Longer durations associated with implanted electrodes may significantly increase risk for infection and prolong costs, duration of hospitalization, and delay recovery.[40,41]

6.3.2 Evoked Potentials

Evoked potential (EP) monitoring has been used diagnostically to localize the central sulcus in patients undergoing surgery near the motor strip.[42] Somatosensory evoked potentials (SSEPs) are normally used to evaluate the integrity of the somatosensory system. The EPs comprise a series of negative and

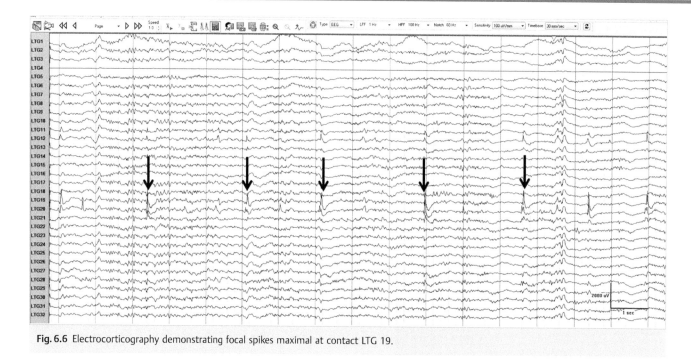

Fig. 6.6 Electrocorticography demonstrating focal spikes maximal at contact LTG 19.

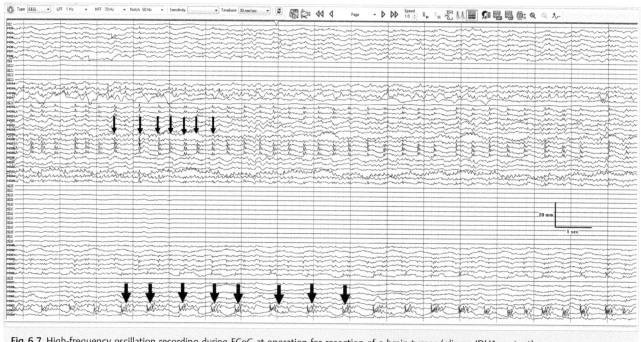

Fig. 6.7 High-frequency oscillation recording during ECoG at operation for resection of a brain tumor (glioma-IDH1 mutant).

positive waveform deflections. Electrical stimulation of Ia afferents peripheral nerves in the upper (median nerve: Erb's point/N9, N13, P14, N20) or lower (tibial nerve: lumbar potential, P31, N34, N37) limbs conduct activity through the dorsal columns in the spinal cord and medial lemniscus in the brainstem to the contralateral primary somatosensory cortex. Intraopera-

tive ECoG recording from an electrode array containing at least eight contacts placed across the area anticipated to contain the central sulcus is performed to guide surgical landmarks. The N20 potential is recorded over the somatosensory cortex and P22 potential over motor cortex as far field potentials that are activated following peripheral nerve stimulation to produce a

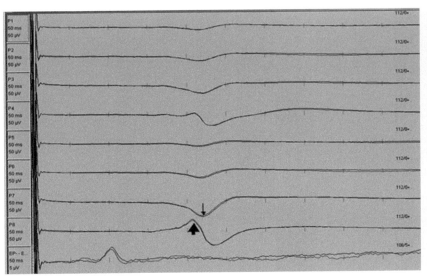

Fig. 6.8 Intraoperative median nerve somatosensory evoked potential performed to localize the central sulcus that lies directly beneath the "pseudo-phase reversal" signified by the N20 (*thick arrow*) and P22 (*thin arrow*) during contralateral median nerve stimulation in the operating room. (Reproduced with permission from Demos Medical Publishing, LLC. In: Handbook of EEG Interpretation. Tatum WO, Husain AM, Benbadis SR, Kaplan PW, eds. 2008:243.)

"pseudo-phase reversal" (▸ Fig. 6.8). The central sulcus lies directly beneath. Additionally, SSEPs may localize sensory deficits, identify silent lesions, and monitor sensory pathway changes during other forms of surgery (e.g., carotid and spinal).[43] Nearly four decades ago, noninvasive brain stimulation, transcranial electrical stimulation (TES), was used as a brief, single, high-voltage electrical current that produced a synchronous motor response eliciting motor EPs from peripheral muscles.

TES uses single- or repetitive-pulse stimulation of the scalp (between 2 and 9) to produce an electrical volley that propagates via the spinal cord to recording electrodes placed over the small muscles in the hand. During TES, high-intensity stimuli are delivered to the scalp in order to stimulate the cortex through an intact skull.[44] The stimulus voltage and current are used at levels far above those necessary to elicit SSEPs and are often used in conjunction during intraoperative monitoring, particularly during spinal surgery. However, some investigators have noted inaccurate results between those obtained from motor evoked potentials (MEP) monitoring and postoperative neurological outcome.[45,46]

Corticocortical evoked potential (CCEP) may be utilized in assessing language connectivity. CCEP involves stimulating one cortical area while recording an averaged response of a signal that is generated in another area to assess functional interconnections.[47,48] In a study of 13 patients, CCEP monitoring was utilized during resection of a tumor located in the dominant cerebral hemisphere, in or around the language-related area.[14] Subdural strip electrodes were placed over the frontal and temporal language areas for recording with potentials that were identified using cortical DES via an adjacent subdural grid. Results indicated that the presence of CCEP responses correlated with the occurrence of postoperative language function, and time to recovery for speech function was significantly associated with changes observed on CCEP as *unchanged*, *decreased*, or *disappeared* when resected at 1.8 ± 1.0 months, 5.5 ± 1.0 months, and 11.0 ± 3.6 months, respectively ($p < 0.01$). Given that CCEP does not require patient input, monitoring speech function under general anesthesia (GA) was possible without an AC.[49]

6.3.3 Magnetoencephalography

MEG is a noninvasive, accurate functional neuroimaging modality for brain mapping by recording magnetic fields of the electrophysiological brain-generated activity and is a direct measurement of cortical activity. It provides precise temporal details about brain activity, in the range of femtotesla to picotesla, as well as accurate spatial localization of neuronal activity. In the United States, MEG is currently approved for preoperative FBM and epilepsy surgery, and accuracy of MEG has been confirmed using intraoperative DES for functional motor mapping.[50] MEG is often combined with MRI and is called magnetic source imaging (MSI) for direct visualization of electromagnetic dipole clusters. While scalp EEG requires at least 6 to 20 cm^2 of synchronized area of neuronal activity for spike detection, MEG require only 3 to 4 cm^2 of cortical area to generate a waveform.[51] Similarly, MEG offers greater spatial resolution of source localization (2–3 mm), as compared to EEG (7–10 mm).[51] Furthermore, magnetic fields are not distorted by conduction of activity through the tissues, whereas electrical fields in EEG are often distorted on recording.[51] Sensorimotor, language, auditory, and visual FBM can be done using MEG.[52] However, it has also been used to measure the presence of tumor infiltration.[53] Further, MEG has been used to evaluate the aggressiveness of a tumor and influence treatment.[54] Remarkably, preoperative resting-state MEG connectivity analysis has been proposed to be a useful noninvasive method to evaluate the functionality connectivity of the tissue surrounding tumors within eloquent areas, potentially contributing to surgical planning.[55] In one study using MEG, maps associated with decreased resting-state functional connectivity in the entire tumor area had a negative predictive value of 100% for absence of eloquent cortex during intraoperative electrical stimulation relative to language, motor, or sensory mapping.[55] MEG studies have also demonstrated functional brain tissue inside low-grade gliomas,[56] and after gross total resection, patients experienced onset of new neurological deficits, and this correlated with the predictive accuracy of MEG.

6.3.4 Transcranial Magnetic Stimulation

TMS mapping has been used successfully in FBM as it applies to measuring central motor conduction time. By varying stimulation techniques and parameters, TMS can excite or inhibit the underlying cortex to facilitate organizational brain maps, which can be coregistered to other imaging and electrophysiological techniques such as fMRI to provide complementary information on motor control.[57] During TMS, disruptive magnetic stimuli are delivered noninvasively from outside the cranial cavity. By placing a coil over the scalp, alternative current flows through the coil to trigger a magnetic field, which further triggers action potentials within the cortical regions. TMS may be limited by its lack of precision/accuracy when placing the coil, leading to variable FBM results. However, navigated TMS (nTMS) has gained interest as an alternative technique to DES, particularly during presurgical mapping of the motor cortex and language areas.[58],[59] nTMS is used with MRI images that are coregistered with a coil placement system to limit placement errors and is now FDA approved as a sole technique. Further, TMS has also been considered as a replacement for intracarotid sodium amobarbital (Wada) for language lateralization.[60]

6.3.5 Future Noninvasive Techniques

HGA between 80 and 140 Hz has shown to reflect local cortical activity, and passive techniques using ECoG spectral analysis of broadband gamma frequencies have recently been described. In a study of five patients with language deficits, passive HGA mapping with CCEP recording during an AC was performed during excision of intra-axial dominant hemisphere brain tumors.[61] HGA mapping of receptive language areas by providing linguistic sounds, while simultaneously delivering electrical pulses to the receptive language area, was used to identify CCEPs within the frontal lobe and was validated by DES.

FBM using artificial intelligence or deep machine learning is an emerging area of interest. State-of-the-art machine learning techniques are increasingly used within neuroimaging (e.g., fMRI), and provide a noninvasive mean of visualizing the human brain from within and identifying the functional organization of cortical structures. Machine learning methods utilize information distributed across multiple voxels (multivoxel fMRI) and can be represented as points in a multidimensional space given the inherent multivariate nature of human brain activity.[62] However, the utility of machine learning models in neuroimaging has chiefly been based on multivoxel analysis, without much consideration given to the brain physiology or technical/mathematical expertise.[62] Thus, a multidisciplinary approach is required to develop and integrate machine learning techniques utilizing neuroimaging with clinical neurophysiological procedures to the field of FBM.

6.4 Direct Electrical Stimulation

Early work to identify a functional brain map of the human motor cortex was outlined by Fedor Krause using DES[63] and sensory responses evoked by DES of the postcentral gyrus were demonstrated by Cushing.[64] Today, direct cortical and subcortical electrical stimulation remains *gold standard* for FBM during

AC; however, the technique has yet to be standardized worldwide. A thorough understanding of the spatial relationship between the electrode and the surrounding brain structures is required. Additionally, important landmarks in the brain must be identified in reference to the stimulating and recording electrodes to help guide the DES and interpretation of results.[65] Accurate localization using neuronavigational systems is helpful in governing the brain–electrode relationship by identifying sites in a grid (▶ Fig. 6.2, lower insert) or depth. Further, identifying baseline function prior to the study for comparison to function during the procedure is particularly important when assessing language and for reliable recognition of stimulation-induced changes.[77] Taking breaks between stimulations or performing DES over several days may be needed if the patient becomes fatigued.[77] Additionally, to overcome subject bias, the patient should not be told when they are being stimulated; however, sham stimulations may be required to differentiate between physiological versus nonphysiological behavioral responses.[77] To validate these results, the patient should be able to reproduce the same response when given repeated stimulations to the same region (see **Video 6.1**).[77] Moreover, a skilled team is required to effectively perform the tasks required during FBM. These tasks range from operating the stimulator probe and the EEG recording equipment to administering and observing patient responses to behavioral and language stimulations. Keeping a watchful eye for subtle muscular contractions and after-discharges on EEG channels is crucial to identify positive motor response or to predict development of seizures. Any EEG patterns concerning for prolonged after-discharges or electrographic seizures should warrant prompt termination of continued DES.

DES may be performed under GA or as an AC under sedation. GA is often used when assessing motor function whereby stimulating a motor site generates involuntary muscular activity. Nonetheless, an AC is necessary when assessing sensory functions, including somatosensory, cognitive, language, memory, reading, and writing, such that when transient stimulation is applied, the patient can provide immediate feedback in real-time. Further, anatomical and functional cerebral connectivity can also be assessed through direct stimulation of white matter tracts and subcortical structures that can potentially limit postoperative neurological deficits.[67]

Commonly used electrodes during DES include subdural grid/strip or depth/penetrating electrodes.[68] Stereo-EEG intracortical electrodes have been implemented in some institutes due to applicability for multisite recording, tolerability, and subcortical sampling of inaccessible, deeply situated regions in the brain, including the insula as well as ventral and medial neocortices.[69] However, a limitation of stereo-EEG includes limited sampling area compared to subdural grid coverage, as well as more limited experience with DES to detect lateral current propagation spread across the neocortical structures. These electrodes have been summarized in ▶ Table 6.2.

DES is readily available, safe using appropriate parameters, and a low-cost procedure.[35] In a study of 250 patients, less than 2% experienced postoperative language deficits after DES.[75] In another study, when DES was used to map motor function, 87% demonstrated no postoperative deficits at 1 month after resecting tumors near the corticospinal tract.[76] When DES induces repeated functional disturbance, an area of eloquence is

Table 6.2 Types of electrodes utilized for DES during FBM[a]

Electrode type	Description
Subdural electrodes	• Linear strips and grids (4–64 electrodes): placed onto the subdural surface of the brain • Advantage: covers large contiguous areas of the neocortical surface; favorable spatial resolution; useful in FBM of eloquent cortex • Disadvantages: requires craniotomy, greater risk of infection/bleeding, poorer tolerability, mass effect, focal neurologic deficits • Prevalence of complications (hemorrhage, infections, focal deficits, electrode malfunction): 5–40.5%[b]
Depth electrodes	• Intracortical electrodes (4–10 contacts): surgically implanted through the parenchyma of the brain • Advantages: useful to approximate deep structures (e.g., mesial temporal lobe); stereotactic placement, potential for diagnostic FBM and therapeutic stimulation (e.g., thalamus, hippocampus, etc.) • Disadvantages: bleeding, limited spatial resolution, cranial access for each electrode utilized • Prevalence of complications (hemorrhage, infections, focal deficits, electrode malfunction): 1–6.4%[70,72,73]
Stereo-EEG	• Intracortical electrodes (8–10 contacts): surgically implanted through multiple small (2.5 mm) twist-drill burr holes into the skull • Advantages: localizes and lateralizes regional and hemispheric seizures in epilepsy surgery evaluation; identifies deep structures (e.g., insular and cingulate cortex), better tolerability, no craniotomy required • Disadvantages: risk of bleeding, stroke, time required for multiple placement (robotics may speed procedure of placement); may necessitate preoperative visualization of blood vessels • Prevalence of complications (hemorrhage, infection, mortality, surgical complications related to electrode insertion): pooled prevalence 0.3–1.3%[74]

Abbreviations: DES, direct electrical stimulation; FBM, functional brain mapping.
[a]Number of contacts used vary in commercially available electrodes.
[b]Number of contacts increase risk of complications.[70,71,72,73]

Table 6.3 Parameters for intraoperative electrical stimulation mapping[a]

Type of pulse	Biphasic
Stimulation	Bipolar/monopolar
Pulse frequency	50 Hz
Pulse width	0.2–0.3 ms
Stimulus duration	3–5 s; 5 s for language testing; up to 10 s when testing for negative motor response
Current intensity	Start at 1 or 2 mA
Current titration	Increments of 0.5–1 mA
Maximum current	Limited by machine; usually 10–20 mA

[a]These parameters are for cortical stimulation using grid or strip subdural electrodes and should not be used for stimulating depth or stereo-EEG electrodes due to risk of tissue damage.

ters for FBM is crucial. If the intensity is too low, stimulation sites will not be adequately activated/inactivated (false negatives). If the stimulus intensity is too high, even normal regions will produce after-discharges or even seizures (false positives). Brain mapping using DES should be performed just below after-discharges threshold. Further, it is important to control the amount of charge density to minimize tissue damage during DES. Charge density is determined by the relationship between the charge per phase delivered and the surface area of the stimulating contact. The amount of charge per phase is relative to the stimulating current coupled with the duration of the single phase of a bipolar/biphasic pulse. The units are expressed as microcoulombs per phase, which is delivered to the brain over an area (cm^2) usually 100 g of tissue. Prior recommendations suggest that a charge density of > 30 $\mu C/cm^2$ may compromise safety and can lead to neural injury.[78] Further, DES parameters may need to be altered depending on the patient, such that a patient with proficient language and cognitive abilities may only require stimulation of 5-second duration, while this may need to be longer in patients with deficits or in children.

A few risks need to be considered with DES. Electrical stimulation may trigger after-discharges (▶ Fig. 6.9) and may collectively produce a seizure, leading to increase in morbidity and delay in FBM due to a postictal period.[35] DES can also be time intensive, ranging from several hours to a few days when performed extraoperative (e.g., EMU) as it usually includes electrical stimulation of each contact in an implanted electrode array in an organized manner using more than a single trial. By contrast, given the time constraints and anesthetic challenges during AC, there is limited time for testing that can be performed safely in the operating room. In addition, patients may experience pain due to cephalalgia and discomfort from prolonged positioning on the surgical table.[31]

suspected, and 1 cm distance should be avoided in the surgical resection. Furthermore, electrical stimulation parameters vary depending upon the type of electrode utilized for DES. Parameters should be followed closely to ensure that DES does not create tissue damage through supraoptimal stimulation. ▶ Table 6.3 outlines stimulation parameters used during DES for subdural electrodes[77] and ▶ Table 6.4 compares parameters for various electrode types.[2] Selecting the appropriate parame-

Table 6.4 Parameters of commonly used electrodes for electrical cortical stimulation

Electrode	Contact size (mm)	Contact interspace (mm)	Effective surface area (mm²)	Current (mA)	Pulse width (ms)	Pulse frequency (Hz)	Train duration (s)
Subdural	2.4–4	10	1.26–4.5	1–15	0.2–0.3	50	3–10
Intracortical/depth	3.5	2	5	0.5–2.5	1	50	3–5
Probe/wand	1	5	1.6	1–10	1	50	3–5

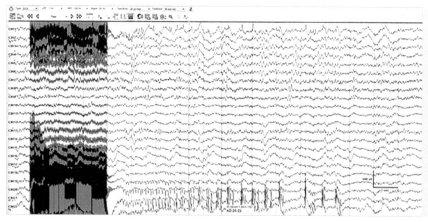

Fig. 6.9 After-discharges on electrocorticography (box) following DES (artifact present in 2–5 s) during functional brain mapping prior to resection of a grade 2 glioma adjacent to the precentral gyrus.

The role of DES has extended beyond FBM for localization of eloquent cortex prior to neurosurgery. Therapy using intermittent direct brain electrocortical stimulation (e.g., thalamic stimulation and RNS) is commercially available. Recently, continuous subthreshold electrical stimulation has shown suppression of interictal epileptiform discharges (IEDs) and improvement in clinical seizures (frequency, intensity, and duration) following extraoperative DES.[79] This suggests that IEDs can be used as a biomarker for identifying parameters of treatment. [79]

6.5 Neurophysiological Approach to Functional Brain Mapping

Electrocortical stimulation of the brain in humans, in and out of the operating room, has increasingly been utilized as a tool for FBM. The approach to FBM depends on the lesion and goals for treatment. In nontumoral epilepsy surgery, the goal is to determine the epileptogenic zone initially, and then map surrounding eloquent cortex, which can effectively take place in the EMU.[80] By contrast, lesional surgery has goals that are distinct and must consider maximizing the boundaries and extent of tumor resection while minimizing postoperative neurological deficits to improve median survival time.[80] In patients with infiltrating tumors traversing white matter tracts, intraoperative mapping with DES would be warranted to effectively map both cortical and subcortical functions.[80] Nonetheless, both extra- and intraoperative techniques encompass a set of inherent risks and benefits that need to be considered when choosing the most effective technique for FBM (▶ Table 6.5). During intraoperative FBM, a handheld probe guided by the surgeon provides electrical stimuli to the implanted electrode to create a map of function. When demarcating areas involved with movement, mapping may be performed under GA; however, when assessing functions related to language, sensation, or vision, AC is warranted to ensure active participation by the patient. If during extraoperative mapping eloquent regions are identified, further intraoperative FBM can be performed to confirm the extraoperative map prior to resection.

Techniques used during FBM have significantly evolved with time. Identification of sensorimotor areas was previously done using EPs.[81,82] However, EPs were incompletely reliable as 6 to

Table 6.5 Indications, risks, and benefits of extraoperative and intraoperative FBM

	Extraoperative	Intraoperative
Indication	Nontumoral epilepsy surgery	Tumoral/epilepsy surgery
Risks	• Prolonged EMU admission • Risk of acquiring hospital acquired infections • Requires special safety equipment and specialized nurses/EEG technologists • High risk for seizures during DES; ASDs warranted • Time consuming (hours to days)	• Severe time constraints limit the list of cognitive tasks that can be performed • Anesthetic challenges of awake craniotomy • High risk for perioperative seizures; ASDs warranted during DES • Patient fatigue/poor cooperation may require early termination of procedure • Perioperative seizures and postictal period delays FBM
Benefits	• No time constraints • May be entirely noninvasive or performed as a staged procedure • Triggering seizures by closely tapering ASDs when determining an epileptogenic focus • Video EEG recordings in the EMU allow for clarification if needed at a later time	• Cortical and subcortical functional mapping of infiltrating tumors migrating along white matter tracts achieved • Diagnostic functional mapping and therapeutic resection of the lesion performed during single setting

Abbreviations: ASD, anti-seizure drugs; DES, direct electrical stimulation; EEG, electroencephalogram; EMU, epilepsy monitoring unit; FBM, functional brain mapping.

9% of localizations of the central sulcus were inaccurate.[83] This resulted in more patients experiencing postoperative functional deficits (20%), likely arising from the resection of subcortical tissue near primary sensory motor cortex involving the pyramidal

Table 6.6 Functional brain mapping of eloquent areas

Eloquent area	Anatomical stimulation	Function produced
Motor	• Primary motor cortex (Brodmann area 4): precentral gyrus, 10 mm anterior to the central sulcus, area posterior to the central sulcus	Contraction of contralateral muscle groups
	• Supplementary sensorimotor area: dorsal convexity of the superior frontal gyrus	Movements or posturing of extremities, vocalization, and contralateral head movements
	• Primary negative motor area: inferior or middle frontal gyrus • Supplementary negative motor area: mesial surface of the superior frontal gyrus, paracentral lobule, and cingulate gyrus	Negative motor response inhibits motor activity or behavior while awareness is preserved
Sensory	• Primary sensory area (Brodmann areas 1, 2, 3): postcentral gyrus	Contralateral tingling, numbness, buzzing, and burning
Language	• Expressive language (Broca area): posterior portion of the inferior frontal gyrus of the dominant hemisphere, posterior portion of the middle frontal gyrus, and anterior portion of the superior temporal gyrus of the dominant hemisphere	Involves a negative response and disrupts ongoing language function when patient is asked to read out-loud, count numbers, or repeat familiar sentences
	• Receptive language (Wernicke area): dominant posterior temporoparietal area or the basal temporal language area (inferior temporal, fusiform, or parahippocampal gyrus)	Involves a negative response and disrupts ongoing language function when performing tasks involving auditory, visual confrontation, and picture naming
Visual	• Primary visual cortex (Brodmann area 17): medial aspect of the occipital lobe	Contralateral phosphenes and unformed shapes, colors, and lines
	• Secondary visual cortex (Brodmann area 18) and visual association cortex (Brodmann area 19)	Visual illusions
Auditory	• Primary auditory cortex (Brodmann area 22) • Posterior perisylvian region	• Buzzing or blunting/distortion of normal hearing • Complex auditory experiences

tract.[84] FBM of eloquent areas has been summarized in ▶ Table 6.6.[77]

6.6 Conclusion

Preservation of essential human functions is essential for maintaining an independent lifestyle. Extra- and intraoperative FBM to delineate eloquent areas of brain involved with critical functions allows the neurosurgeon to optimize the extent of resection for targeted brain tissue and minimize the risk for postoperative long-term neurological deficits. Despite the different brain mapping techniques, limitations exist for each. DES with ECoG has been the gold standard for delineating functional brain tissue through parameter selection. Noninvasive techniques are evolving (e.g., scalp-EEG, motor EPs, MEG, nTMS, MEPs, and passive ECoG of HGA), though they will need to overcome limitations of temporal and spatial constraints to map higher brain functions. In contrast to other forms of neurophysiological brain mapping techniques, DES is available as a practical technique at many tertiary care institutions, and is effective, safe, and cost efficient to accurately outline eloquent areas of brain function.

References

[1] Schuele SU, Lüders HO. Intractable epilepsy: management and therapeutic alternatives. Lancet Neurol. 2008; 7(6):514–524

[2] Ritaccio AL, Brunner P, Schalk G. Electrical stimulation mapping of the brain: basic principles and emerging alternatives. J Clin Neurophysiol. 2018; 35(2): 86–97

[3] Duffau H. Lessons from brain mapping in surgery for low-grade glioma: insights into associations between tumour and brain plasticity. Lancet Neurol. 2005; 4(8):476–486

[4] Duffau H, Fontaine D. Successful resection of a left insular cavernous angioma using neuronavigation and intraoperative language mapping. Acta Neurochir (Wien). 2005; 147(2):205–208, discussion 208

[5] Penfield W, Rasmussen T. The Cerebral Cortex of Man: A Clinical Study of Localization of Function. New York, NY: Macmillan; 1950

[6] Bonini CP. Simulation of Information and Decision Systems in the Firm. Englewood Cliffs, NJ: Prentice-Hall; 1963

[7] Anyanwu C, Motamedi GK. Diagnosis and surgical treatment of drug-resistant epilepsy. Brain Sci. 2018; 8(4):E49

[8] Tatum WO, Dionisio JB, Vale FL. Subdural electrodes in focal epilepsy surgery at a typical academic epilepsy center. J Clin Neurophysiol. 2015; 32(2):139–146

[9] Britton JW. Electrical stimulation mapping with stereo-EEG electrodes. J Clin Neurophysiol. 2018; 35(2):110–114

[10] Shih JJ, Fountain NB, Herman ST, et al. Indications and methodology for video-electroencephalographic studies in the epilepsy monitoring unit. Epilepsia. 2018; 59(1):27–36

[11] Wiebe S, Blume WT, Girvin JP, Eliasziw M, Effectiveness and Efficiency of Surgery for Temporal Lobe Epilepsy Study Group. A randomized, controlled trial of surgery for temporal-lobe epilepsy. N Engl J Med. 2001; 345(5):311–318

[12] Struck AF, Cole AJ, Cash SS, Westover MB. The number of seizures needed in the EMU. Epilepsia. 2015; 56(11):1753–1759

[13] Chang EF, Clark A, Smith JS, et al. Functional mapping-guided resection of low-grade gliomas in eloquent areas of the brain: improvement of long-term survival. Clinical article. J Neurosurg. 2011; 114(3):566–573

[14] Saito T, Tamura M, Muragaki Y, et al. Intraoperative cortico-cortical evoked potentials for the evaluation of language function during brain tumor resection: initial experience with 13 cases. J Neurosurg. 2014; 121(4):827–838

[15] De Witt Hamer PC, Robles SG, Zwinderman AH, Duffau H, Berger MS. Impact of intraoperative stimulation brain mapping on glioma surgery outcome: a meta-analysis. J Clin Oncol. 2012; 30(20):2559–2565

[16] Al-Shamy G, Sawaya R. Management of brain metastases: the indispensable role of surgery. J Neurooncol. 2009; 92(3):275–282

[17] Zhang X, Zhang W, Cao WD, Cheng G, Liu B, Cheng J. A review of current management of brain metastases. Ann Surg Oncol. 2012; 19(3):1043–1050

[18] Fernández Coello A, Moritz-Gasser S, Martino J, Martinoni M, Matsuda R, Duffau H. Selection of intraoperative tasks for awake mapping based on relationships between tumor location and functional networks. J Neurosurg. 2013; 119(6):1380–1394

[19] Sanmillan JL, Fernández-Coello A, Fernández-Conejero I, Plans G, Gabarrós A. Functional approach using intraoperative brain mapping and neurophysio-

logical monitoring for the surgical treatment of brain metastases in the central region. J Neurosurg. 2017; 126(3):698–707

[20] Tong X, Wu J, Cao Y, Zhao Y, Wang S. New predictive model for microsurgical outcome of intracranial arteriovenous malformations: study protocol. BMJ Open. 2017; 7(1):e014063

[21] Lin F, Zhao B, Wu J, et al. Risk factors for worsened muscle strength after the surgical treatment of arteriovenous malformations of the eloquent motor area. J Neurosurg. 2016; 125(2):289–298

[22] Shimamura N, Ohkuma H, Ogane K, et al. Displacement of central sulcus in cerebral arteriovenous malformation situated in the peri-motor cortex as assessed by magnetoencephalographic study. Acta Neurochir (Wien). 2004; 146(4):363–368, discussion 368

[23] Roux FE, Ibarrola D, Lazorthes Y, Berry I. Chronic motor cortex stimulation for phantom limb pain: a functional magnetic resonance imaging study: technical case report. Neurosurgery. 2008; 62(6) Suppl 3:978–985

[24] Casey KL, Lorenz J, Minoshima S. Insights into the pathophysiology of neuropathic pain through functional brain imaging. Exp Neurol. 2003; 184 Suppl 1: S80–S88

[25] Chan AY, Rolston JD, Rao VR, Chang EF. Effect of neurostimulation on cognition and mood in refractory epilepsy. Epilepsia Open. 2018; 3(1):18–29

[26] Gall C, Schmidt S, Schittkowski MP, et al. Alternating current stimulation for vision restoration after optic nerve damage: a randomized clinical trial. PLoS One. 2016; 11(6):e0156134

[27] Minassian K, Hofstoetter U, Tansey K, Mayr W. Neuromodulation of lower limb motor control in restorative neurology. Clin Neurol Neurosurg. 2012; 114(5):489–497

[28] Lewis PM, Rosenfeld JV. Electrical stimulation of the brain and the development of cortical visual prostheses: an historical perspective. Brain Res. 2016; 1630:208–224

[29] Korostenskaja M, Chen PC, Salinas CM, et al. Real-time functional mapping: potential tool for improving language outcome in pediatric epilepsy surgery. J Neurosurg Pediatr. 2014; 14(3):287–295

[30] Roland J, Brunner P, Johnston J, Schalk G, Leuthardt EC. Passive real-time identification of speech and motor cortex during an awake craniotomy. Epilepsy Behav. 2010; 18(1-2):123–128

[31] Su DK, Ojemann JG. Electrocorticographic sensorimotor mapping. Clin Neurophysiol. 2013; 124(6):1044–1048

[32] Feyissa AM, Worrell GA, Tatum WO, et al. High-frequency oscillations in awake patients undergoing brain tumor-related epilepsy surgery. Neurology. 2018; 90(13):e1119–e1125

[33] Crone NE, Miglioretti DL, Gordon B, Lesser RP. Functional mapping of human sensorimotor cortex with electrocorticographic spectral analysis. II. Event-related synchronization in the gamma band. Brain. 1998; 121(Pt 12):2301–2315

[34] Crone NE, Sinai A, Korzeniewska A. High-frequency gamma oscillations and human brain mapping with electrocorticography. Prog Brain Res. 2006; 159: 275–295

[35] Taplin AM, de Pesters A, Brunner P, et al. Intraoperative mapping of expressive language cortex using passive real-time electrocorticography. Epilepsy Behav Case Rep. 2016; 5:46–51

[36] Crone NE, Miglioretti DL, Gordon B, et al. Functional mapping of human sensorimotor cortex with electrocorticographic spectral analysis. I. Alpha and beta event-related desynchronization. Brain. 1998; 121(Pt 12):2271–2299

[37] Leuthardt EC, Miller K, Anderson NR, et al. Electrocorticographic frequency alteration mapping: a clinical technique for mapping the motor cortex. Neurosurgery. 2007; 60(4) Suppl 2:260–270, discussion 270–271

[38] Vansteensel MJ, Bleichner MG, Dintzner LT, et al. Task-free electrocorticography frequency mapping of the motor cortex. Clin Neurophysiol. 2013; 124 (6):1169–1174

[39] Tatum WO, Rubboli G, Kaplan PW, et al. Clinical utility of EEG in diagnosing and monitoring epilepsy in adults. Clin Neurophysiol. 2018; 129(5):1056–1082

[40] Eseonu CI, Rincon-Torroella J, ReFaey K, et al. Awake craniotomy vs craniotomy under general anesthesia for perirolandic gliomas: evaluating perioperative complications and extent of resection. Neurosurgery. 2017; 81(3):481–489

[41] Eseonu CI, Rincon-Torroella J, ReFaey K, Quiñones-Hinojosa A. The cost of brain surgery: awake vs asleep craniotomy for perirolandic region tumors. Neurosurgery. 2017; 81:307–314

[42] Husain AM. Neurophysiologic intraoperative monitoring. In: Tatum WO, Husain AM, Benbadis SR, Kaplan PW, eds. Handbook of EEG Interpretation. New York, NY: Demos Publishers LLC; 2008

[43] Passmore SR, Murphy B, Lee TD. The origin, and application of somatosensory evoked potentials as a neurophysiological technique to investigate neuroplasticity. J Can Chiropr Assoc. 2014; 58(2):170–183

[44] Legatt AD, Emerson RG, Epstein CM, et al. ACNS guideline: transcranial electrical stimulation motor evoked potential monitoring. J Clin Neurophysiol. 2016; 33(1):42–50

[45] Krieg SM, Shiban E, Droese D, et al. Predictive value and safety of intraoperative neurophysiological monitoring with motor evoked potentials in glioma surgery. Neurosurgery. 2012; 70(5):1060–1070, discussion 1070–1071

[46] Suzuki K, Mikami T, Sugino T, et al. Discrepancy between voluntary movement and motor-evoked potentials in evaluation of motor function during clipping of anterior circulation aneurysms. World Neurosurg. 2014; 82(6): e739–e745

[47] Enatsu R, Kubota Y, Kakisaka Y, et al. Reorganization of posterior language area in temporal lobe epilepsy: a cortico-cortical evoked potential study. Epilepsy Res. 2013; 103(1):73–82

[48] Kubota Y, Enatsu R, Gonzalez-Martinez J, et al. In vivo human hippocampal cingulate connectivity: a corticocortical evoked potentials (CCEPs) study. Clin Neurophysiol. 2013; 124(8):1547–1556

[49] Matsumoto R, Nair DR, LaPresto E, et al. Functional connectivity in the human language system: a cortico-cortical evoked potential study. Brain. 2004; 127 (Pt 10):2316–2330

[50] Tarapore PE, Tate MC, Findlay AM, et al. Preoperative multimodal motor mapping: a comparison of magnetoencephalography imaging, navigated transcranial magnetic stimulation, and direct cortical stimulation. J Neurosurg. 2012; 117(2):354–362

[51] Singh SP. Magnetoencephalography: basic principles. Ann Indian Acad Neurol. 2014; 17 Suppl 1:S107–S112

[52] Nakasato N, Yoshimoto T. Somatosensory, auditory, and visual evoked magnetic fields in patients with brain diseases. J Clin Neurophysiol. 2000; 17(2): 201–211

[53] de Jongh A, de Munck JC, Baayen JC, Jonkman EJ, Heethaar RM, van Dijk BW. The localization of spontaneous brain activity: first results in patients with cerebral tumors. Clin Neurophysiol. 2001; 112(2):378–385

[54] de Jongh A, Baayen JC, de Munck JC, Heethaar RM, Vandertop WP, Stam CJ. The influence of brain tumor treatment on pathological delta activity in MEG. Neuroimage. 2003; 20(4):2291–2301

[55] Martino J, Honma SM, Findlay AM, et al. Resting functional connectivity in patients with brain tumors in eloquent areas. Ann Neurol. 2011; 69(3):521–532

[56] Schiffbauer H, Ferrari P, Rowley HA, Berger MS, Roberts TP. Functional activity within brain tumors: a magnetic source imaging study. Neurosurgery. 2001; 49(6):1313–1320, discussion 1320–1321

[57] Lefaucheur JP, André-Obadia N, Antal A, et al. Evidence-based guidelines on the therapeutic use of repetitive transcranial magnetic stimulation (rTMS). Clin Neurophysiol. 2014; 125(11):2150–2206

[58] Picht T, Frey D, Thieme S, Kliesch S, Vajkoczy P. Presurgical navigated TMS motor cortex mapping improves outcome in glioblastoma surgery: a controlled observational study. J Neurooncol. 2016; 126(3):535–543

[59] Sollmann N, Kubitscheck A, Maurer S, et al. Preoperative language mapping by repetitive navigated transcranial magnetic stimulation and diffusion tensor imaging fiber tracking and their comparison to intraoperative stimulation. Neuroradiology. 2016; 58(8):807–818

[60] Pelletier I, Sauerwein HC, Lepore F, Saint-Amour D, Lassonde M. Non-invasive alternatives to the Wada test in the presurgical evaluation of language and memory functions in epilepsy patients. Epileptic Disord. 2007; 9(2):111–126

[61] Tamura Y, Ogawa H, Kapeller C, et al. Passive language mapping combining real-time oscillation analysis with cortico-cortical evoked potentials for awake craniotomy. J Neurosurg. 2016; 125(6):1580–1588

[62] Bjornsdotter M. Machine learning for functional brain mapping. In: Zhang Y, ed. Application of Machine Learning. InTech; 2010:280

[63] Krause F. Surgery of the Brain and Spinal Cord Based on Personal Experience. Vol. 2. New York, NY: Rebman; 1912

[64] Cushing H. A note upon the faradic stimulation of the postcentral gyrus in conscious patients. Brain. 1909; 32:44–53

[65] Voorhies JM, Cohen-Gadol A. Techniques for placement of grid and strip electrodes for intracranial epilepsy surgery monitoring: pearls and pitfalls. Surg Neurol Int. 2013; 4:98

[66] Gonen T, Gazit T, Korn A, et al. Intra-operative multi-site stimulation: expanding methodology for cortical brain mapping of language functions. PLoS One. 2017; 12(7):e0180740

[67] Duffau H, Capelle L, Sichez N, et al. Intraoperative mapping of the subcortical language pathways using direct stimulations. An anatomo-functional study. Brain. 2002; 125(Pt 1):199–214

[68] Lesser RP, Crone NE, Webber WRS. Subdural electrodes. Clin Neurophysiol. 2010; 121(9):1376–1392

[69] Trébuchon A, Chauvel P. Electrical stimulation for seizure induction and functional mapping in stereoelectroencephalography. J Clin Neurophysiol. 2016; 33(6):511–521

[70] Hedegärd E, Bjellvi J, Edelvik A, Rydenhag B, Flink R, Malmgren K. Complications to invasive epilepsy surgery workup with subdural and depth electrodes: a prospective population-based observational study. J Neurol Neurosurg Psychiatry. 2014; 85(7):716–720

[71] Kim YH, Kim CH, Kim JS, Lee SK, Chung CK. Resection frequency map after awake resective surgery for non-lesional neocortical epilepsy involving eloquent areas. Acta Neurochir (Wien). 2011; 153(9):1739–1749

[72] Sweet JA, Hdeib AM, Sloan A, Miller JP. Depths and grids in brain tumors: implantation strategies, techniques, and complications. Epilepsia. 2013; 54 Suppl 9:66–71

[73] Wellmer J, von der Groeben F, Klarmann U, et al. Risks and benefits of invasive epilepsy surgery workup with implanted subdural and depth electrodes. Epilepsia. 2012; 53(8):1322–1332

[74] Mullin JP, Shriver M, Alomar S, et al. Is SEEG safe? A systematic review and meta-analysis of stereo-electroencephalography-related complications. Epilepsia. 2016; 57(3):386–401

[75] Sanai N, Mirzadeh Z, Berger MS. Functional outcome after language mapping for glioma resection. N Engl J Med. 2008; 358(1):18–27

[76] Nossek E, Korn A, Shahar T, et al. Intraoperative mapping and monitoring of the corticospinal tracts with neurophysiological assessment and 3-dimensional ultrasonography-based navigation. Clinical article. J Neurosurg. 2011; 114(3):738–746

[77] So EL, Alwaki A. A guide for cortical electrical stimulation mapping. J Clin Neurophysiol. 2018; 35(2):98–105

[78] Gordon B, Lesser RP, Rance NE, et al. Parameters for direct cortical electrical stimulation in the human: histopathologic confirmation. Electroencephalogr Clin Neurophysiol. 1990; 75(5):371–377

[79] Lundstrom BN, Van Gompel J, Britton J, et al. Chronic subthreshold cortical stimulation to treat focal epilepsy. JAMA Neurol. 2016; 73(11): 1370–1372

[80] Duffau H. Brain mapping in tumors: intraoperative or extraoperative? Epilepsia. 2013; 54 Suppl 9:79–83

[81] Neuloh G, Pechstein U, Cedzich C, Schramm J. Motor evoked potential monitoring with supratentorial surgery. Neurosurgery. 2004; 54(5):1061–1070, discussion 1070–1072

[82] Romstöck J, Fahlbusch R, Ganslandt O, Nimsky C, Strauss C. Localisation of the sensorimotor cortex during surgery for brain tumours: feasibility and waveform patterns of somatosensory evoked potentials. J Neurol Neurosurg Psychiatry. 2002; 72(2):221–229

[83] Wiedemayer H, Sandalcioglu IE, Armbruster W, Regel J, Schaefer H, Stolke D. False negative findings in intraoperative SEP monitoring: analysis of 658 consecutive neurosurgical cases and review of published reports. J Neurol Neurosurg Psychiatry. 2004; 75(2):280–286

[84] Cedzich C, Taniguchi M, Schäfer S, Schramm J. Somatosensory evoked potential phase reversal and direct motor cortex stimulation during surgery in and around the central region. Neurosurgery. 1996; 38(5):962–970

7 Extraoperative Mapping for Epilepsy Surgery: Epilepsy Monitoring, Wada, and Electrocorticography

Emily L. Johnson and Eva K. Ritzl

Abstract

Extraoperative mapping with electroencephalography, Wada, electrocorticography, or electrical stimulation mapping helps guide epilepsy surgical planning. For patients with medically refractory focal seizures, epilepsy surgery can be a curative and even life-saving procedure. However, seizure foci may occur in or close to primary motor, sensory, or language areas, or in the hippocampus, putting patients at risk for postoperative deficits. Extraoperative mapping can help identify indispensable eloquent cortex, and help tailor surgical resection so that the patient does not have unintended consequences from the surgery.

Keywords: epilepsy surgery, Wada, epilepsy monitoring unit, electrocorticography, electrical stimulation mapping

7.1 Introduction

A seizure is a transient neurologic event, caused by abnormally synchronous or excess brain activity.[1] Epilepsy is the condition in which a patient has two or more unprovoked seizures, or is at high risk for recurrent seizures.[2] While approximately two-thirds of patients with epilepsy can have their seizures controlled with medications, the remaining one-third are medically refractory,[3,4,5] and the chance of achieving seizure freedom is relatively low with additional medications tried. Epilepsy is considered medically refractory if a patient has seizures despite adequate trials of two or more appropriate antiseizure drugs (ASDs) at therapeutic doses.[5] For patients with medically refractory focal epilepsy, seizure surgery should be considered. Two randomized controlled trials demonstrated that surgery for epilepsy results in seizure freedom for 60 to 85% of qualifying patients with temporal lobe surgery, while continued medical management results in seizure freedom in only 0 to 8% of refractory epilepsy patients.[6,7]

The most common type of epilepsy surgery is the temporal lobectomy, as temporal lobe epilepsy (particularly mesial temporal lobe epilepsy, originating in the hippocampus or amygdala) is the most common type of focal epilepsy.[8] In recent years, laser interstitial thermal ablation therapy has been used for specific focal lesions (most commonly hippocampal sclerosis) in which the neurosurgeon places a probe under magnetic resonance imaging (MRI) guidance, then uses heat to ablate the tissue of interest.[9]

Rates of complete seizure freedom range from 50 to 85% after temporal lobe surgery or ablation.[6,7,10] After surgery in extratemporal locations, seizure freedom rates may be 29 to 55%, with higher rates observed in patients with a known lesion on MRI or positron emission tomography (PET) imaging.[11,12] Resection of epileptic tissue in any lobe may be performed with careful planning to ensure the patient is not left with major deficits. After seizure monitoring with scalp electrodes, a Wada test or intracranial electrocorticography (ECoG) monitoring and mapping may be needed.

Extraoperative mapping for epilepsy, therefore, comprises epilepsy monitoring to determine the seizure onset zone as well as functional mapping to help delineate eloquent brain regions that need to be spared during seizure surgery.

7.2 Epilepsy Monitoring with Scalp Electrodes

7.2.1 Purpose

To identify the seizure focus as a target for resection, patients are admitted to an epilepsy monitoring unit (EMU) for continuous video electroencephalography (vEEG). The goal of vEEG monitoring is to record at least three to four of the patient's typical seizures,[13] to determine the seizure onset based on scalp EEG.

7.2.2 Procedure

Patients are admitted to the EMU for 5 to 8 days, and electrodes are placed on the head according to a standardized montage. Often, the patient's ASDs are lowered to facilitate recording seizures in a week-long admission.[14,15] Epileptologists identify seizures from the patient's symptoms and from the EEG, and use visual inspection of the seizures to determine the location of onset. In some cases, particularly if the patient fits into a defined epilepsy syndrome and has a known lesion on imaging, the information obtained on scalp EEG may be sufficient to proceed with surgery.

7.2.3 Additional Testing

Focal findings on MRI or PET that correspond to the patient's seizure onset on scalp EEG are predictive of a better outcome after surgery.[16] Additional testing, such as magnetoencephalography (MEG) or ictal single-photon emission computed tomography (SPECT) can be supportive if no lesion is found on MRI or PET.[17,18] Neuropsychology testing revealing deficits corresponding to the suspected seizure onset zone is also supportive, and is predictive of less cognitive decline after surgery.[19,20]

If the seizure onset zone is suspected to be close to eloquent cortex or in the dominant hemisphere, additional brain "mapping" with Wada, functional MRI (fMRI), or ECoG may be required prior to surgery to ensure that the resection would not result in major deficits.

7.3 Wada Test

In 1964, epileptologist Juhn Wada introduced the intracarotid sodium amytal test to help determine language lateralization in patients with brain tumors.[21] Today, language mapping can be done with fMRI,[22] but the Wada retains a utility for predicting memory deficits after temporal lobectomy. During the procedure, a short-acting anesthetic is introduced to one side of the anterior circulation at a time, and the resulting language and memory deficits are assessed. The test is meant to mimic the effects of a temporal lobectomy on memory (when the side under consideration for surgery is anesthetized) and to test the "functional reserve" of the hippocampus to be removed (when the side contralateral to the surgical side is anesthetized).[23,24]

7.3.1 Technique

Prior to a Wada test, the patient has EEG electrodes placed on the head (so that any seizures during the procedure can be detected). During the test, after local anesthesia to the groin for introduction of the angiography catheter, the neurosurgeon introduces the catheter into the internal carotid artery (generally beginning with the side under consideration for surgery).[25] Contrast is injected, and placement confirmed radiographically. The patient raises his or her arms and may be asked to count. Then the anesthetic is administered through the catheter at a rate of 25 mg every 5 seconds (typical dose 75–150 mg sodium amytal, though occasionally more is needed) until contralateral motor hemiparesis is observed. Typically, an epileptologist or neurologist in the case assesses motor strength to determine when the hemiparesis develops. EEG slowing of the affected hemisphere can be observed at the same time. Excess anesthetic can result in oversedation of the patient, making test results invalid.

Once the hemisphere has been anesthetized based on motor findings, the catheter is partially withdrawn and the neuropsychologist or neuropsychometrist uses a standard battery of tests to assess language production and reception, and gives the patient verbal lists and nonverbal items to remember. Throughout the test, motor function is assessed intermittently to ensure the hemisphere remains anesthetized.

After the effects of the anesthetic wear off (typically after 10–15 minutes), the neuropsychologist tests the patient for free recall and for recognition of the verbal and nonverbal items. The same procedure is then repeated on the opposite hemisphere.[21,25]

7.3.2 Complications

Complications of the Wada test can include seizures, carotid vasospasm, encephalopathy, and stroke in up to 5 to 11% of patients.[26,27]

7.4 Electrocorticography

In some cases, scalp EEG monitoring and supportive noninvasive tests are insufficient to localize the seizure onset zone accurately enough for surgical planning. In those situations, intracranial monitoring with ECoG can help localize the seizure onset.[28] In ECoG, the neurosurgeon places strip or grid electrodes directly on the surface of the brain and may place depth electrodes into the amygdala or hippocampus. Seizure recording then takes place from the implanted electrodes. In some cases, stereo EEG (sEEG) is used instead, in which the neurosurgeon places multiple depth electrodes to sample seizure propagation along anatomico-functional connections.[29] It should also

be noted that while ECoG allows for better spatial resolution of the electrical brain activity in the area monitored, a seizure focus outside of the brain region covered with electrodes may go undetected. Careful planning of intracranial electrode placement based on scalp EEG monitoring is therefore essential.

7.4.1 Technique

The patient is typically under general anesthesia for the placement of the intracranial electrodes. Approach is determined based on the desired location of electrodes, and must be tailored to the patient's anatomy. After electrode placement, the connecting wires from the electrodes are maintained outside the dura and may be tunneled through a subcutaneous plane to exit separately from the surgical site.[30] When the patient recovers and is transferred to the EMU, the electrode wires are connected to EEG monitoring hardware for ECoG. Prophylactic antibiotics may be given.

7.4.2 Complications

The major complications of intracranial electrode placement are hemorrhage, intracranial or superficial infection, elevated intracranial pressure, new neurologic deficits, and stroke, with risks of 2 to 23% for each complication and a total complication rate of 19% (prior to 1997).[29] Higher numbers of electrodes and longer monitoring periods are associated with an increased risk of complications.[30]

7.4.3 Seizure Monitoring

The patient is monitored in the EMU for approximately 7 days of vEEG monitoring, and ASDs may be reduced to facilitate seizures. Once seizures have been recorded, epileptologists use visual inspection and computer-assisted analysis to determine the seizure onset location on the intracranial electrodes. The seizure onset zone is then used to make a proposed resection plan. After monitoring is finished, the neurosurgeon removes the electrodes in the operating room under general anesthesia. If a craniotomy was performed to place the subdural grid or strip electrodes, and if sufficient information has been obtained, the neurosurgeon may perform the planned resection during the same operation as electrode removal. In sEEG cases, the resective surgery will be planned for a later date.

7.4.4 Functional Mapping with Stimulation

ECoG provides a unique opportunity to map cortical function directly from the brain with electrical stimulation mapping (ESM). During ESM, epileptologists use pulses of electricity to stimulate cortical electrodes to elicit or disrupt normal cortical function at specific points, and observe the effects on language, motor, and sensory functions. These results are recorded and a "map" of cortical function is drawn, which is compared to the proposed surgical resection to determine whether any deficits are predicted (▶ Fig. 7.1). Identifying primary motor, language, and sensory areas is a major goal as these areas must be spared during resection whenever possible. While cortical function

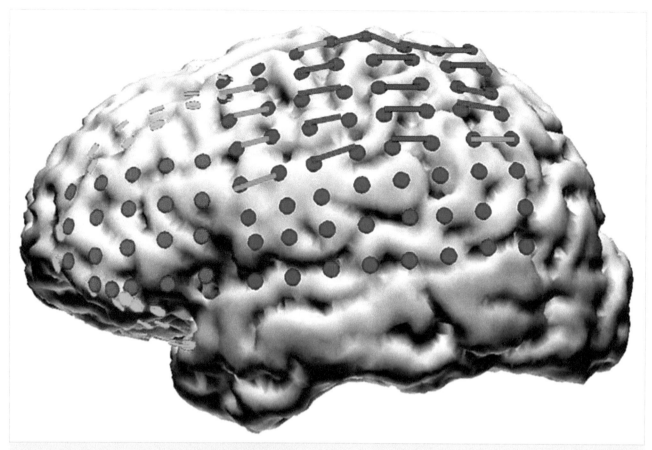

Fig. 7.1 Cortical stimulation map. The cortical stimulation results can be displayed as a map of the brain. For this purpose, a presurgically obtained 3D MRI is stripped to display the brain only and overlaid with a postoperatively obtained 3D CT of the electrode array. The electrodes are colored based on which electrode grid they belong to (Curry software by Compumedics Neuroscan, Charlotte, NC). Electrode pairs in this image are marked as *red* if stimulation resulted in motor activity and as *green* if stimulation did not activate eloquent cortex.

Table 7.1 Commonly used stimulation parameters for electrical stimulation mapping[31,32]

Type of electrode	Effective surface area (mm²)	Current (mA): initial	Current (mA): increasing	Pulse width (ms)	Train duration (s)	Pulse frequency (Hz)
Grid or strip, 2.4 mm diameter with 10 mm spacing	4.5	1–2	1 mA steps up to 15–17 mA	0.2–0.3	3–10	50/60
Depth, 2 mm electrode with 3.5 mm spacing	5.0	0.5	0.5 mA steps up to 2.5 mA	1	3–5	50/60

follows general organizational principles (such as the homunculus taught in medical schools around the world), lesions such as brain tumors or epileptic tissue can lead to reorganization, and there is also some degree of normal interindividual variability.[31]

ESM has been developed over many decades, and no standardized protocols exist for stimulation parameters. Commonly used settings are shown in ▶ Table 7.1. These parameters depend on the size of the electrodes used (effective surface area) and on the brain region tested. The procedure runs the risk of inducing seizures in susceptible patients, and therefore, is commonly performed near the end of EMU monitoring and after the patient has resumed ASDs.[32] During ESM, the neurologist and stimulation team explain the procedure to the patient

and ensure a quiet environment without interruptions. The neurologist makes a plan for ESM based on the expected function near the proposed resection area.

For motor mapping, the patient is asked to rest quietly. The stimulation team then introduces the desired initial current to the electrodes of interest, and if no clinical or EEG response is seen, the stimulation is increased gradually with successive stimulations. The stimulation team observes the patient for any unintended motor activity (positive motor response) and records specific responses with the electrode number and current at which the responses occur. Once the motor response (or lack thereof, at maximal stimulation) is determined, the next set of electrodes is stimulated, again starting with low current. Negative (inhibitory) motor responses can also be observed, such as from the inferior or middle frontal gyri, while the patient is asked to do tasks requiring sustained motor activity.[32]

For sensory mapping, the patient is asked to rest quietly and to report any sensations that he or she feels during stimulation. Again, the stimulation team introduces current at a low level to the electrodes under study, increasing gradually with successive stimulations. The patient's sensory response (or lack thereof) is recorded with the electrode numbers and stimulation parameters.

Language mapping requires active patient participation. For testing of speech production, the patient is asked to repeat phrases while stimulation is applied. Reading, listening, and comprehension via token tests (e.g., "point to the blue triangle") are tested during stimulation for other aspects of language function. The stimulation team observes the patient for pauses in speech, impaired comprehension, and impaired reading during the stimulation, which indicates interruption of language function and involvement of the cortical area under study.

Standard practice is to leave at least 10 to 20 mm "margin" adjacent to the nearest ESM-defined language area before resection, which has resulted in improved postoperative language outcomes.[31]

The stimulation team must monitor the patient's ECoG during stimulation sessions to identify the presence of after-discharges. This stimulation-induced irritability of the cortex is important because it may (1) lead to a seizure and (2) affect the observed mapping results. Electrical discharges induced by stimulation may spread to adjacent or distant cortex and interrupt the function of cortex beyond the stimulated electrodes. Thus, if a clinical response is observed, the cortical location responsible may not be at the stimulated electrodes. Sometimes, the monitoring team is able to terminate after-discharges by administering short pulses of stimulation at the electrodes that were originally stimulated. If the after-discharges persist and spread and cause a clinical seizure, standard seizure safety should be observed (e.g., turning the patient on his or her side and providing supportive oxygen, if necessary). Additional ASD or a benzodiazepine may be necessary if the patient has recurrent after-discharges.

7.4.5 Passive Mapping

New techniques such as high-gamma detection and mapping may offer a passive method of mapping to supplement or eventually replace ESM. This technique examines the power modulations in the high gamma (> 40 Hz) band of ECoG activity while the patient carries out tasks such as picture naming.[33] This technique has the benefit of being able to be carried out at any time during the patient's ECoG, rather than (as is typical for ESM) after seizures have been recorded and the patient has resumed ASDs. A recent meta-analysis found that modulations in high-gamma activity were highly specific (79%) but not sensitive (61%) for language localization, compared to ESM as a gold standard.[33]

7.4.6 Seizure Network Mapping

Cortico-cortical evoked potentials explore connectivity between brain regions using low-frequency (< 0.25–2 Hz) electrical stimulation.[34] Stimulation at a defined point propagates preferentially via axonal tracts, and the response at other electrodes is measured to determine the connectivity between sites. Networks with many bidirectional connections and tight clusters are likely to be pathologic, and abnormal connectivity can help identify the seizure onset location for surgical planning.[34,35]

7.5 Conclusion

In surgical planning for epilepsy, extraoperative mapping to determine the seizure onset location (via EMU scalp monitoring and sometimes ECoG) is vitally important. For many patients, functional mapping (with Wada, fMRI, or ESM) is necessary to ensure that no eloquent tissue from primary language, sensory, or motor areas is resected. The Wada test can help assess hippocampal function, but is becoming replaced in many cases by fMRI for language and neuropsychology assessment for memory assessment. Neurosurgeons should be aware of the available techniques for assessing predicted deficits after surgery.

References

[1] Fisher RS, van Emde Boas W, Blume W, et al. Epileptic seizures and epilepsy: definitions proposed by the International League Against Epilepsy (ILAE) and the International Bureau for Epilepsy (IBE). Epilepsia. 2005; 46(4):470–472

[2] Fisher RS, Acevedo C, Arzimanoglou A, et al. ILAE official report: a practical clinical definition of epilepsy. Epilepsia. 2014; 55(4):475–482

[3] Brodie MJ, Barry SJ, Bamagous GA, Norrie JD, Kwan P. Patterns of treatment response in newly diagnosed epilepsy. Neurology. 2012; 78(20):1548–1554

[4] Kwan P, Brodie MJ. Early identification of refractory epilepsy. N Engl J Med. 2000; 342(5):314–319

[5] Kwan P, Arzimanoglou A, Berg AT, et al. Definition of drug resistant epilepsy: consensus proposal by the ad hoc Task Force of the ILAE Commission on Therapeutic Strategies. Epilepsia. 2010; 51(6):1069–1077

[6] Engel J, Jr, McDermott MP, Wiebe S, et al. Early Randomized Surgical Epilepsy Trial (ERSET) Study Group. Early surgical therapy for drug-resistant temporal lobe epilepsy: a randomized trial. JAMA. 2012; 307(9):922–930

[7] Wiebe S, Blume WT, Girvin JP, Eliasziw M, Effectiveness and Efficiency of Surgery for Temporal Lobe Epilepsy Study Group. A randomized, controlled trial of surgery for temporal-lobe epilepsy. N Engl J Med. 2001; 345(5):311–318

[8] Sperling MR, O'Connor MJ, Saykin AJ, Plummer C. Temporal lobectomy for refractory epilepsy. JAMA. 1996; 276(6):470–475

[9] Wicks RT, Jermakowicz WJ, Jagid JR, et al. Laser interstitial thermal therapy for mesial temporal lobe epilepsy. Neurosurgery. 2016; 79 Suppl 1:S83–S91

[10] Kang JY, Wu C, Tracy J, et al. Laser interstitial thermal therapy for medically intractable mesial temporal lobe epilepsy. Epilepsia. 2016; 57(2):325–334

[11] Xue H, Cai L, Dong S, Li Y. Clinical characteristics and post-surgical outcomes of focal cortical dysplasia subtypes. J Clin Neurosci. 2016; 23:68–72

[12] Noe K, Sulc V, Wong-Kisiel L, et al. Long-term outcomes after nonlesional extratemporal lobe epilepsy surgery. JAMA Neurol. 2013; 70(8):1003–1008

[13] Struck AF, Cole AJ, Cash SS, Westover MB. The number of seizures needed in the EMU. Epilepsia. 2015; 56(11):1753–1759

[14] Rizvi SAA, Hernandez-Ronquillo L, Wu A, Téllez Zenteno JF. Is rapid withdrawal of anti-epileptic drug therapy using video EEG monitoring safe and efficacious? Epilepsy Res. 2014; 108(4):755–764

[15] Henning O, Baftiu A, Johannessen SI, Landmark CJ. Withdrawal of antiepileptic drugs during presurgical video-EEG monitoring: an observational study for evaluation of current practice at a referral center for epilepsy. Acta Neurol Scand. 2014; 129(4):243–251

[16] Ramey WL, Martirosyan NL, Lieu CM, Hasham HA, Lemole GM, Jr, Weinand ME. Current management and surgical outcomes of medically intractable epilepsy. Clin Neurol Neurosurg. 2013; 115(12):2411–2418

[17] Englot DJ, Nagarajan SS, Imber BS, et al. Epileptogenic zone localization using magnetoencephalography predicts seizure freedom in epilepsy surgery. Epilepsia. 2015; 56(6):949–958

[18] Devous MD, Sr, Thisted RA, Morgan GF, Leroy RF, Rowe CC. SPECT brain imaging in epilepsy: a meta-analysis. J Nucl Med. 1998; 39(2):285–293

[19] Dulay MF, Busch RM. Prediction of neuropsychological outcome after resection of temporal and extratemporal seizure foci. Neurosurg Focus. 2012; 32(3):E4

[20] Chelune GJ, Naugle RI, Lüders H, Awad IA. Prediction of cognitive change as a function of preoperative ability status among temporal lobectomy patients seen at 6-month follow-up. Neurology. 1991; 41(3):399–404

[21] Taussig D, Montavont A, Isnard J. Invasive EEG explorations. Neurophysiol Clin. 2015; 45(1):113–119

[22] Benjamin CFA, Dhingra I, Li AX, et al. Presurgical language fMRI: technical practices in epilepsy surgical planning. Hum Brain Mapp. 2018; 39(10): 4032–4042

[23] Mani J, Busch R, Kubu C, Kotagal P, Shah U, Dinner D. Wada memory asymmetry scores and postoperative memory outcome in left temporal epilepsy. Seizure. 2008; 17(8):691–698

[24] Chiaravalloti ND, Glosser G. Material-specific memory changes after anterior temporal lobectomy as predicted by the intracarotid amobarbital test. Epilepsia. 2001; 42(7):902–911

[25] Powell GE, Polkey CE, Canavan AGM. Lateralisation of memory functions in epileptic patients by use of the sodium amytal (Wada) technique. J Neurol Neurosurg Psychiatry. 1987; 50(6):665–672

[26] Loddenkemper T, Morris HH, Möddel G. Complications during the Wada test. Epilepsy Behav. 2008; 13(3):551–553

[27] Beimer NJ, Buchtel HA, Glynn SM. One center's experience with complications during the Wada test. Epilepsia. 2015; 56(8):e110–e113

[28] Weinand ME, Wyler AR, Richey ET, Phillips BB, Somes GW. Long-term ictal monitoring with subdural strip electrodes: prognostic factors for selecting temporal lobectomy candidates. J Neurosurg. 1992; 77(1):20–28

[29] Kovac S, Vakharia VN, Scott C, Diehl B. Invasive epilepsy surgery evaluation. Seizure. 2017; 44:125–136

[30] Arya R, Mangano FT, Horn PS, Holland KD, Rose DF, Glauser TA. Adverse events related to extraoperative invasive EEG monitoring with subdural grid electrodes: a systematic review and meta-analysis. Epilepsia. 2013; 54(5): 828–839

[31] Ritaccio AL, Brunner P, Schalk G. Electrical stimulation mapping of the brain: basic principles and emerging alternatives. J Clin Neurophysiol. 2018; 35(2): 86–97

[32] So EL, Alwaki A. A guide for cortical electrical stimulation mapping. J Clin Neurophysiol. 2018; 35(2):98–105

[33] Arya R, Horn PS, Crone NE. ECoG high-gamma modulation versus electrical stimulation for presurgical language mapping. Epilepsy Behav. 2018; 79:26–33

[34] Prime D, Rowlands D, O'Keefe S, Dionisio S. Considerations in performing and analyzing the responses of cortico-cortical evoked potentials in stereo-EEG. Epilepsia. 2018; 59(1):16–26

[35] Mouthaan BE, van 't Klooster MA, Keizer D, et al. Single pulse electrical stimulation to identify epileptogenic cortex: clinical information obtained from early evoked responses. Clin Neurophysiol. 2016; 127(2):1088–1098

8 Neuropsychologist's Role in the Management of Brain Tumor Patients

David S. Sabsevitz, Kathleen H. Elverman, Kyle Noll, and Jeffrey Wefel

Abstract

Brain tumors represent a dynamic disease in which neuropsychological functioning can change dramatically throughout the disease course. High rates of cognitive dysfunction have been reported in brain tumor patients and the presence of cognitive impairment is associated with decreased quality of life and functional independence, and shorter survival time. Neuropsychologists are becoming increasingly involved in the assessment and management of brain tumor patients at all stages of care. This chapter provides an overview of the neuropsychologist's role in the management of patients with brain tumors with specific focus on the intraoperative stage.

Keywords: neuropsychological testing, intraoperative brain mapping, brain tumors

8.1 The Neuropsychological Exam

Neuropsychology is a specialized field within clinical psychology that focuses on evaluating brain–behavioral relationships or the effects of disease or injury on cognitive and emotional functions. A neuropsychological evaluation provides important information about the structural and functional integrity of the brain through careful clinical interview and the administration of a series of standardized tests that are compared relative to a normative sample or to the patient's own previous performance in the case of longitudinal follow-up. The domains often evaluated include intelligence, memory, attention, processing speed, learning and memory, language, spatial abilities, executive functions, and sensorimotor abilities in addition to assessment of mood and quality of life. It is essential to broadly sample across neurocognitive domains when evaluating patients with brain tumors, as patients may present with broad and nonlocalizing deficits in addition to more focal features.

The typical structure of a neuropsychological exam includes a record review and clinical interview to obtain relevant history followed by administration of paper-and-pencil, question-and-answer, and computerized cognitive and emotional measures. Testing can range from 15 to 30 minutes using brief, bedside screening tools (e.g., Mini-Mental State Examination [MMSE] and Montreal Cognitive Assessment [MoCA]) to more comprehensive assessment lasting up to several hours where multiple cognitive domains are evaluated in detail. While the brevity and ease of administration of screening tools are appealing, they tend to lack sensitivity in detecting more mild cognitive impairment. Specifically, when comparing the MMSE to a more comprehensive neuropsychological test battery in a sample of brain tumor patients, the MMSE showed a sensitivity of only 0.50.[1] Further, screening tools also lack sensitivity in detecting longitudinal change in cognitive functioning associated with treatment effect.[2] Accordingly, more comprehensive testing batteries sampling across cognitive domains is preferred, though test selection and battery length must be

carefully considered given the propensity for fatigue in this patient population. The extent of testing is often dictated by the clinical questions being asked and the patient's functional level. Use of measures that are repeatable with multiple forms and minimal practice effects are preferred since patients are typically reevaluated postoperatively and often at regular intervals throughout the disease course. Assessment of mood, quality of life, and symptoms common to patients with brain tumors is also important.

8.2 Neuropsychology in the Preoperative Stage

The pattern of neuropsychological deficits in patients with brain tumors can vary greatly depending upon lesion location and other patient and tumor characteristics.[3] While deficits can be observed in a variety of domains, memory and executive functions seem particularly vulnerable (▶ Fig. 8.1).[4,5,6] Patients with tumors in the dominant hemisphere tend to have more cognitive deficits than patients with tumors in the nondominant hemisphere,[7] and while focal syndromes (e.g., aphasia with left perisylvian tumors) can be seen, cognitive dysfunction can also be more mild and nonfocal than typical of other neurologic insults such as stroke.[8] This may be explained by more widespread effects of the tumor via its infiltrative nature and associated edema and mass effect, which can disrupt broader cerebral networks and cause impairments in domains more distal to tumor location. Growth momentum also plays an important role in a patient's cognitive presentation with greater neuropsychological impairment observed in patients with rapidly growing tumors compared to slow-growing tumors.[3,9,10] It is likely that the slow growth rate mitigates the impairment that might be expected based purely on lesion location and size in part by allowing for greater functional reorganization and neural compensation. In fact, there are numerous case examples in the literature where large amounts of tissue can be surgically removed in patients with low-grade gliomas in expected eloquent regions without any observed functional consequences.[11]

Obtaining a comprehensive neuropsychological evaluation prior to surgery is ideal and provides the medical team with a better understanding of the unique impact of the tumor on cognition. This allows for better differentiation between the cognitive effects of the tumor versus surgery and other therapies (e.g., radiation and chemotherapy) as a patient is being followed over time. Obtaining a preoperative neuropsychological evaluation also captures individual differences that can influence cognition, such as preexisting cognitive weaknesses from learning or developmental delays, cognitive changes from preexisting medical problems (e.g., vascular risk factors and seizure disorder), and the impact of cultural differences on test performance. Without having a pretreatment baseline, abnormal test performances attributed to these factors can sometimes be misinterpreted as related to the disease. It is not always feasible to

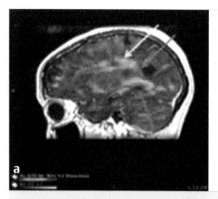 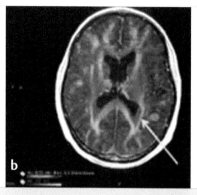 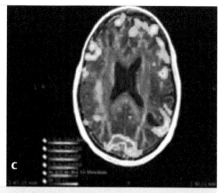

Fig. 8.1 Diffusion anisotropy color coded maps (**a** and **b**) with superimposed fMRI language mapping results (**c**). Arrows identify the superior longitudinal fasciculus (SLF) (*yellow arrow*) and AF (*red arrow*) and inferior frontal occipital fasciculus (IFOF) (*blue arrow*) in panel **a** and a bundle of fibers containing the inferior longitudinal fasciculus, IFOF, and optic radiation (*yellow arrow*) in panel **b**.

obtain a comprehensive evaluation prior to surgery given the medical urgency and short time frame to proceed to surgery, especially in high-grade glioma patients, and in such cases baselining a patient after surgery but prior to initiation of adjuvant therapies is a reasonable alternative. Establishing a baseline is also critical to monitoring disease status over time. Studies have shown that changes in neuropsychological status can predict tumor recurrence,[12] in some cases even before evidence of radiographic progression.[13] Being able to detect such changes over time is dependent on having a baseline or benchmark for longitudinal comparison.

Neuropsychological testing can also inform surgical risk to cognitive functioning. Preoperative neuropsychological testing has been shown to be a strong predictor of postoperative outcomes in specific cognitive domains with greater preoperative memory and language performance associated with greater postoperative declines in these areas.[14] The duration or persistence of a presenting deficit can also be used to assess risk. Consider, for example, a patient presenting with a transient aphasia that resolves with steroid treatment. The transient nature suggests lesion proximity to language areas, presumably from edema or mass effect, but the fact that it resolved indicates that those systems have not been irreversibly damaged by the tumor and that with careful surgical planning risk can be mitigated. This is in contrast to a patient who presents with a persisting deficit where predictive value is less clear.

Preoperative neuropsychological testing adds further value to the broader presurgical workup in determining the feasibility of brain mapping procedures, whether pre- or intraoperative. Patients presenting with severe deficits such as profound aphasia may be poor candidates for functional magnetic resonance imaging (fMRI) or intraoperative mapping. If brain mapping is deemed feasible, this preoperative assessment is highly beneficial for determining specific domains for intraoperative focus and identifying situations in which paradigms need to be modified (e.g., to meet the ability level of the patient). Given that patients vary considerably with respect to functional level, it is important to take a highly individualized approach to selecting testing materials for intraoperative mapping. Baselining a patient on intraoperative mapping protocols during the preoperative assessment familiarizes the patient with the testing protocols they may be exposed to during surgery and allows

the examiner to select only those items that each individual patient can reliably and accurately respond to, thus creating a set of test stimuli that are specific to that patient. By doing so, the examiner can have greater confidence that errors occurring during surgery represent potential surgical effects or true disruption from stimulation rather than lack of knowledge or preexisting deficits.

8.3 Neuropsychology in the Intraoperative Stage

Intraoperative mapping requires a coordinated effort across disciplines (▸ Fig. 8.2). There is considerable variability across institutions in the personnel used to perform behavioral and cognitive testing during awake surgery. Speech pathologists, neurologists, neurosurgical fellows or residents, anesthesiologists, and surgical nurses have all been used in this capacity. Neuropsychologists are particularly well suited for this role given their expertise in psychometrics and test design, functional neuroanatomy, and their high-level conceptual understanding of cognitive functions, which allows for more informed task development, task selection, and interpretation of mapping results. In fact, recent evidence suggests higher rates of gross total resection, shorter duration of surgery, and lower rates of unexpected residual tumor when neuropsychologists are used for intraoperative mapping.[15]

There is also significant variability in the extent and timing of cognitive testing during surgery. Direct cortical stimulation (DCS) is often used to explore the cortical surface for eloquence prior to starting surgical resection and for targeted mapping of white matter tracts and deep subcortical gray matter structures. However, DCS constitutes a relatively small portion of the overall surgery and there is often significant time during which resections are performed without stimulation. During these times, intraoperative cognitive monitoring (IOCM) can be conducted wherein the patient is continuously tested and assessed for cognitive change or evolving deficits. When changes in performance are observed, the neurosurgeon is notified, and surgical decisions are made accordingly. IOCM is particularly valuable in the context of negative mapping when DCS produces no disruptions or responses. Negative mapping is quite

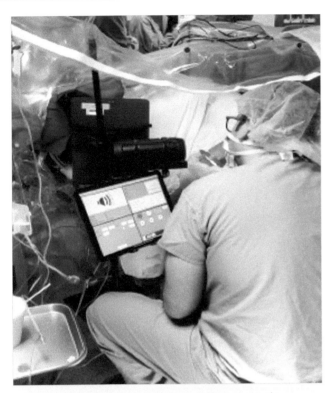

Fig. 8.2 NeuroMapper dual iPad testing platform setup in the operating room. The iPad facing the patient displays stimuli and captures video recording of each trial. The iPad facing the examiner is used to select tasks, control the delivery of the stimuli, record accuracy and monitor reaction time relative to baseline performance, and enter electrocorticography parameters.

common and can be due to factors such as small craniotomy with minimal exposed cortex, individual variability in functional organization, inadequate stimulation parameters (e.g., mA limited by after-discharges), functional reorganization associated with the brain lesion, use of inappropriate tasks to assess the target area, and neural connectivity engaging a distributed network that cannot be sufficiently disrupted by stimulation of a small area.[16] Negative mapping does not negate the possibility of postoperative deficits, and IOCM can help mitigate this risk as it can capture cumulative or additive effects of active resection on cognitive networks.

A highly individualized approach to task selection for DCS and IOCM is advocated. Tasks should be selected based on knowledge of functional neuroanatomy and the proximity of the tumor to known eloquent areas, localization data obtained from functional neuroimaging studies and diffusion tensor imaging (DTI), and review of presenting symptoms and baseline neuropsychological test performance. Testing should also be multidimensional in nature as tumors can be located in areas where more than one function has proximity to the tumor border. Take for example the patient shown in ▶ Fig. 8.3 where there is a lesion located in the posterior left middle temporal gyrus. This lesion has proximity on its posterior border to the angular gyrus, indicating possible risk to semantics, reading, and other dominant parietal functions (e.g., writing, math, right–left orientation, and finger localization); immediate

proximity at the anterior border to the arcuate fasciculus (AF), suggesting risk to phonological retrieval systems; and immediate proximity on its medial border to a bundle of fibers containing the inferior longitudinal fasciculus (ILF), inferior frontal occipital fasciculus (IFOF), and optic radiations (OR), indicating possible risk to semantics (from the ILF and IFOF) and vision (from the OR). In this case, vascular anatomy complicated the surgical pathway to the lesion and fMRI showed robust language activation around the lesion. Mapping this type of case requires testing of multiple functions, DCS to inform the approach and particular high-risk areas, as well as continuous IOCM to monitor for moment-to-moment fluctuations in neurocognitive functioning.

Awake craniotomies have historically focused on sensorimotor and language mapping. Sensorimotor mapping is relatively straightforward with respect to anatomic localization and technique and is discussed in detail in another chapter of this book. Mapping language is far more complex both conceptually and anatomically. It is widely accepted that language involves a more distributed network than Broca and Wernicke areas and that there are anatomically dissociable regions that are specialized in processing specific linguistic aspects of language. See Hickok and Poeppel,[17] Chang et al,[18] and Binder[19] for a review of eloquent regions associated with critical language functions. For example, there are regions in the ventral temporal occipital, or fusiform area, that are specialized in processing orthographic or written letter content, areas in the mid-superior temporal gyrus and sulcus dedicated to processing phonology or speech sounds, areas more posterior in the superior temporal gyrus and inferior parietal lobule involved in phonological access and retrieval, and areas in lateral middle and inferior temporal lobe, posterior inferior parietal lobe (angular gyrus), and dorsolateral frontal cortex that are involved in processing semantics (i.e., the meaning of pictures, words, phrases, etc.).

Language mapping often involves administration of relatively simple tasks to test basic, automatic speech functions, such as counting or reciting overlearned phrases (e.g., days of the week, alphabet, and Pledge of Allegiance), and if a disruption is observed, the examiner can further explore the basis for the deficit by having the patient phonate or repeat sounds such as "pa-pa-pa," "la-la-la," and "ga-ga-ga" to evaluate mouth, tongue, and palate movements. Object naming is considered the "gold standard" for mapping language. Naming objects engages a number of language processes, including phonological access, lexical–semantic retrieval, and speech motor functions, allowing for broad sampling of the language network with one task. There is significant individual variability in the location of object naming sites when tested with DCS, with disruptions seen over a wide area of left lateral cortex including temporal, parietal, and frontal regions.[18] Other naming paradigms have been developed that differ in input modality and semantic category. For example, auditory naming has been associated with more anterior temporal localization than visual naming,[20,21,22] greater verb than object naming specific sites have been reported in the prefrontal cortex,[23,24] and naming proper nouns has been associated with the temporal pole and uncinate fasciculus.[25,26] Repeating nonwords has been shown to be effective in mapping phonology systems in the vicinity of the AF[27] and nonverbal semantics using a picture semantic association task (i.e., selecting which picture from two choices is

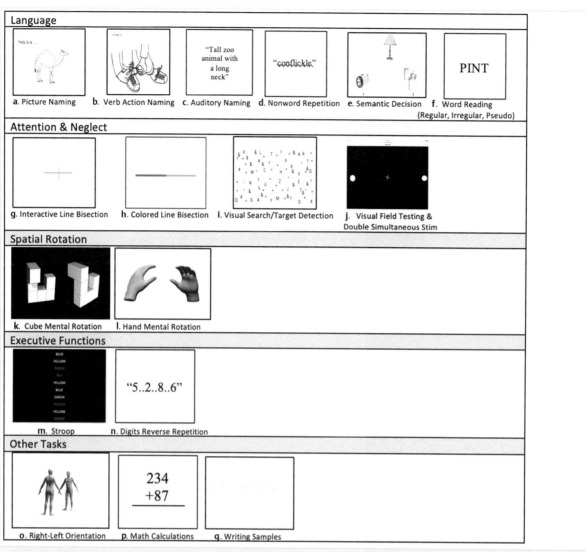

Fig. 8.3 Sample of tasks used in the NeuroMapper testing platform. (**a**) Object naming requires the patient to name a series of line drawings from the series of Snodgrass and Vanderwalt. (Snodgrass and Vanderwalt. A standardized set of 260 pictures: norms for name agreement, image agreement, familiarity, and visual complexity. J. Exp Psychol Hum Learn 1980;6(2):174–215.). (**b**) Verb action naming consists of naming an action being depicted in a series of line drawings. Items were obtained with permission from the test developer (Druks J, Masterson J. An Object and Action Naming Battery. Hove: Psychology Press; 2000). (**c**) Auditory naming consists of naming objects based on their verbal description. Stimuli were selected from a set of stimuli created by Pillay et al. (Pillay et al. Lesion localization of speech comprehension deficits in chronic aphasia. Neurology 2017;88(9):970–975). (**d**) Nonword repetition consists of repeating a series of pseudowords ranging from one to four syllables. Stimuli created by J. R. Binder at the Medical College of Wisconsin. (**e**) Semantic decision consists of viewing a triad of pictures and selecting one of two pictures presented at the bottom that is most like the picture at the top in meaning from Binder et al. Surface errors without semantic impairment in acquired dyslexia: a voxel-based lesion symptom mapping study. Brain 2016;139(5):1517–1526). (**f**) Word reading consists of reading a series of regular and irregular (or exception) words and pseudowords. (**g**) Interactive line bisection requires the patient to bisect a series of lines shown on the iPad with their finger. (**h**) Colored line bisection requires the patient to indicate whether the two-colored segments of the line are equal in length or not. This task does not require a motor response. (**i**) Visual search and target detection require the patient to scan an array of letters and symbols and identify which numbered quadrant a specified target letter is located. (**j**) Visual field testing requires the patient to fixate on a rotating cross and identify whether they see a flashing dot on the left, right, or on both sides in the upper, mid, and lower visual fields. (**k**) Cube rotation requires the patient to view pairs of three-dimensional cubes and determine whether they are the same or different by mentally rotating the second stimuli. Stimuli were acquired from Ganis and Kievit (free use stimuli). (Ganis and Kievit. A new set of three-dimensional shapes for investigating mental rotation processes: Validation data and stimulus set. Journal of Open Psychology Data; 2015). (**l**) Hand rotation is another type of mental rotation task. The patient is presented two hands on the screen and has to determine if the second hand (hand on the right) is the same or different than the first hand by mentally rotating the second stimuli. (**m**) Stroop test requires the patient to inhibit reading the word and indicate the color of the printed color word. (**n**) Digit repetition requires the patient to repeat back a string of digits in reverse order. (**o**) Right–left orientation requires the patient to identify whether the shaded limb on a person is on the right or left side of their body. (**p**) Math calculations consist of a series of arithmetic operations presented horizontally and vertically stacked with and without carryover operations. (**q**) Writing samples require the patient to spontaneously generate a sentence or write a sentence to dictation using their finger or a stylus pen.

most related to a target in meaning) has been shown to be useful in mapping the ventral semantic stream (IFOF) in the left but also right hemisphere.[28,29,30] Further research and discussion regarding language mapping is presented in Chapter 11 (Speech Mapping).

While risk for cognitive complications is often assumed to be lower in nondominant hemisphere resections, declines in cognition have been reported following these resections[31] and the concept of noneloquence in brain areas beyond dominant hemisphere language regions should be challenged. The right hemisphere is known to play an important role in visuoperception, attention, and social cognition[32] and there is increasing focus on developing tasks to assess these functions during awake surgery, which frequently involves adaptation of traditional neuropsychological measures to the operating room (OR) environment. For example, unilateral spatial neglect whereby the patient cannot attend to one side of space (most often the left side with right-sided lesions) can result from right parietal, frontal, or even subcortical damage. Line bisection tasks are commonly used to assess neglect; however, physical positioning of the patient in the OR often prohibits a precise written response. Adapted line bisection tasks can circumvent motoric requirements, such as a colored line bisection task used by the authors of this chapter. In this task, the patient is shown a horizontal line divided into two colored segments (e.g., half in red and half in green) and they indicate verbally if the two segments are equal in length or one is longer. Neglect should be suspected if the patient states that the color on the left is shorter than the color on the right when they are actually equal in length (i.e., the patient is neglecting a portion of the color segment on the left). We have also adapted cancellation tasks (which typically require patients to cross out target letters/symbols within an array of distractors) for the operating room. In these visual search tasks, the patient is presented an array of letters among distractor symbols on a screen divided into four labeled quadrants and verbally indicates the quadrant of the target letter. Accuracy and reaction time are monitored and omissions and/or slowing when searching the left side of space may indicate neglect. Double simultaneous stimuli presentation can also be used where the patient fixates on a central crosshair and stimuli (flashing dot or numbers) are presented unilateral or bilaterally and the patient has to indicate on which side they see the stimuli. Conditions where they perceive unilateral stimuli but not stimuli on the left during bilateral or simultaneous presentation may indicate neglect.

Mental rotation tasks can also be used to test the nondominant parietal lobe. In these tasks, patients identify whether two objects are the same or different by mentally rotating them. In a meta-analysis and review of neuroimaging studies, Zacks[33] found that regions in the superior parietal, frontal, and inferotemporal cortices were consistently activated during these tasks. While activation was bilateral in most areas, parietal activity was more common in the nondominant, right hemisphere (specifically posterior parietal cortex). Math tasks (e.g., basic calculation) can also be used to test parietal functioning. Acalculia can result from damage to the dominant angular gyrus, and fMRI studies have shown activation along the intraparietal sulcus, parietal lobe as well as prefrontal cortex and other regions, with laterality differences based on the nature of the task.[34] Social cognition tasks (e.g., facial emotion recogni-

tion, emotional prosody, empathy, and theory of mind tasks) have also shown to activate regions including the supramarginal gyrus, angular gyrus, superior temporal gyrus, middle temporal gyrus, and aspects of the frontal lobes[35] and deficits have been reported following right inferior frontal surgery.[36,37]

Executive functioning is an umbrella term used to describe higher order cognitive processes such as planning, shifting from one mental set to another, updating and monitoring of information, and inhibitory control that commonly localize to frontal regions of the brain.[38] Monitoring of executive functions is, thus, particularly important during frontal resections, though executive functioning also involves more distributed corticocortico and cortico-subcortical networks and executive deficits can develop with damage outside the frontal lobes. Tasks to assess executive abilities intraoperatively include those assessing inhibitory control (e.g., Stroop color–word interference tests, Go/No Go tests such as squeeze if examiner taps on hand twice, do nothing if examiner taps on hand once), working memory (e.g., reverse digit sequencing), verbal fluency (e.g., saying as many words starting with a particular letter within a short period of time), and mental flexibility (e.g., Oral Trails Test requiring alternating recitation of ascending numbers and letters).

As depicted earlier, there is a growing range of testing paradigms that can be utilized for brain mapping and it is neither feasible nor clinically indicated for all patients to be administered all tests within this large range. Again, we reiterate the importance of taking an individualized and functional anatomically informed approach to task selection to optimize mapping/monitoring for any given patient. In addition to greater focus on task development, there is also increased attention on identifying the most effective and innovative methods for administering testing in the OR where efficiency is critical and surgical progress should not be slowed by cumbersome testing procedures. Laptop- and tablet-based systems are increasingly utilized to display stimuli to patients (e.g., PowerPoint presentations) and allow for extensive stimuli to be stored and displayed electronically, rather than needing hard copies of stimuli in the OR. However, the transition to computers alone does not address the often unstructured and highly variable testing methods used across institutions. Increased consensus in this regard would be valuable in allowing for more comprehensive research endeavors with larger samples across collaborating institutions and further identification of best practices. Consensus is becoming increasingly possible through development of specific surgical brain mapping software packages/applications that can be used in a standardized fashion across institutions. One such testing platform is NeuroMapper, which was developed by the lead author of this chapter. It utilizes dual iPads to administer a variety of cognitive paradigms to patients in a highly customized and flexible manner, allows for highly individualized mapping by using baseline performance to select stimulus sets for the operating room, allows examiners to quickly and easily code patient responses (e.g., correct/incorrect and types of errors made) and monitor changes in task accuracy and reaction times in real time, and video records patients responses for later review. ▶ Fig. 8.2 shows the NeuroMapper testing platform setup in the operating room and ▶ Fig. 8.3 shows examples of some of the tasks included in the package.

8.4 Postoperative Stage

Over 60% of patients with brain tumors show cognitive decline on neuropsychological testing in the near postoperative period despite the use of modern brain mapping and microsurgical techniques.[31,39] Deficits may be more focal than seen preoperatively, as resection of brain tumors may damage localized healthy tissue surrounding the tumor. For instance, resections involving eloquent regions important to speech and memory tend to be associated with declines in these specific functions in particular, though broader impairments across other domains are also common. Additionally, tumors in the left hemisphere show greatest risk of postoperative worsening,[31] though decline is relatively common following resection of right hemisphere tumors. Importantly, patients with right hemisphere tumor resection can even show decline in language and verbal memory, functions more often associated with the left hemisphere. Such changes likely relate to disruption of distributed networks and potential nonspecific effects of surgery such as postoperative edema. Postoperative neurocognitive functioning also has significant prognostic value, as reductions in overall and progression free survival time are associated with the presence of neurocognitive impairment.[12,40]

Emotional functioning represents another important consideration in the management of patients with primary brain tumors, with depression representing the most prevalent problem.[41] In addition to comprising the single largest influence upon quality of life in patients with malignant glioma,[31] evidence indicates that depression also has been associated with reduced survival time.[42,43] Identification of neurocognitive and emotional symptoms via neuropsychological evaluation may facilitate early intervention, which may improve quality of life and potentially even prolong survival.

Proper timing of postoperative neuropsychological assessment is critical. Patient performances during evaluations conducted shortly following neurosurgical intervention may be impacted by transient issues, such as edema and medication side effects. Indeed, patients tend to show rapid improvement in cognition in the weeks after brain tumor resection despite initial postoperative worsening.[44,45] However, patients with brain tumors, especially malignant glioma, typically begin chemotherapy and/or radiation in the weeks following neurosurgical resection. These therapies can adversely impact neurocognitive functioning. Accordingly, the timing of neuropsychological evaluation in the postoperative period is largely dictated by the referral question and goals of assessment. In cases in which postoperative cognitive change is of interest, neuropsychological reevaluation within 3 to 5 weeks after resection likely allows for early stages of spontaneous recovery as well as assessment of functioning prior to initiation of therapies with potential adverse impact on neuropsychological status.

Ultimately, the objective of well-planned and executed postoperative neuropsychological evaluations in a neurosurgical setting is to provide outcome information and resources to preserve or improve patient functioning and quality of life. As such, personalized recommendations are as crucial as the identification of any existing impairments. Patients can benefit from education and instruction regarding implementation of various compensatory strategies, including environmental modifications, external aids, and internal strategies.[46,47] For those with more severe postoperative neurocognitive decline, neurorehabilitation is often beneficial. While studies are mixed, a variety of pharmacotherapies (e.g., donepezil, memantine, methylphenidate, and modafinil) can be trialed to prevent and/or treat neurocognitive dysfunction.[48,49,50]

8.5 Conclusion

Cognitive impairment is common in brain tumor patients and the ability to effectively assess and monitor cognitive functioning and minimize deficits in this patient population is important for optimizing quality of life. Neuropsychological assessment during the preoperative stage can help guide surgical planning and facilitate other neuromedical procedures such as preoperative and intraoperative brain mapping. Neuropsychological testing during awake craniotomy can mitigate risk for cognitive complications and optimize extent of surgical resection. Postoperatively, neuropsychological assessment is often used to guide rehabilitation efforts and monitor disease course and response to treatment. As such, neuropsychologists are increasingly considered essential members of the neurosurgical team, vital to ensuring valid and effective brain mapping, and critical for comprehensively assessing cognition, mitigating the impact of impairment, and maximizing patient's quality of life throughout the disease course.

References

[1] Meyers CA, Wefel JS. The use of the mini-mental state examination to assess cognitive functioning in cancer trials: no ifs, ands, buts, or sensitivity. J Clin Oncol. 2003; 21(19):3557–3558

[2] Meyers CA, Kudelka AP, Conrad CA, Gelke CK, Grove W, Pazdur R. Neurotoxicity of CI-980, a novel mitotic inhibitor. Clin Cancer Res. 1997; 3(3):419–422

[3] Wefel JS, Noll KR, Scheurer ME. Neurocognitive functioning and genetic variation in patients with primary brain tumours. Lancet Oncol. 2016; 17(3):e97–e108

[4] Tucha O, Smely C, Preier M, Lange KW. Cognitive deficits before treatment among patients with brain tumors. Neurosurgery. 2000; 47(2):324–333, discussion 333–334

[5] Dwan TM, Ownsworth T, Chambers S, Walker DG, Shum DH. Neuropsychological assessment of individuals with brain tumor: comparison of approaches used in the classification of impairment. Front Oncol. 2015; 5:56

[6] Talacchi A, Santini B, Savazzi S, Gerosa M. Cognitive effects of tumour and surgical treatment in glioma patients. J Neurooncol. 2011; 103(3):541–549

[7] Taphoorn MJ, Heimans JJ, Snoek FJ, et al. Assessment of quality of life in patients treated for low-grade glioma: a preliminary report. J Neurol Neurosurg Psychiatry. 1992; 55(5):372–376

[8] Anderson SW, Damasio H, Tranel D. Neuropsychological impairments associated with lesions caused by tumor or stroke. Arch Neurol. 1990; 47(4):397–405

[9] Hom J, Reitan RM. Neuropsychological correlates of rapidly vs. slowly growing intrinsic cerebral neoplasms. J Clin Neuropsychol. 1984; 6(3):309–324

[10] Kayl AE, Meyers CA. Does brain tumor histology influence cognitive function? Neuro-oncol. 2003; 5(4):255–260

[11] Duffau H, Capelle L, Denvil D, et al. Functional recovery after surgical resection of low grade gliomas in eloquent brain: hypothesis of brain compensation. J Neurol Neurosurg Psychiatry. 2003; 74(7):901–907

[12] Armstrong TS, Wefel JS, Wang M, et al. Net clinical benefit analysis of radiation therapy oncology group 0525: a phase III trial comparing conventional adjuvant temozolomide with dose-intensive temozolomide in patients with newly diagnosed glioblastoma. J Clin Oncol. 2013; 31(32):4076–4084

[13] Meyers CA, Hess KR, Yung WK, Levin VA. Cognitive function as a predictor of survival in patients with recurrent malignant glioma. J Clin Oncol. 2000; 18 (3):646–650

[14] Gehring K, et al. Prediction of memory outcomes after resection of high-grade glioma. Neuro-oncol. 2011; 13 Suppl 3:75–75

[15] Kelm A, Sollmann N, Ille S, Meyer B, Ringel F, Krieg SM. resection of gliomas with and without neuropsychological support during awake craniotomy—effects on surgery and clinical Outcome. Front Oncol. 2017; 7:176

[16] Skrap M, Marin D, Ius T, Fabbro F, Tomasino B. Brain mapping: a novel intra-operative neuropsychological approach. J Neurosurg. 2016; 125(4):877–887

[17] Hickok G, Poeppel D. Dorsal and ventral streams: a framework for understanding aspects of the functional anatomy of language. Cognition. 2004; 92 (1–2):67–99

[18] Chang EF, Raygor KP, Berger MS. Contemporary model of language organization: an overview for neurosurgeons. J Neurosurg. 2015; 122(2):250–261

[19] Binder JR. fMRI of language systems: methods and applications. In: Functional Neuroradiology. Springer; 2011: 393–417

[20] Hamberger MJ, McClelland S, III, McKhann GM, II, Williams AC, Goodman RR. Distribution of auditory and visual naming sites in nonlesional temporal lobe epilepsy patients and patients with space-occupying temporal lobe lesions. Epilepsia. 2007; 48(3):531–538

[21] Hamberger MJ, Seidel WT. Auditory and visual naming tests: normative and patient data for accuracy, response time, and tip-of-the-tongue. J Int Neuropsychol Soc. 2003; 9(3):479–489

[22] Hamberger MJ, Seidel WT. Localization of cortical dysfunction based on auditory and visual naming performance. J Int Neuropsychol Soc. 2009; 15(4):529–535

[23] Havas V, Gabarrós A, Juncadella M, et al. Electrical stimulation mapping of nouns and verbs in Broca's area. Brain Lang. 2015; 145–146:53–63

[24] Ojemann JG, Ojemann GA, Lettich E. Cortical stimulation mapping of language cortex by using a verb generation task: effects of learning and comparison to mapping based on object naming. J Neurosurg. 2002; 97(1):33–38

[25] Middlebrooks EH, Yagmurlu K, Szaflarski JP, Rahman M, Bozkurt B. A contemporary framework of language processing in the human brain in the context of preoperative and intraoperative language mapping. Neuroradiology. 2017; 59(1):69–87

[26] Papagno C, Miracapillo C, Casarotti A, et al. What is the role of the uncinate fasciculus? Surgical removal and proper name retrieval. Brain. 2011; 134(Pt 2):405–414

[27] Sierpowska J, Gabarrós A, Fernandez-Coello A, et al. Words are not enough: nonword repetition as an indicator of arcuate fasciculus integrity during brain tumor resection. J Neurosurg. 2017; 126(2):435–445

[28] Herbet G, Maheu M, Costi E, Lafargue G, Duffau H. Mapping neuroplastic potential in brain-damaged patients. Brain. 2016; 139(Pt 3):829–844

[29] Herbet G, Moritz-Gasser S, Boiseau M, Duvaux S, Cochereau J, Duffau H. Converging evidence for a cortico-subcortical network mediating lexical retrieval. Brain. 2016; 139(11):3007–3021

[30] Moritz-Gasser S, Herbet G, Duffau H. Mapping the connectivity underlying multimodal (verbal and non-verbal) semantic processing: a brain electrostimulation study. Neuropsychologia. 2013; 51(10):1814–1822

[31] Noll KR, Weinberg JS, Ziu M, Benveniste RJ, Suki D, Wefel JS. Neurocognitive changes associated with surgical resection of left and right temporal lobe glioma. Neurosurgery. 2015; 77(5):777–785

[32] Bernard F, Lemée JM, Ter Minassian A, Menei P. Right hemisphere cognitive functions: from clinical and anatomic bases to brain mapping during awake craniotomy part I: clinical and functional anatomy. World Neurosurg. 2018; 118:348–359

[33] Zacks JM. Neuroimaging studies of mental rotation: a meta-analysis and review. J Cogn Neurosci. 2008; 20(1):1–19

[34] Arsalidou M, Taylor MJ. Is 2+2=4? Meta-analyses of brain areas needed for numbers and calculations. Neuroimage. 2011; 54(3):2382–2393

[35] Lemée J-M, Bernard F, Ter Minassian A, Menei P. Right hemisphere cognitive functions: from clinical and anatomical bases to brain mapping during awake craniotomy part II: neuropsychological tasks and brain mapping. World Neurosurg. 2018; 118:360–367

[36] Herbet G, Lafargue G, Bonnetblanc F, Moritz-Gasser S, Duffau H. Is the right frontal cortex really crucial in the mentalizing network? A longitudinal study in patients with a slow-growing lesion. Cortex. 2013; 49(10):2711–2727

[37] Herbet G, Lafargue G, Bonnetblanc F, Moritz-Gasser S, Menjot de Champfleur N, Duffau H. Inferring a dual-stream model of mentalizing from associative white matter fibres disconnection. Brain. 2014; 137(Pt 3):944–959

[38] Miyake A, Friedman NP, Emerson MJ, Witzki AH, Howerter A, Wager TD. The unity and diversity of executive functions and their contributions to complex "frontal lobe" tasks: a latent variable analysis. Cognit Psychol. 2000; 41(1): 49–100

[39] Satoer D, Vork J, Visch-Brink E, Smits M, Dirven C, Vincent A. Cognitive functioning early after surgery of gliomas in eloquent areas. J Neurosurg. 2012; 117(5):831–838

[40] Johnson DR, Sawyer AM, Meyers CA, O'Neill BP, Wefel JS. Early measures of cognitive function predict survival in patients with newly diagnosed glioblastoma. Neuro-oncol. 2012; 14(6):808–816

[41] Acquaye AA, Vera-Bolanos E, Armstrong TS, Gilbert MR, Lin L. Mood disturbance in glioma patients. J Neurooncol. 2013; 113(3):505–512

[42] Gathinji M, McGirt MJ, Attenello FJ, et al. Association of preoperative depression and survival after resection of malignant brain astrocytoma. Surg Neurol. 2009; 71(3):299–303, discussion 303

[43] Litofsky NS, Farace E, Anderson F, Jr, Meyers CA, Huang W, Laws ER, Jr, Glioma Outcomes Project Investigators. Depression in patients with high-grade glioma: results of the Glioma Outcomes Project. Neurosurgery. 2004; 54(2): 358–366, discussion 366–367

[44] Duffau H, Taillandier L, Gatignol P, Capelle L. The insular lobe and brain plasticity: lessons from tumor surgery. Clin Neurol Neurosurg. 2006; 108(6):543–548

[45] Rostomily RC, Berger MS, Ojemann GA, Lettich E. Postoperative deficits and functional recovery following removal of tumors involving the dominant hemisphere supplementary motor area. J Neurosurg. 1991; 75(1):62–68

[46] Ferguson RJ, Ahles TA, Saykin AJ, et al. Cognitive-behavioral management of chemotherapy-related cognitive change. Psychooncology. 2007; 16(8):772–777

[47] Gehring K, Aaronson NK, Taphoorn MJ, Sitskoorn MM. Interventions for cognitive deficits in patients with a brain tumor: an update. Expert Rev Anticancer Ther. 2010; 10(11):1779–1795

[48] Boele FW, Douw L, de Groot M, et al. The effect of modafinil on fatigue, cognitive functioning, and mood in primary brain tumor patients: a multicenter randomized controlled trial. Neuro-oncol. 2013; 15(10):1420–1428

[49] Brown PD, Pugh S, Laack NN, et al. Radiation Therapy Oncology Group (RTOG). Memantine for the prevention of cognitive dysfunction in patients receiving whole-brain radiotherapy: a randomized, double-blind, placebo-controlled trial. Neuro-oncol. 2013; 15(10):1429–1437

[50] Day J, Zienius K, Gehring K, et al. Interventions for preventing and ameliorating cognitive deficits in adults treated with cranial irradiation. Cochrane Database Syst Rev. 2014(12):CD011335

Section II

Intraoperative Brain Mapping

9 Awake Craniotomy Operating Room Setup and Surgical Instruments

Karim ReFaey, Shashwat Tripathi, Sanjeet S. Grewal, Kaisorn L. Chaichana, and Alfredo Quinones-Hinojosa

Abstract

Awake craniotomy with direct cortical/subcortical stimulation facilitates the safe resection of the eloquent brain lesions such as motor, language cortical, and subcortical areas. Due to the complexity and the challenges during the awake craniotomies, the operating room setup and used instrumentations for awake craniotomy are slightly different from any other neurological brain surgery, which aims to allow for patient comfort, perform and visualize intraoperative without reducing the patient's ability to cooperate with their tasks.

Keywords: awake craniotomy, surgical instruments, operating room setup

9.1 Introduction

An awake craniotomy can facilitate more effective surgery especially when a lesion is located in eloquent brain regions such as the motor or language cortical and subcortical areas.[1,2,3,4,5,6,7,8,9,10,11,12,13,14,15,16,17,18,19,20,21,22,23,24,25,26,27,28,29,30,31,32,33,34,35,36,37,38,39,40,41] It has also been advocated for cortical and subcortical regions that were historically considered noneloquent, but now has been shown to be important for functions such as decision making and facial recognition. During surgery, patients are asked to perform tasks to map important functional regions in the brain. Effective mapping is paramount to maximizing resection while minimizing the risk of iatrogenic deficits.[12,13,14,18,20,21,22,23,24,25,42] In brain tumor cases through greater extent of resection (EOR), awake craniotomies can improve length of survival while maintaining or increasing quality of life for patients.[12,13,14,18,20,21,22,23,24,25,42] While brain stimulation is performed for functional mapping of cortical and subcortical structures, when combined with an awake craniotomy, surgeons are able to create a more thorough and accurate map of eloquent cortical and subcortical regions.[3,4,12,13,14,19,24,28,29,30]

Awake craniotomies vary slightly from normal neurosurgical cases. From a neuroanesthesia perspective, medications must be carefully titrated throughout the procedure to allow for patient comfort, without reducing the patient's ability to cooperate with their tasks. In terms of operating room (OR) setup, the patient must be positioned and draped correctly to perform and visualize intraoperative tasks. Finally, awake craniotomies require additional equipment, personnel, and supplies. The goal of this chapter is to review basic OR setup for awake craniotomies with brain mapping including patient positioning, intraoperative imaging, and neuronavigation.

9.2 Awake Craniotomy Operating Room Setup

Surgical efficiency can be improved through correct OR layout including positioning of the patient and anesthesia, navigation equipment, and critical and noncritical personnel (▶ Fig. 9.1). Most ORs have an operating table in the center of the OR that should be adjusted for correct patient positioning and for surgeon preference (see section "Patient Positioning" for more details).[39] Within the sterile field and opposite the door to the OR, there should be a Mayo stand and a back/scrub table (▶ Fig. 9.1). Due to its mobility, a Mayo stand provides increased accessibility to necessary equipment throughout the procedure. The height and location of the Mayo stand will be adjusted according to patient positioning and surgeon preference.

Direct visualization of the patient's face is required during the procedure. An unobstructed, preferably transparent tent is made with the sterile surgical drape to allow for the visualization of not only the patient's face but also the patient's arms and legs as needed for monitoring (▶ Fig. 9.1, ▶ Fig. 9.2). By creating the tent, it also minimizes the patient's potential for anxiety from claustrophobia. Consoles for surgical equipment such as mono- and bipolar coagulation units, drills, and suction containers and electrophysiological monitoring machines are located at the foot of the operating table to reduce wire tangling and obstruction of the sterile field.[39,43] The OR microscope and chair should be draped and positioned at the head of the operating table, ready for use when required. There should be multiple monitors placed throughout the OR for use by surgeons, OR personnel, and anesthesiologists; these can be used by nonsurgical staff, including students, for observation. During surgery, these allow the surgeon to view the patient's face and limbs and navigational imaging, which helps the surgeon to dynamically adjust the approach.[39,40,43]

In awake neurosurgical cases, primary surgeon, assistant surgeon, a scrub technician, a circulating nurse, anesthesiologist, and an examiner (preferably a qualified neurologist or neuropsychologist) are required. At academic centers, a neurosurgery resident, an anesthesia resident, certified registered nurse anesthetist (CRNA), and/or medical and undergraduate students are generally available in the OR. Additionally, an electrophysiological technician may be present when neurophysiological monitoring is required. Given the ease with which the OR can become crowded, an optimal OR setup is necessary to maintain the flow and efficiency during the operation. It is also important to keep the number of personnel and the noise level to a minimum as the patient is awake, and the surgeon must be able to hear and examine the patient carefully at all times.

The lead surgeon will be at the head of the OR table with the scrub technician on the patient side within arm's reach of the Mayo stand, back/scrub table, and the surgeon and typically opposite to the side of the patient being evaluated (▶ Fig. 9.1). The anesthesiologist will be positioned on the contralateral side from the site of surgery and near the head and chest area of the patient. This allows for access to all anesthesia equipment, the endotracheal tube, and the intravenous/intra-arterial lines. The anesthesia machines should be placed close to the head of the OR table (▶ Fig. 9.1). The examiner (neurologist or neuropsychologist) will be positioned in front of the patient with a

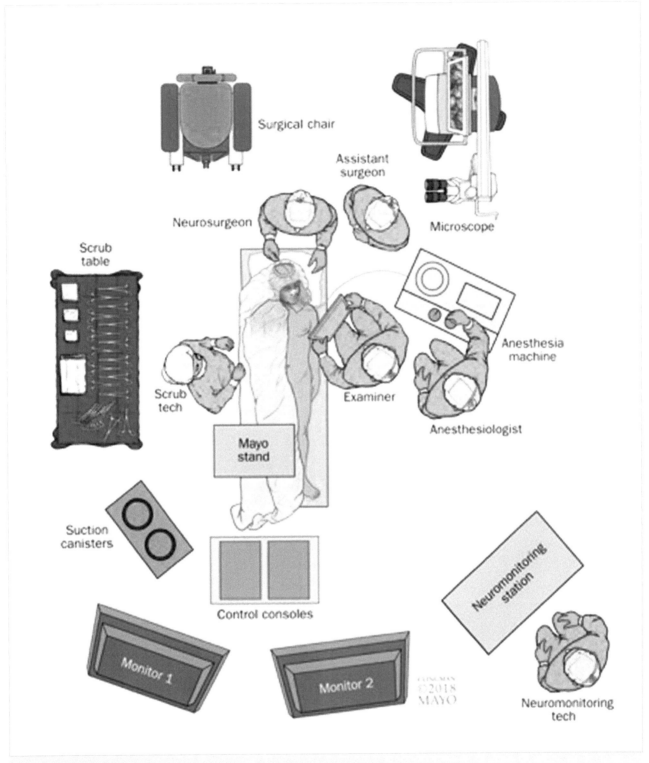

Fig. 9.1 Operating room setup.

clear view of the face, arm, and legs. To ensure a proper place for the examiner, all monitoring machines should be placed far away from the patient (▶ Fig. 9.1).

It should be noted that an alternative is to position the patient 180 degrees away from the anesthesia machine. This setup has been preferred by several surgeons, as it increases the working space around the patient's head. However, the disadvantage is that the patient's airway is further away from the anesthesia machine, which can make it difficult to access during emergency situations.

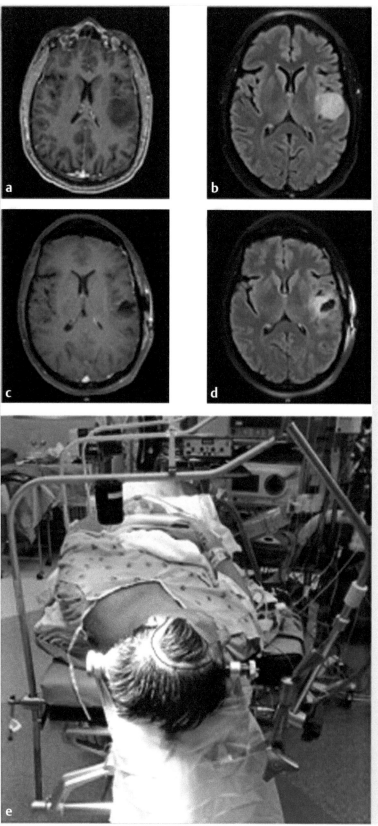

Fig. 9.2 Example of an awake mapping case and setup. **(a)** Axial T1-weighted MRI with contrast showing left-sided hypointense lesion in the left frontal lobe. **(b)** Axial T2 FLAIR MRI showing left-sided hyperintense lesion in the frontal lobe. **(c–d)** Postoperative axial T1-weighted MRI with contrast and T2 FLAIR, respectively, showing the extent of resection of the left-sided frontal lesion. **(e)** Showing patient in the supine position with skin incision marked and prepped.

9.3 Awake Anesthesia

There are two main anesthetic techniques for awake craniotomies: monitored anesthesia care (MAC) and "asleep, awake, asleep" (AAA).[7,15,16,17,26,27] During MAC, the patient is kept in a state of conscious sedation.[7] The AAA method, on the other hand, uses a partial or fully protected airway often with a laryngeal mask airway (LMA).[7,15,16,17,26,27] There is a paucity of literature and class I data highlighting the superiority of either technique over the other.

At our institution, patients receive a complete scalp block to the bilateral supraorbital, pre- and postauricular, and lesser and greater occipital nerves, as well as supplementation to the pin sites with lidocaine and/or bupivacaine in the preoperative holding area. An alternative for more precision is to use high-frequency ultrasound to identify the nerves for blocking. Intravenous anesthetics should be chosen with the following criteria: short acting, fast onset and offset, amnesia and adequate pain management, and easy to titrate.[7] The decision for pursuing either anesthetic technique should be taken to determine the anesthetic phases and agents before and after cortical mapping. Supporters of the AAA technique advocate that the first phase should include general anesthesia with LMA for positive ventilation, due to low risk of hypertension and/or excessive use of sedation.[44,45] In this phase, the combination of remifentanil and propofol is preferred as it provides adequate ventilation and rapid transition to awakening. MAC technique, on the other hand, aims to utilize a combination of rapid-onset and short-acting sedative analgesics with high therapeutic index and low risk for cardiorespiratory depression.[46] Several sedative agents have been used for the MAC technique, such as droperidol/alfentanil,[47] propofol-fentanyl,[48] propofol-remifentanil,[49] and dexmedetomidine.[50,51,52] The anticipated surgical duration plays a crucial role in the selection of the technique of choice. In a previous study by Lobo et al,[46] it was suggested that AAA technique should be used in surgeries with durations exceeding 4 hours, as patients tend to cooperate better in longer surgeries by minimizing their awake time. The type of anesthesia technique also depends on the type of mapping being done. For more intricate mapping including phonetics, semantics, and nonverbal semantics, AAA technique is preferred because patient fatigue can interfere with precise examination. The MAC technique can be done when less precise mapping is needed, such as when language output and motor/somatosensory function are being mapped. Regardless, Eseonu et al documented that there was no difference between MAC and AAA techniques as both provide safe and efficient anesthetic techniques.[7]

Awake craniotomy has gained popularity for the neurosurgical treatment for gliomas and epilepsy and tends to be very well tolerated.[16] However, anxiety is a commonly associated response to any surgical intervention,[53] but the concept of being consciously awake during brain surgery in particular can be fraught with a range of fear and anxieties.[54,55] Sounds and scenes from the OR are known as stressors for patients, which can be the leading cause of anxiety.[56] Literature has revealed that there is a consistent relation between intraoperative surgical anxieties and postoperative pain,[57,58] which leads to increase in analgesic needs[59] and delayed recovery.[60] A previous study by Legrain et al[61] hypothesized that pain perception could be interrupted by applying attention-grapping stimuli for distraction. Thus, the utilization of music,[62] comforting words,[63] audiovisual stimuli, and touch has shown to be effective in the reduction of pain and anxiety before and during the surgical procedure. Therefore, our surgical team is partnering with the Mayo Clinic Robert D. and Patricia E. Kern Center for the Science of Health Care Delivery to conduct several studies exploring the role of music in improving patient experience in the OR during awake craniotomies.

9.4 Microscope Setup

During the intradural portion of the craniotomy, the surgeon may need to use an operating microscope. The microscope has several surgical benefits including greater visualization of important structures, increased illumination of deeper brain regions, better ability to differentiate lesional tissue from nonlesional tissue, and improved accuracy of coagulation, thus preserving surrounding neural and vascular structures.[38,39,43,64,65,66] However, the microscope also decreases the surgeon's awareness of surrounding structures outside the microscope's view and can potentially limit the ability for the assistant surgeon to help with the case.

Owing to high sensitivity and magnification, the operating microscope must be balanced before every case. The correct lens, eyepiece, mouthpiece, lighting, and zoom speed must be adjusted based on craniotomy location and surgeon preference (▶ Fig. 9.1). For educational and research purposes, video-recording equipment can be activated on the microscope. If intraoperative imaging and navigation is available, the microscope should be synced with the stereotactic neuronavigation.[19,24,38,39,40,43,64] This will provide the surgeon a reconstructed image on the focal point of the surgeon's microscopic view to assist with surgical planning. A foot panel, placed under the surgeon's left or right foot on the floor stand, can be used to control the angle, focus, and zoom of the microscope so that the surgeon can keep his or her hands in the surgical field.

The observer's eyepiece varies with the location of the craniotomy. For intracranial cases, the observer's eyepiece will typically be positioned on the opposite side as the surgical technician. The position of the eyepiece must not obstruct the coordination between the surgeon and the scrub technician; the surgical tech and surgical and anesthesia equipment must be considered when positioning the observer's eyepiece.

Given the duration of certain cranial operations, a microscope chair will help prevent surgeon fatigue. The chair must be properly draped prior to use to ensure sterility is maintained. Loose-fitting sterile drapes should be placed around the microscope and microscope chair. Constrictive draping will limit the range of motion and prevent utilization of the mouthpiece.[38,39] The operating chair moves in either the horizontal or vertical direction and should be locked into place to prevent movement. The height and armrests of the chair must be adjusted correctly for the surgeon. The microscope foot pedal and bipolar coagulation pedal should be placed on the floor stand attached to the chair. The microscope controller is typically placed on the surgeon's left foot, whereas the coagulation controller is placed on the surgeon's right foot.

To increase ease of microscope positioning, a mouthpiece attachment allows hands-free control of the microscope, where the surgeon can reposition the microscope using only his or her mouth to reduce unnecessary hand movements.[38,39] After preoperatively balancing the microscope, the mouthpiece should be adjusted to the surgeon's face. The surgeon's top teeth should be placed on the adjustment mouth plate and while biting down, the surgeon must ensure that he or she does not lose line of sight.[38,39] The surgeon can now move the microscope with his or her teeth by biting down on the mouth switch. The microscope can move in either the horizontal or vertical direction. The microscope should be moved into position and then the surgeon can adjust the position using the mouthpiece to maximize his or her comfort as well as visualization.

9.5 Patient Positioning

For awake craniotomies, patients are positioned in one of the two ways: supine or direct lateral. Importantly, for frontal, anterior parietal, or cranial base neoplasms, the supine positioning should be utilized; for occipital or posterior parietal, the direct lateral positioning should be utilized.[41,43] Attention should be taken while positioning the head to ensure that the airway is secured, and the patient's face can be seen by the neurologist/neuropsychologist on the screen monitor (**Video 9.1**, **Video 9.2**). Awake craniotomies are rarely done for infratentorial tumors, and therefore not discussed here.

9.6 Head Fixation

Proper head fixation helps maximize access to the surgical site. A three-pin skull clamp should be positioned at the equator of the skull. To decrease risk of infection, antibiotic ointment should be placed on each pin prior to insertion in the skull. Most importantly, the pin should not impede the surgical field or view of the face, or be inserted into thin bone, frontal sinus, any prior shunts, mastoid sinus, cranial defects, and/or thick temporalis muscle.[41,43] Pinning of any of these structures can result in unsecure positioning, as well as potential epidural hematoma.

Clamp use and tension varies between adult and pediatric cases. Tension on the clamp should be around 60 lb in adults and lesser pressures for pediatric patients.[43]

9.7 General Craniotomy Techniques

For operative planning, the patient's hair is minimally shaved using electric clippers around the desired incision site. The incision should be continuous and placed behind the hairline, avoiding any relevant vascular supply of the scalp. Intersecting incision lines should be avoided as they lead to poor wound healing. For preoperative planning, the previously placed incision is preferably used and extended if necessary. The ear is plugged with Xeroform gauze (Covidien) to prevent fluid accumulation in the external auditory canal during wound sterilization but must be removed during the awake position so that the patient's hearing is not impeded. The surgical site is sterilized using povidone iodine scrub for 5 minutes and dried with sterile towels; Chloraprep is used in patients who are allergic to iodine.

A marking pen is used to mark the planned surgical incision, with prep applied to the desired surgical field and left to dry. After the surgeon is scrubbed in, a timeout should be performed with neurosurgeon, neuroanesthesiologist, and nursing staff to validate the patient's information and correct procedure title and site, preoperatively administered medications, and allergies. Before skin incision, the surgical site is injected with local anesthetics preferably lidocaine with epinephrine for both pain and hemostasis. Surgical incision should be performed using a scalpel and monopolar cauterization. Depending on surgeon's preference, scalp clips can be used to achieve scalp hemostasis. Care should be taken around superficial temporal artery to avoid compromising the vascular supply.

A scalpel or monopolar cautery in the cutting setting is used to cut the fascial layer. The underlying temporalis muscle should be dissected bluntly from the skull to preserve the vascular blood supply. The muscle and skin flap are retracted using fishhooks or self-retraining retractors. The muscle can also be anesthetized with local anesthetics to help with patient comfort. In addition, a rolled-up gauze should be placed under the flap to prevent vascular kinking and patient discomfort due to pressure on the eye.

Burr holes can be made with a perforator drill bit and connected using a footplate craniotomy. The bone flap is then removed to achieve the craniotomy. It is important to leave the dura intact especially in the AAA, as it may lead to brain herniation by the dural defects in patients who wake up combative. Prior to waking the patient up, cauterizing dural bleeding, and opening the dura, the dura is anesthetized with a local anesthetic between the two leaves of dura on both sides of the meningeal artery branches to minimize dural-related pain. The dural incision can be made using a no. 15 blade and fine-toothed forceps. The dural flap is then made with fine scissors to expose the lesion. A dural cuff approximately 0.5 cm near the bone edges should be left for closure. The flap can be made in a cruciate or semicircular fashion depending on the surgeon's preference.

Once the desired cortex is exposed, the surgeon proceeds with cortical brain stimulation using the Ojemann Stimulator (Integra Lifesciences), Nicolet Cortical Stimulator (Natus Medical Incorporation), or other bipolar stimulators depending on his or her preference. Stimulation endpoints are considered when maximal stimulation is reached without functional response and/or identification of intraoperative after discharges on the electrocorticography. Intraoperative cortical stimulation during brain mapping may lead to induced seizures which are treated using cold-water irrigation when not self-limited and intravenous administration of antiepileptic agents if necessary. In cases of persistent seizure activity despite cold-water irrigation and administration of drugs, longer acting medications such as benzodiazepines or barbiturates may be given with the understanding that brain stimulation will no longer be effective in mapping eloquence.

Once resection is completed or the desired areas disconnected, the patient can be put back to sleep. Hemostasis can be achieved using saline irrigation, Gelfoam, and/or oxidized cellulose polymer. The dura is then closed in a watertight fashion with 4–0 Nurolon interrupted or running sutures (Ethicon). Dural defects can be repaired using muscle, pericranial fascia, or synthetic dural graft. For prevention of cerebrospinal fluid leakage, DuraSeal (Integra) or fibrin sealant can also be used. The bone flap is put back in place and secured with titanium plates and miniscrews. The muscle and fascia are closed with sutures. The skin can be closed using either staples or sutures. The surgery for various brain lesions will be discussed in other chapters.

9.8 Operative Modifications for Specialized Cases

Based on surgeon's preference, pathology, tumor location, and patient's comorbidities, specialized procedures may be performed using different instruments. First, a craniotomy set including drill, microinstrument set, and the basic neurosurgical soft tissue set should be available. Monopolar and bipolar cauteries are used in all cases and should be set up as mentioned earlier. For tumor cases, frameless stereotactic instruments, craniotomy drape, cranial titanium plates, biopsy forceps, cottonoids, cotton balls, bone wax, and hemostatic agents may be utilized. Should the tumor involve the cranial nerves or the brainstem, microdissectors, hooks, microscissors, arachnoid knives, and a nerve stimulator can also be used to preserve the delicate structures. Postresection, synthetic dural grafts for dural closure when pericranium is not available may be placed.

9.9 Imaging

9.9.1 Neuronavigation

Neuronavigation allows surgeons to increase EOR by guiding the surgeon to the lesion and evaluating EOR. A computer detection system (normally light-emitting diodes) tracks the location of a registered pointer and projects it onto a monitor with the desired pre- or intraoperative images.[19,24,28,29,30,31,40,43,67,68] The surgeon can use the pointer to correlate the surgical field with images on the screen, allowing the surgeon to plan approaches and identify internal landmarks.[9,19,24,28,29,30,31,40,43,67,68] The common sequences that are utilized include T1-weighted images with contrast for contrast-enhancing lesions and/or T2-weighted images for low-grade lesions that do not enhance with contrast. T2 images allow the surgeon to see the extent of edema caused by the lesion(s) and better identify sulcal anatomy.[31,40,68] Oftentimes, the T2 provides better visualization of the brain anatomy including the sulcus and cranial nerves. It should be noted that neuronavigation can be prone to errors particularly with increasing brain shifts during and throughout the course of surgery.

9.9.2 Intraoperative Ultrasound

Recent improvements in image quality and reduction of hand-piece sizes have allowed the use of intraoperative ultrasound (IoUS). Advantages of IoUS include dynamic, real-time visualization of the parenchyma and detection of lesions.[9,10,28,29,30,31,40,43,68,69] Further integration of IoUS with navigation systems and 3D US have increased the applicability of IoUS.[9,10,69] These systems are, however, limited due to unfamiliarity with techniques and a perceived difficulty to differentiate tissue except through differences in density.

9.9.3 Intraoperative Computed Tomography/Magnetic Resonance Imaging

Intraoperative imaging provides dynamic and pertinent information during surgery. The imaging systems are normally located in a room attached to the OR, and a roof-mounted rail system is used to bring the imager into the OR.[70] Intraoperative MRIs (iMRI) help determine EOR and monitor possible complications.[19,28,29,30,31,40,68,70,71] Moreover, the navigational system can be updated to account for brain shifts. Due to low image quality and radiation exposure, the current CTs remain inferior to MRIs. Despite the limitations of CTs, modern OR suites often have mounted-CT systems, similar to the MRIs. Additional preoperative planning is required in cases with intraoperative imaging, as the patient must be positioned correctly to fit into the scanner and the site of interest must be exposed to the scanner. Of note, surgeons should not rely on imaging, as it is often inaccurate due to various intraoperative changes (brain shift).[9,28,29,30,31,68]

9.10 Conclusion

Preoperative OR setup is paramount to maximizing efficiency and outcomes during awake surgery. For awake craniotomies, anesthesia must be adjusted to ensure relaxed and cooperative patients. Personnel should ensure all required equipment is available prior to surgery. The surgical microscope should be draped and ready for use when required. Patient positioning should account for tumor location, surgeon preference, and intraoperative imaging. Neuronavigation and intraoperative imaging help surgeons better visualize internal landmarks, monitor possible complications, and determine EOR; however, surgeons must be aware of possible intraoperational changes (i.e., brain shift). Awake craniotomies for tumors and seizure foci can help increase EOR while limiting the risk of loss of function, and thus should be used when tumors are located in cortical and subcortical eloquent areas.

References

[1] Madriz-Godoy MM, Trejo-Gallegos SA. Anaesthetic technique during awake craniotomy. Case report and literature review. Rev Med Hosp Gen (Mex). 2016; 79(3):155–160

[2] July J, Manninen P, Lai J, Yao Z, Bernstein M. The history of awake craniotomy for brain tumor and its spread into Asia. Surg Neurol. 2009; 71(5):621–624, discussion 624–625

[3] Duffau H. Acute functional reorganisation of the human motor cortex during resection of central lesions: a study using intraoperative brain mapping. J Neurol Neurosurg Psychiatry. 2001; 70(4):506–513

[4] Szelényi A, Bello L, Duffau H, et al. Workgroup for Intraoperative Management in Low-Grade Glioma Surgery within the European Low-Grade Glioma Network. Intraoperative electrical stimulation in awake craniotomy: methodological aspects of current practice. Neurosurg Focus. 2010; 28(2):E7

[5] Penfield P. Combined regional and general anesthesia for craniotomy and cortical exploration. Part I. Neurosurgical considerations. Int Anesthesiol Clin. 1986; 24(3):1–11

[6] Bulsara KR, Johnson J, Villavicencio AT. Improvements in brain tumor surgery: the modern history of awake craniotomies. Neurosurg Focus. 2005; 18 (4):e5

[7] Eseonu CI, ReFaey K, Garcia O, John A, Quiñones-Hinojosa A, Tripathi P. Awake craniotomy anesthesia: a comparison of the monitored anesthesia care and asleep-awake-asleep techniques. World Neurosurg. 2017; 104:679–686

[8] Nimsky C, Ganslandt O, Cerny S, Hastreiter P, Greiner G, Fahlbusch R. Quantification of, visualization of, and compensation for brain shift using intraoperative magnetic resonance imaging. Neurosurgery. 2000; 47(5):1070–1079, discussion 1079–1080

[9] Koivukangas J, Louhisalmi Y, Alakuijala J, Oikarinen J. Ultrasound-controlled neuronavigator-guided brain surgery. J Neurosurg. 1993; 79(1):36–42

[10] Unsgaard G, Rygh OM, Selbekk T, et al. Intra-operative 3D ultrasound in neurosurgery. Acta Neurochir (Wien). 2006; 148(3):235–253, discussion 253

[11] Tronnier VM, Wirtz CR, Knauth M, et al. Intraoperative diagnostic and interventional magnetic resonance imaging in neurosurgery. Neurosurgery. 1997; 40(5):891–900, discussion 900–902

[12] Boetto J, Bertram L, Moulinié G, Herbet G, Moritz-Gasser S, Duffau H. Electrocorticography is not necessary during awake brain surgery for gliomas. World Neurosurg. 2016; 91:656–657

[13] Chan-Seng E, Moritz-Gasser S, Duffau H. Awake mapping for low-grade gliomas involving the left sagittal stratum: anatomofunctional and surgical considerations. J Neurosurg. 2014; 120(5):1069–1077

[14] De Benedictis A, Moritz-Gasser S, Duffau H. Awake mapping optimizes the extent of resection for low-grade gliomas in eloquent areas. Neurosurgery. 2010; 66(6):1074–1084, discussion 1084

[15] Deras P, Moulinié G, Maldonado IL, Moritz-Gasser S, Duffau H, Bertram L. Intermittent general anesthesia with controlled ventilation for asleep-awake-asleep brain surgery: a prospective series of 140 gliomas in eloquent areas. Neurosurgery. 2012; 71(4):764–771

[16] Beez T, Boge K, Wager M, et al. European Low Grade Glioma Network. Tolerance of awake surgery for glioma: a prospective European Low Grade Glioma Network multicenter study. Acta Neurochir (Wien). 2013; 155(7):1301–1308

[17] Duffau H. The usefulness of the asleep-awake-asleep glioma surgery. Acta Neurochir (Wien). 2014; 156(8):1493–1494

[18] Duffau H. Indications of awake mapping and selection of intraoperative tasks. In; Duffau H. Brain Mapping. Vienna: Springer; 2011:321–334

[19] Berger MS. Minimalism through intraoperative functional mapping. Clin Neurosurg. 1996; 43:324–337

[20] Hervey-Jumper SL, Berger MS. Maximizing safe resection of low- and high-grade glioma. J Neurooncol. 2016; 130(2):269–282

[21] Hervey-Jumper SL, Berger MS. Technical nuances of awake brain tumor surgery and the role of maximum safe resection. J Neurosurg Sci. 2015; 59(4):351–360

[22] Hervey-Jumper SL, Li J, Lau D, et al. Awake craniotomy to maximize glioma resection: methods and technical nuances over a 27-year period. J Neurosurg. 2015; 123(2):325–339

[23] Lau D, Hervey-Jumper SL, Han SJ, Berger MS. Intraoperative perception and estimates on extent of resection during awake glioma surgery: overcoming the learning curve. J Neurosurg. 2018; 128(5):1410–1418

[24] Krieg SM, Tarapore PE, Picht T, et al. Optimal timing of pulse onset for language mapping with navigated repetitive transcranial magnetic stimulation. Neuroimage. 2014; 100:219–236

[25] Magill ST, Han SJ, Li J, Berger MS. Resection of primary motor cortex tumors: feasibility and surgical outcomes. J Neurosurg. 2018; 129(4):961–972

[26] Meng L, McDonagh DL, Berger MS, Gelb AW. Anesthesia for awake craniotomy: a how-to guide for the occasional practitioner. Can J Anaesth. 2017; 64 (5):517–529

[27] Meng L, Berger MS, Gelb AW. The potential benefits of awake craniotomy for brain tumor resection: an anesthesiologist's perspective. J Neurosurg Anesthesiol. 2015; 27(4):310–317

[28] Quiñones-Hinojosa A, Ojemann SG, Sanai N, Dillon WP, Berger MS. Preoperative correlation of intraoperative cortical mapping with magnetic resonance imaging landmarks to predict localization of the Broca area. J Neurosurg. 2003; 99(2):311–318

[29] Racine CA, Li J, Molinaro AM, Butowski N, Berger MS. Neurocognitive function in newly diagnosed low-grade glioma patients undergoing surgical resection with awake mapping techniques. Neurosurgery. 2015; 77(3):371–379, discussion 379

[30] Sanai N, Berger MS. Operative techniques for gliomas and the value of extent of resection. Neurotherapeutics. 2009; 6(3):478–486

[31] Southwell DG, Hervey-Jumper SL, Perry DW, Berger MS. Intraoperative mapping during repeat awake craniotomy reveals the functional plasticity of adult cortex. J Neurosurg. 2016; 124(5):1460–1469

[32] Benzagmout M, Gatignol P, Duffau H. Resection of World Health Organization Grade II gliomas involving Broca's area: methodological and functional considerations. Neurosurgery. 2007; 61(4):741–752, discussion 752–753

[33] Boetto J, Bertram L, Moulinié G, Herbet G, Moritz-Gasser S, Duffau H. Low rate of intraoperative seizures during awake craniotomy in a prospective cohort with 374 supratentorial brain lesions: electrocorticography is not mandatory. World Neurosurg. 2015; 84(6):1838–1844

[34] Boissonneau S, Duffau H. Identifying clinical risk in low grade gliomas and appropriate treatment strategies, with special emphasis on the role of surgery. Expert Rev Anticancer Ther. 2017; 17(8):703–716

[35] Surbeck W, Hildebrandt G, Duffau H. The evolution of brain surgery on awake patients. Acta Neurochir (Wien). 2015; 157(1):77–84

[36] Blazier C. Operating room requirements for neurosurgical procedures. Oper Techn Neurosurg. 1998; 1(1):2–13

[37] Connolly ES. Fundamentals of Operative Techniques in Neurosurgery. 2nd ed. New York: Thieme; 2010

[38] Holly EH. Mouth guide for operating microscope. Technical note. J Neurosurg. 1976; 44(5):642–643

[39] Kobayashi S, Sugita K, Matsuo K. An improved neurosurgical system: new operating table, chair, microscope and other instrumentation. Neurosurg Rev. 1984; 7(2–3):75–80

[40] Nabavi A, Stark AM, Dörner L, Mehdorn HM. Surgical navigation with intraoperative imaging: special operating room concepts. In: Quiñones-Hinojosa A, ed. Schmidek & Sweet: Operative Neurosurgical Techniques: Indications, Methods and Results. 6th ed. Philadelphia, PA: Saunders, Elsevier Inc.; 2012:12–20

[41] Rozet I, Vavilala MS. Risks and benefits of patient positioning during neurosurgical care. Anesthesiol Clin. 2007; 25(3):631–653, x

[42] Bloch O, Han SJ, Cha S, et al. Impact of extent of resection for recurrent glioblastoma on overall survival: clinical article. J Neurosurg. 2012; 117(6):1032–1038

[43] Eseonu CI, Rincon-Torroella J, Refaey K, Quiñones-Hinojosa A. Operating Room Requirements for Brain Tumor Surgery. Video Atlas of Neurosurgery: Contemporary Tumor and Skull Base Surgery. Cortical/Subcortical Motor Mapping for Gliomas. Vol. 1. Philadelphia, PA: Elsevier; 2016

[44] Sarang A, Dinsmore J. Anaesthesia for awake craniotomy–evolution of a technique that facilitates awake neurological testing. Br J Anaesth. 2003; 90(2): 161–165

[45] Deras P, Moulinié G, Maldonado IL, Moritz-Gasser S, Duffau H, Bertram L. Intermittent general anesthesia with controlled ventilation for asleep-awake-asleep brain surgery: a prospective series of 140 gliomas in eloquent areas. Neurosurgery. 2012; 71(4):764–771

[46] Lobo FA, Wagemakers M, Absalom AR. Anaesthesia for awake craniotomy. Br J Anaesth. 2016; 116(6):740–744

[47] Welling EC, Donegan J. Neuroleptanalgesia using alfentanil for awake craniotomy. Anesth Analg. 1989; 68(1):57–60

[48] Sinha PK, Koshy T, Gayatri P, Smitha M, Abraham M, Rathod RC. Anesthesia for awake craniotomy: a retrospective study. Neurol India. 2007; 55(4):376–381

[49] Lobo F, Beiras A. Propofol and remifentanil effect-site concentrations estimated by pharmacokinetic simulation and bispectral index monitoring during craniotomy with intraoperative awakening for brain tumor resection. J Neurosurg Anesthesiol. 2007; 19(3):183–189

[50] Ard JL, Jr, Bekker AY, Doyle WK. Dexmedetomidine in awake craniotomy: a technical note. Surg Neurol. 2005; 63(2):114–116, discussion 116–117

[51] Rozet I. Anesthesia for functional neurosurgery: the role of dexmedetomidine. Curr Opin Anaesthesiol. 2008; 21(5):537–543

[52] Garavaglia MM, Das S, Cusimano MD, et al. Anesthetic approach to high-risk patients and prolonged awake craniotomy using dexmedetomidine and scalp block. J Neurosurg Anesthesiol. 2014; 26(3):226–233

[53] Hudson BF, Ogden J, Whiteley MS. Randomized controlled trial to compare the effect of simple distraction interventions on pain and anxiety experienced during conscious surgery. Eur J Pain. 2015; 19(10):1447–1455

[54] Mitchell M. Patient anxiety and modern elective surgery: a literature review. J Clin Nurs. 2003; 12(1):806–815

[55] Wetsch WA, Pircher I, Lederer W, et al. Preoperative stress and anxiety in day-care patients and inpatients undergoing fast-track surgery. Br J Anaesth. 2009; 103(2):199–205

[56] Mitchell M. Conscious surgery: influence of the environment on patient anxiety. J Adv Nurs. 2008; 64(3):261–271

[57] Carr EC, Nicky Thomas V, Wilson-Barnet J. Patient experiences of anxiety, depression and acute pain after surgery: a longitudinal perspective. Int J Nurs Stud. 2005; 42(5):521–530

[58] Ip HY, Abrishami A, Peng PW, Wong J, Chung F. Predictors of postoperative pain and analgesic consumption: a qualitative systematic review. Anesthesiology. 2009; 111(3):657–677

[59] Powell R, Johnston M, Smith WC, et al. Psychological risk factors for chronic post-surgical pain after inguinal hernia repair surgery: a prospective cohort study. Eur J Pain. 2012; 16(4):600–610

[60] Mavros MN, Athanasiou S, Gkegkes ID, Polyzos KA, Peppas G, Falagas ME. Do psychological variables affect early surgical recovery? PLoS One. 2011; 6(5): e20306

[61] Legrain V, Crombez G, Verhoeven K, Mouraux A. The role of working memory in the attentional control of pain. Pain. 2011; 152(2):453–459

[62] Bradt J, Dileo C, Shim M. Music interventions for preoperative anxiety. Cochrane Database Syst Rev. 2013(6):CD006908

[63] Shenefelt PD. Anxiety reduction using hypnotic induction and self-guided imagery for relaxation during dermatologic procedures. Int J Clin Exp Hypn. 2013; 61(3):305–318

[64] Thind H, Hardesty DA, Zabramski JM, Spetzler RF, Nakaji P. The role of microscope-integrated near-infrared indocyanine green videoangiography in the surgical treatment of intracranial dural arteriovenous fistulas. J Neurosurg. 2015; 122(4):876–882

[65] Hanel RA, Nakaji P, Spetzler RF. Use of microscope-integrated near-infrared indocyanine green videoangiography in the surgical treatment of spinal dural arteriovenous fistulae. Neurosurgery. 2010; 66(5):978–984, discussion 984–985

[66] Killory BD, Nakaji P, Gonzales LF, Ponce FA, Wait SD, Spetzler RF. Prospective evaluation of surgical microscope-integrated intraoperative near-infrared indocyanine green angiography during cerebral arteriovenous malformation surgery. Neurosurgery. 2009; 65(3):456–462, discussion 462

[67] Golfinos JG, Fitzpatrick BC, Smith LR, Spetzler RF. Clinical use of a frameless stereotactic arm: results of 325 cases. J Neurosurg. 1995; 83(2):197–205

[68] Southwell DG, Birk HS, Han SJ, Li J, Sall JW, Berger MS. Resection of gliomas deemed inoperable by neurosurgeons based on preoperative imaging studies. J Neurosurg. 2018; 129(3):567–575

[69] Ellegala DB, Leong-Poi H, Carpenter JE, et al. Imaging tumor angiogenesis with contrast ultrasound and microbubbles targeted to alpha(v)beta3. Circulation. 2003; 108(3):336–341

[70] Black PM, Moriarty T, Alexander E, III, et al. Development and implementation of intraoperative magnetic resonance imaging and its neurosurgical applications. Neurosurgery. 1997; 41(4):831–842, discussion 842–845

[71] Jolesz FA. 1996 RSNA Eugene P. Pendergrass New Horizons Lecture. Image-guided procedures and the operating room of the future. Radiology. 1997; 204(3):601–612

10 Anesthetic Considerations for Intraoperative Cerebral Brain Mapping

Elird Bojaxhi and Perry Bechtle

Abstract

Intraoperative mapping is often supplemented by the following techniques: electrocorticography, which helps identify epileptogenic foci; direct electrical stimulation, which directly stimulates the cortex and helps identify regions responsible for motor, language, vision, or sensation; microelectrode recordings, which identify deep brain structures for placement of deep brain stimulators; and neurocognitive testing which requires the patient to be fully awake and able to participate. The integrity of these neurophysiological evaluations is heavily dependent on the anesthetic choice and technique as all anesthetics alter neuronal activity. With the concomitant goals of providing adequate perioperative conditions for surgical exposure, accurate neurophysiological evaluation, and patient comfort and safety, the pharmacology of an anesthetic agent needs careful consideration. Differentiated by use of different anesthetic agents and airway management, the commonly utilized anesthetic techniques have been broadly defined as general anesthesia ("asleep"), regional anesthesia ("awake"), or combined techniques. It is important to note that there is no ideal anesthetic or technique, as each approach has distinct advantages and disadvantages described primarily through case series due to a lack of randomized control trials on this topic. With various patient needs, risks, and comorbidities, different anesthetic guidelines for intraoperative brain mapping exist in clinical practice, but each technique abides by certain basic principles.

Keywords: scalp block, craniotomies, regional anesthesia, cerebral mapping, total intravenous anesthesia, intraoperative complications

10.1 Pharmacology of Common Anesthetic Agents and Cerebral Mapping

10.1.1 Inhaled Anesthetics

Inhaled volatile anesthetics (sevoflurane, desflurane, and isoflurane) are the most commonly used maintenance agents for general anesthesia (GA) due to their ease of delivery and reliable, dose-dependent amnesia, hypnosis, and akinesia.[1] Volatile anesthetics have no single site of activity and are agents of mass action and globally depress activity in the brain and spinal cord. The primary hypnotic effect involves gamma-aminobutyric acid (GABA) type A receptors; however, there are many other sites of action such as ion channels, nicotinic, serotonin type 3, glycerin, and glutamate receptors.[2] These agents hinder brain-mapping techniques in a dose-dependent fashion either by depressing epileptogenic foci or hindering their locations by paradoxical neuroexcitatory properties. At high concentrations, sevoflurane

can cause burst suppression and reduce electrocorticography (ECoG) spike activity.[3] However, seizure-like activity and electroencephalography (EEG)-recorded seizures have been described with volatile anesthetics, and they are thought to be due to excitatory neuronal foci stimulated by the global inhibition of the central nervous system.[4] Despite this finding, in general, this neuronal stimulation is unreliable when seeking to identify ECoG spike activity during epileptic surgery.[5] For these reasons, although some authors will describe the use of volatile anesthetics as a way to potentially stimulate epileptogenic foci during ECoG while under GA, it is most common to limit these agents to 0.5 MAC with higher doses of opioids as an adjunct to the anesthetic, as the effect on ECoG recording is negligible.[6]

Similarly, nitrous oxide has also been used in the neurosurgical population and has been shown to attenuate the frequency of spike in epileptic patients,[7] but is thought to not interfere with ECoG when combined with high doses of opioids alone.[6] Nitrous oxide is significantly less potent when compared to volatile anesthetics during GA and has several limitations, such as expansion of gas-filled spaces (i.e., potential for pneumocephalus[8]) and diffusion hypoxia.[9] Nitrous oxide/opioid technique can be associated with a higher risk of nausea and vomiting, which has resulted in its decreased popularity over the years and replacement with intravenous (IV) anesthetic techniques.

The neuroinhibitory effects of vapor anesthetics can also significantly hinder cerebral mapping using direct electrical stimulation (DES) of the motor cortex. As inhaled anesthetics are used only under GA with a secured airway, DES is the only type of cortical mapping that can be performed in this setting, typically with an observer looking for motor movement in the face and extremities. Moreover, even low concentrations of inhaled anesthetic of 0.5 MAC can result in inadequate or failed mapping.[10,11] Because of these reasons, vapor anesthetics are often replaced by IV anesthetic agents in cases where motor evoked potentials are used intraoperatively, and it is thought to be due to less interference of alpha motor neurons from IV agents.[12]

10.1.2 Intravenous Hypnotic and Analgesic Agents

Intravenous anesthetic agents (propofol, dexmedetomidine, ketamine, remifentanil, and sufentanil) are often utilized as an adjunct to inhaled anesthetics or as part of a total intravenous anesthesia (TIVA) technique with the intent of minimizing interference with cortical mapping and, in some situations, enhancing it.

Propofol is the most commonly used induction and IV maintenance agent in GA cases under TIVA. Low doses of propofol are also titrated to achieve moderated sedation in surgical procedures under a nerve block or local anesthetic infiltration with special care in maintaining the patient's natural airway. It is also a preferred anesthetic in ambulatory settings due to its rapid emergence and decreased risk of postoperative nausea and vomiting (PONV). Propofol has significant dose-dependent anxiolytic, hypnotic, and antiepileptic effects due primarily to it being a GABA type A receptor agonist.[13] Similar to inhaled anesthetics, propofol causes a dose-dependent initial increase in EEG activity with low doses, but progresses to inhibition of epileptic foci, burst suppression, and isoelectricity with higher doses.[14] In the setting of epileptic surgery, ECoG recording can be a challenge when propofol is used in general anesthetic doses. However, because of rapid metabolism and redistribution, reliable ECoG recording can be obtained within 20 to 30 minutes after the discontinuation of the infusion.[15,16]

Ketamine and dexmedetomidine are unique, as they produce hypnosis via non-GABA mechanism of action and have analgesic properties. Ketamine is an N-methyl-D-aspartate (NMDA) receptor antagonist and is useful in procedure sedation, as it provides hypnosis and dissociative analgesia but with less respiratory depression. Although the medication functions by inhibiting glutamatergic neurotransmission, it also increases the release of excitatory amino acids such as glutamate and aspartate.[17] Therefore, ketamine has the potential to enhance EEG recording and motor cortex excitability, making it a useful anesthetic in ECoG and DES for motor mapping. A significant drawback of using ketamine, especially with conscious sedation or in an awake craniotomy, is that the anesthetic can cause psychosis-like side effects.[18] Thus, dexmedetomidine has largely replaced the use of ketamine for procedure sedation in the neurosurgical population. Dexmedetomidine is a selective α2-adrenergic agonist which indirectly increases activation of GABA neurons and produces sedation mirroring physiological sleep.[19] When combined as an analgesic adjunct to GA, dexmedetomidine has minimal effect to ECoG and adequate mapping can take place without discontinuing the infusion.[20] A significant advantage of dexmedetomidine at low doses is that it causes minimal respiratory depression and maintains a relaxed but a cooperative patient, making it ideal for awake craniotomies.[21]

Opioids play a unique and vital role in neuroanesthesia particularly during cerebral mapping. During GA, maintenance anesthetics, such as propofol or inhaled anesthetics, are reduced to minimal amnestic doses in order to prevent interference with cerebral mapping. Therefore, high doses of opioids are used to avoid patient discomfort and movement, such as coughing on the endotracheal tube. Opioids generally do not interfere with EEG recording, ECoG, DES, or microelectrode recording (MER). Short-acting opioids, such as sufentanil or remifentanil infusions, are commonly used, as they are easily titratable and allow for a rapid emergence upon their discontin-

uation. Remifentanil infusion can also be titrated with conscious sedation in awake craniotomy as an analgesic adjunct,[21] and respiratory depression can be quickly reversed with its discontinuation due to rapid breakdown of remifentanil in the plasma.[22] However, opioids have a few unique considerations in this surgical population. A rapid bolus of fentanyl can cause centrally mediated muscle rigidity that is not epileptic in nature.[23] High doses of opioids can also stimulate EEG seizure activity and this property has been utilized intraoperatively to facilitate ECoG recording.[24,25,26] It is important to consider that high doses and prolonged infusions of short-acting opioids can lead to postoperative hyperalgesia and poor pain management, as made evident in both animal models[27] and clinical practice.[28,29]

10.2 Anesthetic Techniques

A balanced integration of anesthetic and analgesic agents depends on multiple factors such as patient selection, comorbidities, surgical needs, and the expertise of the anesthesia team. A broad categorization of anesthetic techniques for craniotomies includes GA ("asleep"), regional anesthesia (RA) with intermittent moderate sedation ("awake"), or a combined technique ("asleep–awake–asleep"). These terms are used almost interchangeably in the neuroanesthesia and neurosurgical literature; however, they should not be considered as completely separate techniques due to their overlap in the clinical setting. Advantages and disadvantages of these anesthetic strategies are briefly summarized in ▶ Table 10.1.

10.2.1 General Anesthesia—"Asleep"

General anesthesia is the most common anesthetic technique as it maximizes patient comfort, immobilization, and surgical exposure. Since the patient's airway is secured prior to the surgery, GA offers the ideal conditions for airway management, oxygenation, and ventilation during surgery. However, as previously discussed in the chapter, anesthetics administered during GA have the greatest interference with cerebral mapping. The following guidelines can help overcome common interferences:
1. Avoid benzodiazepines preoperatively.
2. Titration of an opioid infusion to avoid movement or "bucking" on the ventilator.
   a) Sufentanil 0.2–0.5 μg/kg/h or
   b) Remifentanil 0.1–0.5 μg/kg/h.

Table 10.1 Anesthetic strategies for intraoperative cerebral brain mapping

General anesthesia—"asleep"	Regional anesthesia with intermittent moderate sedation—"awake"	Combined technique—"asleep/awake/asleep"
• Most comfortable for the patient • Does not require intraoperative patient cooperation • Ideal intubation conditions • A secure airway intraoperatively • Immobile patient while in pins • Able to hyperventilate the patient • Versatile for all neurosurgical procedures • Greatest interference with intraoperative mapping • A scalp block is optional	• Requires special attention to patient comfort • Requires intraoperative patient cooperation • Maintain a natural airway with sedation • May require emergent intubation • The patient may move while in pins • Unable to hyperventilate the patient • Limited to supratentorial lesions near the cortex • Ideal for intraoperative mapping • Well-established scalp block prior to pinning	• Improved patient comfort during surgical exposure • Requires intraoperative patient cooperation • Challenges with emerging and extubating while in pins • May require emergent intubation • The patient may move while in pins • Unable to hyperventilate the patient • Limited to supratentorial lesions near the cortex • Less interference with intraoperative mapping • Higher risk of unanticipated scalp block failure

3. Prior to cerebral mapping, decrease the maintenance anesthetic dose to amnestic doses.
   a) Volatile anesthetic at less than 0.5 MAC or
   b) Propofol 100–150 μg/kg/min.
4. Add dexmedetomidine at 0.5–1.0 μg/hg/h to supplement analgesia and hypnosis as it has minimal effect on ECoG.[20]
5. Other pharmacologic agents for enhancing ECoG recording include nitrous oxide,[7] etomidate,[30] methohexital,[31] alfentanil,[25] and remifentanil.[26]
6. During mapping of the motor cortex via DES, neuromuscular blockers and volatile anesthetics are to be avoided.

Performing a "scalp block" as an adjunct to GA is recommended as it improves intraoperative hemodynamic stability, reduces anesthetics requirements, reduces the risk for PONV, and provides postoperative analgesia for up to 24 hours.[32,33,34] A detailed technical description of a scalp block and local anesthetic infiltration during craniotomies is to follow.

10.2.2 Regional Anesthesia with Intermittent Moderate Sedation—"Awake"

Despite advances in imaging, stereotactic navigation system, and fMRI, the ideal intraoperative monitor remains an awake, cooperative patient. Thus, an "awake" craniotomy is considered to be the gold standard for tumor resections in eloquent areas of the brain, mapping and resection of epileptogenic foci via ECoG, and identifying deep brain structures during MER. The foundation of RA is a well-established bilateral scalp block that will cover both the pin sites and the surgical incision. The block is performed in the preoperative holding area under conscious sedation with ample time for rapport to be established between the anesthesiologist and the patient, thus also giving an opportunity to assess the patient's ability in participating in their care. When performing the block, care must be taken to consider the surgical incision and head frame pin site, and the block must be evaluated prior to proceeding with the surgery. To provide surgical anesthesia, long-acting local anesthetics are used, and epinephrine is often added to prolong the block and minimize bleeding at the injection site. The anatomy for the block and injection technique is outlined in ▶ Fig. 10.1 (see also **Video 10.1**).

The decision to perform the surgery awake under RA begins with patient selection and education prior to the surgery, as most patients are not keen at the notion of undergoing surgery "awake." Each patient is to be evaluated on a case-by-case basis via a multidisciplinary team that includes neurosurgeons, anesthesiologist, and neurologist. Although there is no defined age limit, young children might not be suitable candidates, and a child psychiatrist may need to be involved in the preoperative

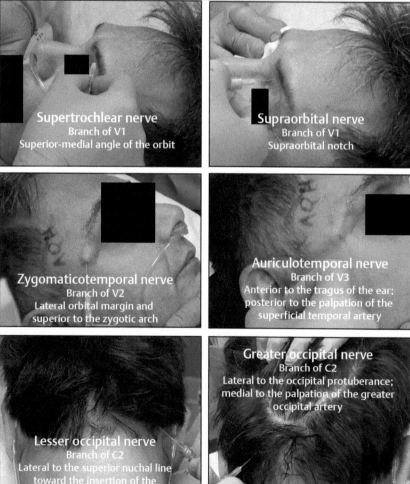

Fig. 10.1 Scalp blocks under landmark technique.

Supertrochlear nerve
Branch of V1
Superior-medial angle of the orbit

Supraorbital nerve
Branch of V1
Supraorbital notch

Zygomaticotemporal nerve
Branch of V2
Lateral orbital margin and superior to the zygotic arch

Auriculotemporal nerve
Branch of V3
Anterior to the tragus of the ear; posterior to the palpation of the superficial temporal artery

Lesser occipital nerve
Branch of C2
Lateral to the superior nuchal line toward the insertion of the sternocleidomastoid muscle

Greater occipital nerve
Branch of C2
Lateral to the occipital protuberance; medial to the palpation of the greater occipital artery

assessment to determine the level of maturity of the patient. Additional contraindications that need to be addressed during patient selection include developmental delay, psychiatric disorder (i.e., overwhelming anxiety), morbid obesity, severe sleep apnea, chronic cough, or inability to lie flat on the operating table.

Each patient needs to be briefed in advance and have a clear understanding of the perioperative course, which includes a scalp block. Patients must also be aware of the level of participation during mapping and reassured that sedatives will be administered intermittently during the surgery when patient participation is not necessary. GA is always a backup plan for which the anesthesia team needs to be ready to set up in advance with appropriate emergency airway equipment.

Different intraoperative protocols include variations in anesthetic agents and doses; however, long-acting sedatives are often avoided and special care must be taken to maintain adequate spontaneous oxygenation and ventilation. Although not as necessarily titratable as propofol, dexmedetomidine is often the preferred sedative in awake craniotomies, as it causes significantly less respiratory depression and is associated with less respiratory events in awake craniotomies.[21,35]

With the exposure of the dura, it should be noted that its innervation originates from meningeal branches of the maxillary and mandibular nerves. The scalp block does not cover stretching and incision upon the dura, and the patient may experience significant discomfort and nausea. It is also at this time that sedatives should be discontinued, as propofol needs to be turned off for at least 20 minutes to prevent interference with ECoG recordings.[16] To alleviate discomfort from opening the dura, local anesthetic-soaked microsponges or direct injection of the dura with 1% lidocaine can be performed in the surgical field (▶ Fig. 10.2). With the dura open and the patient awake, cerebral mapping, neurocognitive testing, and ECoG recording can take place. During this time, the perioperative team needs to be as efficient as possible and conscientious of the patient. It is necessary to have a perioperative staff member establish good rapport with the patient preoperatively; this staff member needs to be as attentive as possible to the patient perioperatively to ensure his or her compliance during the

procedure and prevent any discomfort emotionally and physically. If continuous analgesia and anxiolysis is required during cerebral mapping and resection, dexmedetomidine can be continued at a low dose (0.1–0.5 µg/kg/h) with minimal to no hindrance to monitoring, arousability, or respiratory depression.[36] During closure, pain and discomfort is often minimal compared to the initial surgical exposure. However, sedation with spontaneous ventilation is often resumed at this time for patient comfort.

10.2.3 Combined Technique—"Asleep/ Awake/Asleep"

GA and RA techniques can also be combined in effort to maximize patient comfort while allowing for the opportunity for cerebral mapping and brain tissue resection to be performed awake or in a semiarousable state. In this setting, GA is induced with the airway secured and the patient on a ventilator. The scalp block can be performed while the patient is in pins, and surgical exposure occurs under GA (▶ Fig. 10.3). Once the dura is exposed, the patient is emerged from GA and extubated while still in pins. To facilitate a smooth emergence, a laryngeal masked airway is often used when possible, as it is less stimulating to the airway and the patient is extubated "deep." The time it takes for the patient to become awake enough to participate with neurocognitive testing is likely prolonged when compared to RA with sedation alone. However, once the patient is awake, the perioperative course is similar to the "awake" technique described earlier.

However, the combined approach has certain pitfalls. With emergence from GA and extubation, it can be very difficult to control the patient from coughing. Also, some patients have the propensity to emerge delirious, combative, and are difficult to orient because of having their head in pins while covered with surgical drapes. In this setting, an emergent reintubation might be necessary. The combined approach is also associated with a high primary block failure rate with one study reporting 19% of significant intraoperative incisional pain and, of these patients, there is a 10% risk of emergent reintubation.[37] The likely

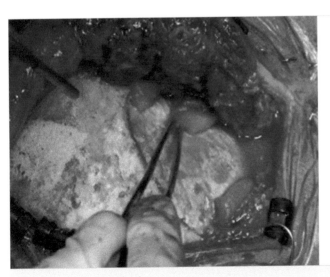
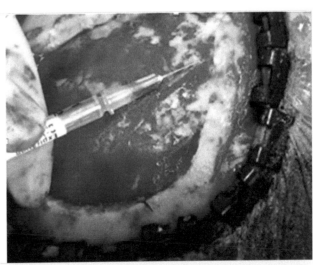

Fig. 10.2 Anesthetizing the dura.

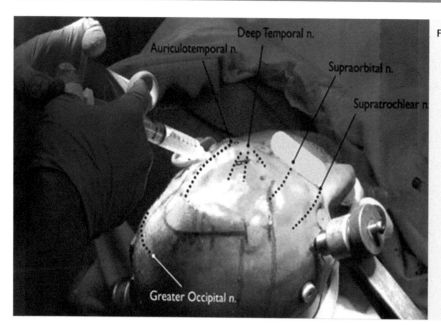

Fig. 10.3 Scalp block under general anesthesia.

10.3 Special Considerations

Regardless if the initial surgical exposure was performed under GA or RA with sedation, there are a few additional considerations to be made toward an "awake" craniotomy.

Hyperventilation is a common strategy during supratentorial craniotomy to reduce intracranial pressure (ICP) and improve surgical access and reduce "brain bulk."[27] However, hyperventilation can only be reliably achieved if the patient is intubated and mechanically ventilated; in an awake patient, the brain might feel "tight" especially if the patient is hypoventilating due to sedatives. Strategies to reduce ICP intraoperatively need to be addressed between the surgical and anesthesia team prior to the surgery and may include elevating the head of the bed, mannitol 0.25 to 1.0 g/kg IV, dexamethasone 4 to 10 mg IV, furosemide 10 to 20 mg IV, or hypertonic saline.[28]

Patients undergoing a craniotomy are prone to develop PONV with the risk as high as 50% in the first 24 hours when GA is used.[29] With a decrease in opioid use, patients undergoing awake craniotomies are significantly less likely to develop PONV.[38] These patients are still at risk of becoming nauseated, and this may occur intraoperatively with the patient on the operating table in the head frame. Commonly, dual prophylactic antiemetics such as dexamethasone 4 mg IV and ondansetron 4 mg IV are administered intraoperatively with droperidol 0.625 mg IV, or promethazine 6.25 to 12.5 mg IV used as breakthrough.[39]

The ability of the anesthesia team to handle challenges rapidly and smoothly any of these techniques is absolutely necessary for the safety and successful outcome of the patient. These challenges include nausea and vomiting in unintubated patients, airway obstruction, hypoxia, intraoperative seizure, sudden onset of severe claustrophobia, anxiety, pain, and surgical bleeding. The risk of intraoperative seizures during a craniotomy has been reported to range from 2.2 to 21.9%[40] and depends on preexisting history of epilepsy to direct stimulation-induced seizures. Preoperatively, these patients often receive antiepileptic pharmacotherapeutics, and select cases may require dual antiepileptic therapy.[41] If an intraoperative seizure was to occur in a sedated or awake patient, the surgeon would stop any direct stimulation to the brain, apply ice-cold saline irrigation, and protect the brain bulk from herniating out of the craniotomy site and the anesthetist would administer propofol. In nearly all cases, the seizure will end quickly and the patient will need several minutes to recover from the postictal state.

Despite a successful RA, there is always a potential need to emergently secure the patient's airway and convert to GA due to intraoperative complications. During a craniotomy, the patient is in a compromising position with head fixed in pins and sterile surgical drapes covering the vital structures (▶ Fig. 10.2). With approximately 25% of anesthesia-related deaths being due to a difficult airway,[42] suboptimal conditions in airway management are an ever-present concern to the anesthesia team. As with all other critical components of the perioperative course, proper airway management involves collaboration and communication between the operating room staff, surgeon, and anesthesiologist.

References

[1] Campagna JA, Miller KW, Forman SA. Mechanisms of actions of inhaled anesthetics. N Engl J Med. 2003; 348(21):2110–2124
[2] Franks NP, Lieb WR. Molecular and cellular mechanisms of general anaesthesia. Nature. 1994; 367(6464):607–614
[3] Endo T, Sato K, Shamoto H, Yoshimoto T. Effects of sevoflurane on electrocorticography in patients with intractable temporal lobe epilepsy. J Neurosurg Anesthesiol. 2002; 14(1):59–62
[4] Modica PA, Tempelhoff R, White PF. Pro- and anticonvulsant effects of anesthetics (Part II). Anesth Analg. 1990; 70(4):433–444

[5] Watts AD, Herrick IA, McLachlan RS, Craen RA, Gelb AW. The effect of sevoflurane and isoflurane anesthesia on interictal spike activity among patients with refractory epilepsy. Anesth Analg. 1999; 89(5):1275–1281

[6] Soriano SG, Bozza P. Anesthesia for epilepsy surgery in children. Childs Nerv Syst. 2006; 22(8):834–843

[7] Kurita N, Kawaguchi M, Hoshida T, Nakase H, Sakaki T, Furuya H. Effects of nitrous oxide on spike activity on electrocorticogram under sevoflurane anesthesia in epileptic patients. J Neurosurg Anesthesiol. 2005; 17(4):199–202

[8] Reasoner DK, Todd MM, Scamman FL, Warner DS. The incidence of pneumocephalus after supratentorial craniotomy. Observations on the disappearance of intracranial air. Anesthesiology. 1994; 80(5):1008–1012

[9] Becker DE, Rosenberg M. Nitrous oxide and the inhalation anesthetics. Anesth Prog. 2008; 55(4):124–130, quiz 131–132

[10] Taniguchi M, Cedzich C, Schramm J. Modification of cortical stimulation for motor evoked potentials under general anesthesia: technical description. Neurosurgery. 1993; 32(2):219–226

[11] Neuloh G, Pechstein U, Cedzich C, Schramm J. Motor evoked potential monitoring with supratentorial surgery. Neurosurgery. 2007; 61(1) Suppl:337–346, discussion 346–348

[12] Macdonald DB. Intraoperative motor evoked potential monitoring: overview and update. J Clin Monit Comput. 2006; 20(5):347–377

[13] Trapani G, Altomare C, Liso G, Sanna E, Biggio G. Propofol in anesthesia. Mechanism of action, structure-activity relationships, and drug delivery. Curr Med Chem. 2000; 7(2):249–271

[14] Wood PR, Browne GP, Pugh S. Propofol infusion for the treatment of status epilepticus. Lancet. 1988; 1(8583):480–481

[15] Herrick IA, Craen RA, Gelb AW, et al. Propofol sedation during awake craniotomy for seizures: electrocorticographic and epileptogenic effects. Anesth Analg. 1997; 84(6):1280–1284

[16] Soriano SG, Eldredge EA, Wang FK, et al. The effect of propofol on intraoperative electrocorticography and cortical stimulation during awake craniotomies in children. Paediatr Anaesth. 2000; 10(1):29–34

[17] Liu J, Moghaddam B. Regulation of glutamate efflux by excitatory amino acid receptors: evidence for tonic inhibitory and phasic excitatory regulation. J Pharmacol Exp Ther. 1995; 274(3):1209–1215

[18] Krystal JH, Karper LP, Seibyl JP, et al. Subanesthetic effects of the noncompetitive NMDA antagonist, ketamine, in humans. Psychotomimetic, perceptual, cognitive, and neuroendocrine responses. Arch Gen Psychiatry. 1994; 51(3):199–214

[19] Huupponen E, Maksimow A, Lapinlampi P, et al. Electroencephalogram spindle activity during dexmedetomidine sedation and physiological sleep. Acta Anaesthesiol Scand. 2008; 52(2):289–294

[20] Oda Y, Toriyama S, Tanaka K, et al. The effect of dexmedetomidine on electrocorticography in patients with temporal lobe epilepsy under sevoflurane anesthesia. Anesth Analg. 2007; 105(5):1272–1277

[21] Elbakry AE, Ibrahim E. Propofol-dexmedetomidine versus propofol-remifentanil conscious sedation for awake craniotomy during epilepsy surgery. Minerva Anestesiol. 2017; 83(12):1248–1254

[22] Kapila A, Glass PS, Jacobs JR, et al. Measured context-sensitive half-times of remifentanil and alfentanil. Anesthesiology. 1995; 83(5):968–975

[23] Scott JC, Sarnquist FH. Seizure-like movements during a fentanyl infusion with absence of seizure activity in a simultaneous EEG recording. Anesthesiology. 1985; 62(6):812–814

[24] Tempelhoff R, Modica PA, Bernardo KL, Edwards I. Fentanyl-induced electrocorticographic seizures in patients with complex partial epilepsy. J Neurosurg. 1992; 77(2):201–208

[25] Cascino GD, So EL, Sharbrough FW, et al. Alfentanil-induced epileptiform activity in patients with partial epilepsy. J Clin Neurophysiol. 1993; 10(4):520–525

[26] Wass CT, Grady RE, Fessler AJ, et al. The effects of remifentanil on epileptiform discharges during intraoperative electrocorticography in patients undergoing epilepsy surgery. Epilepsia. 2001; 42(10):1340–1344

[27] Gelb AW, Craen RA, Rao GS, et al. Does hyperventilation improve operating condition during supratentorial craniotomy? A multicenter randomized crossover trial. Anesth Analg. 2008; 106(2):585–594

[28] Li J, Gelb AW, Flexman AM, Ji F, Meng L. Definition, evaluation, and management of brain relaxation during craniotomy. Br J Anaesth. 2016; 116(6):759–769

[29] Latz B, Mordhorst C, Kerz T, et al. Postoperative nausea and vomiting in patients after craniotomy: incidence and risk factors. J Neurosurg. 2011; 114(2):491–496

[30] Hsieh JC, Shih YS, Hwang LD, et al. Activation of epileptogenic activities by etomidate in electrocorticoencephalography (ECoG) during operation for epilepsy. Ma Zui Xue Za Zhi. 1990; 28(2):127–135

[31] Wyler AR, Richey ET, Atkinson RA, Hermann BP. Methohexital activation of epileptogenic foci during acute electrocorticography. Epilepsia. 1987; 28(5):490–494

[32] Pinosky ML, Fishman RL, Reeves ST, et al. The effect of bupivacaine skull block on the hemodynamic response to craniotomy. Anesth Analg. 1996; 83(6):1256–1261

[33] Ayoub C, Girard F, Boudreault D, Chouinard P, Ruel M, Moumdjian R. A comparison between scalp nerve block and morphine for transitional analgesia after remifentanil-based anesthesia in neurosurgery. Anesth Analg. 2006; 103(5):1237–1240

[34] Guilfoyle MR, Helmy A, Duane D, Hutchinson PJ. Regional scalp block for postcraniotomy analgesia: a systematic review and meta-analysis. Anesth Analg. 2013; 116(5):1093–1102

[35] Goettel N, Bharadwaj S, Venkatraghavan L, Mehta J, Bernstein M, Manninen PH. Dexmedetomidine vs propofol-remifentanil conscious sedation for awake craniotomy: a prospective randomized controlled trial. Br J Anaesth. 2016; 116(6):811–821

[36] Souter MJ, Rozet I, Ojemann JG, et al. Dexmedetomidine sedation during awake craniotomy for seizure resection: effects on electrocorticography. J Neurosurg Anesthesiol. 2007; 19(1):38–44

[37] Chaki T, Sugino S, Janicki PK, et al. Efficacy and safety of a lidocaine and ropivacaine mixture for scalp nerve block and local infiltration anesthesia in patients undergoing awake craniotomy. J Neurosurg Anesthesiol. 2016; 28(1):1–5

[38] Manninen PH, Tan TK. Postoperative nausea and vomiting after craniotomy for tumor surgery: a comparison between awake craniotomy and general anesthesia. J Clin Anesth. 2002; 14(4):279–283

[39] Eberhart LH, Morin AM, Kranke P, Missaghi NB, Durieux ME, Himmelseher S. Prevention and control of postoperative nausea and vomiting in post-craniotomy patients. Best Pract Res Clin Anaesthesiol. 2007; 21(4):575–593

[40] Eseonu CI, Rincon-Torroella J, ReFaey K, et al. Awake craniotomy vs craniotomy under general anesthesia for perirolandic gliomas: evaluating perioperative complications and extent of resection. Neurosurgery. 2017; 81(3):481–489

[41] Eseonu CI, Eguia F, Garcia O, Kaplan PW, Quinones-Hinojosa A. Comparative analysis of monotherapy versus duotherapy antiseizure drug management for postoperative seizure control in patients undergoing an awake craniotomy. J Neurosurg. 2017; 128(6):1661–1667

[42] Cook TM, MacDougall-Davis SR. Complications and failure of airway management. Br J Anaesth. 2012; 109 Suppl 1:i68–i85

11 Speech Mapping

Shawn Hervey-Jumper and Mitchel S. Berger

Abstract

Cytoreduction surgery plays a fundamental role in the management of patients with low- and high-grade glioma. Maximal resection can be difficult to achieve due to tumor proximity to functional cortical and subcortical structures. Current evidence suggests that a more extensive surgical resection is associated with longer survival and improved quality of life, therefore, maximal safe resection is the goal whenever feasible. Intraoperative speech and language mapping using direct cortical and subcortical stimulation is a useful tool to improve extent of tumor resection while minimizing morbidity. This chapter summarizes the evidence supporting the role of surgery for patients with low- and high-grade gliomas within functional areas focused on cortical and subcortical neuroanatomy, preoperative planning, intraoperative language mapping technique, and complication avoidance.

Keywords: glioma, glioblastoma, low-grade glioma, brain mapping, speech

11.1 Introduction

Surgical resection plays a central role in the management of intrinsic brain tumors, and there is a growing body of evidence concerning the value of extent of resection to improve patient outcome and quality of life (QOL). The challenge, however, remains in that many intrinsic brain tumors are within regions of presumed functional significance. This is particularly true when considering cortical and subcortical speech and language areas in proximity to the tumor. Intraoperative brain mapping via the awake craniotomy, functional neuronavigation, and a firm understanding of relevant neuroanatomy are useful tools to improve extent of tumor resection while minimizing morbidity. Current evidence suggests that a more extensive surgical resection is associated with longer survival and improved QOL for patients with either low- or high-grade gliomas. This chapter outlines the evidence supporting the role of surgery for intrinsic brain tumors, surgical neuroanatomy, and techniques for intraoperative speech and language mapping to maximize extent of resection while minimizing morbidity.

11.2 Surgical Neuroanatomy: Dorsal and Ventral Language Pathways

11.2.1 Cerebral Hemispheres and Craniocerebral Relationship

A knowledge of cortical landmarks, anatomy, and subcortical structures is critical when considering speech mapping for intrinsic brain tumors. The adult cerebrum is divided into two hemispheres containing frontal, parietal, temporal, occipital lobes, and the insula. The cerebrum is divided by six principal sulci which are continuous: the sylvian, callosal, parieto-occipital, collateral, central, and calcarine sulci. There are also two interrupted sulci: the precentral and inferior temporal sulci.

The perisylvian language network is critical for speech mapping and is based along the frontal, parietal, temporal lobes in addition to the insula. The frontal lobe is separated by two main sulci: the superior and inferior frontal sulci which divide the lateral surface of the frontal lobe into the superior, middle, and inferior frontal gyri. These extend from the precentral sulcus and are oriented in the anterior-posterior direction. Running parallel to the central sulcus is the precentral sulcus. The inferior frontal gyrus is further divided by the anterior ascending and the posterior rami of the Sylvian fissure into the pars orbitalis, triangularis, and opercularis. Broca motor speech area is classically defined by the pars opercularis and pars triangularis. Along the posterior border of the frontal lobe is a readily recognizable landmark, the Greek letter "Ω" (omega) seen at the intercepting point between the superior frontal and precentral sulci which marks the hand region of the motor cortex.

Boundaries of the parietal lobe include the interhemispheric fissure medially, the Sylvian fissure and temporal-occipital line inferiorly, the central sulcus anteriorly, and the lateral parietal-temporal line posteriorly. There are two main sulci in the parietal lobe: postcentral and intraparietal sulci. The intraparietal sulcus divides the parietal lobe into the superior and inferior parietal lobules. The superior parietal lobule is superomedial and smaller and continues as the precuneus medially, whereas the inferior parietal lobule comprises the supramarginal and angular gyri. The supramarginal gyrus is the posterior continuation of the superior temporal gyrus, and the angular gyrus is the posterior continuation of the middle temporal gyrus (MTG). The temporal lobe is marked superiorly by the Sylvian fissure. The temporal lobe has the superior and inferior temporal sulci which divide the temporal lobe into superior, middle, and inferior temporal gyri. These three temporal gyri converge anteriorly to form the temporal pole.

Separating the frontal, parietal, and temporal lobes is the Sylvian fissure, which is composed of both deep and superficial portions. Deep to the Sylvian fissure lays the insular cortex which is covered by the frontal and temporal operculum. The superficial portion of the Sylvian fissure contains a stem and three rami. The stem extends medially from the uncus to the lateral end of the sphenoid wing, where it divides into the anterior horizontal, anterior ascending, and posterior rami. The deep portion of the Sylvian fissure is divided into sphenoidal and operculoinsular compartments.[1] The sphenoidal compartment arises anteriorly in the region of the limen insulae and extends laterally toward the anterior perforated substance.[1] At the threshold between the carotid cistern medially and the Sylvian fissure laterally is the limen insula. The central sulcus of the insula divides the lateral surface of the insula into three anterior short gyri (anterior, middle, and posterior gyri) and two posterior gyri (anterior and posterior long gyri).[1] Encircling the insula is the circular sulcus (also known as the superior and inferior limiting sulci of the insula) which separates it from the overlying opercula.

11.2.2 White Matter Tracts

A contemporary view of human language has shifted from a rigid organization to a more dynamic view of brain processing.[2] Large-scale subcortical white matter networks facilitate complex functions such as language, movement, and cognition. The primary fasciculi of clinical significance for speech and language are (1) the superior longitudinal fasciculus (SLF), (2) uncinate fasciculus (UF), (3) inferior occipitofrontal fasciculus (IFOF), (4) arcuate fasciculus (AF), (5) middle longitudinal fasciculus (MdLF), and (6) intermediate longitudinal fasciculus (ILF; ▶ Fig. 11.1). The SLF is separated into SLF II, SLF III, and SLF-tp. In general, the SLF curves around the insula and connects the frontal, parietal, and temporal lobes. Specifically, SLF II connects frontal and parietal lobes allowing communication between the dorsal premotor and prefrontal cortices to angular gyrus. SLF II also contains frontal to parietal connections terminating within the supramarginal gyrus. SLF-tp joins temporal and parietal lobes running in the posterior direction from inferior parietal to posterior temporal lobe. The UF lies within the anterior insula

along the limen insulae and connects the basal frontal lobe with the temporal lobe by extending under the Sylvian fissure within the insula. Connecting the frontal and occipital lobes, as well as the posterior portion of the temporal and parietal lobes, is the IFOF. The IFOF runs anterior to posterior passing through the anterior floor of the external capsule medial to the temporal lobe, sending radiations to the MTG, ITG, and occipital lobe. The AF connects frontal-opercular cortical sites with posterior temporal cortex and is thought of classically as connecting Broca with Wernicke regions. MdLF connects anterior and posterior temporal regions while ILF connects the temporal pole to the occipital lobe.

11.3 Evidence-based Clinical Decisions

11.3.1 Preoperative Planning

Preoperative clinical evaluation includes a baseline language assessment performed within 24 hours of surgery. High-quality contrast magnetic resonance imaging (MRI) scans with and without enhancement are vital for developing the optimal

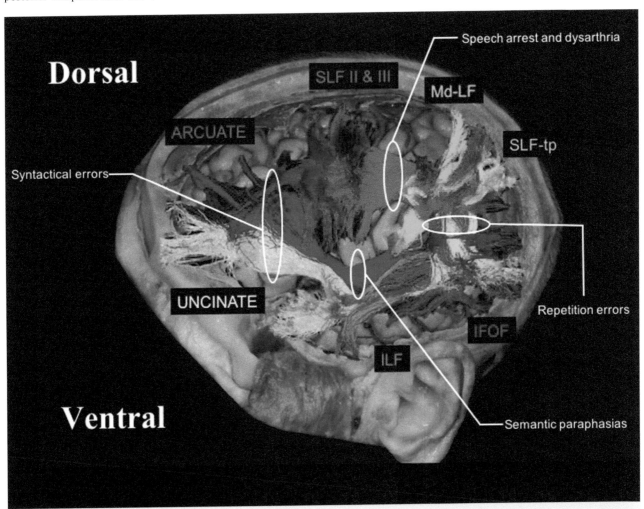

Fig. 11.1 MRI tractography identified dorsal and ventral language pathways including arcuate fasciculus (*red*), superior longitudinal fasciculus (SLF) II and III (*purple*), SLF-tp (*light blue*), middle longitudinal fasciculus (Md-LF; *green*), uncinate fasciculus (*yellow*), intermediate longitudinal fasciculus (ILF; *orange*), inferior occipitofrontal fasciculus (IFOF; *dark blue*).

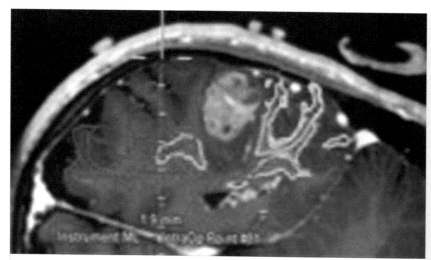

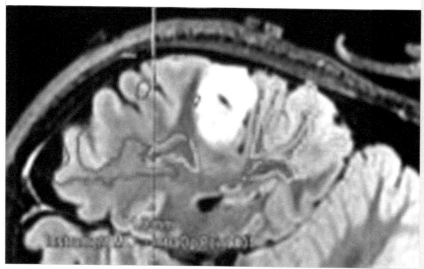

Fig. 11.2 Intraoperative neuronavigation for left parietal glioma. Frameless navigation with associated diffusion tensor imaging tractography permits the surgeon to identify the corticospinal tract (*red*) superior and medial to the mass, in addition to the superior longitudinal fasciculus II (*green*), III (*blue*), arcuate fasciculus (*pink*), and inferior occipitofrontal fasciculus (*yellow*) around the lesion.

operative plan. Diffusion tensor imaging (DTI) for white matter tracts or task-based functional brain MRI (fMRI) are helpful studies to assist with preoperative planning.[3,4] Preoperative MRI provides insight into tumor size, location, focality, vascularity, mass effect, peritumoral edema, and proximity to areas of potential functional significance. The optimal transcortical approach for approaching intrinsic tumors during speech and language mapping is along the equator of the mass.[5] In addition, MRIs can be reconstructed to create three-dimensional models combined with tractography that can be used during surgery (neuronavigation; ▶ Fig. 11.2). DTI tractography, fMRI, and perfusion MRI enable clinicians to make more accurate preoperative diagnoses and provide information regarding the interface of tumor tissue with adjacent functional cortical and subcortical pathways. The fMRI uses the blood-oxygenation-level-dependent (BOLD) signal to identify cortical and subcortical regions of activation to create an operative corridor or plan for resection that minimizes risk to eloquent surrounding structures.[6,7] Perfusion MRI is useful for evaluating tumor angiogenesis, endothelial permeability, and potentially distinguishing between recurrent glioma and treatment-related changes. DTI tractography is used to mark the subcortical dorsal and ventral language tracts surrounding a tumor and is commonly used in surgical planning.[8,9,10] For the brain tumor surgeon, functional

and anatomic image guidance is an essential part of determining the risks associated with surgery and for consulting patients about potential postoperative neurological outcomes. Image guidance also allows for a generalized preoperative impression of where a functional pathway might be displaced in relationship to a space-occupying lesion. Neuronavigation is widely used in brain tumor surgery that can be integrated with DTI tractography, magnetoencephalography (MEG), or fMRI to identify cortical and subcortical areas of potential sensory, motor, language, and visual significance (▶ Fig. 11.1 and ▶ Fig. 11.2).[11] Neuronavigation can, therefore, generate individualized maps of functional areas and their relationship with mass lesions within the brain. These studies, however, lack sensitivity, given the variability in individual patient's neuroanatomy, distortion due to mass lesions, and functional reorganization caused by plasticity make classic anatomic identification of functional areas insufficient.[12,13] Compared with direct cortical stimulation, fMRI has a sensitivity and specificity of 91 and 64% for identification of Broca area, 93 and 18% for identification of Wernicke area, and 100 and 100% in motor areas, respectively.[14] Resting state coherence measured with MEG is capable of mapping functional connectivity of the brain. Intrinsic brain tumors with decreased resting state connectivity have a relatively low risk of postoperative language deficits, while those with increased resting state connectivity are associated with higher risk of postoperative aphasia.[15] Identification of subcortical pathways is critical to prevent injury to white matter pathways and preserve function.[16] The gold standard approach for resection of intrinsic brain tumors within speech areas is cortical and subcortical intraoperative brain mapping.

11.3.2 Medical Management

Prior to speech mapping, preoperative clinical evaluation includes baseline language and sensorimotor assessment performed 24 to 48 hours prior to surgery.[17] Corticosteroids are commonly used preoperatively to reduce symptoms of mass effect and peritumoral vasogenic edema. Timing and dose of corticosteroids vary based on tumor size, vasogenic edema, and mass effect; however, a common regimen for adult patients is 4 to 6 mg of dexamethasone every 6 or 8 hours. Patients presenting with seizures should be started on an anticonvulsant with an initial loading dose. However, with few exceptions, there is no data to suggest that the prophylactic use of anticonvulsants reduces the risk of new-onset seizures in patients with intrinsic brain tumors.[18,19,20]

11.4 Surgical Techniques

11.4.1 Evidence in Support of Extent of Resection

Given the natural history of gliomas, clinical observation of surgically treatable gliomas is rarely encouraged, even when considering tumors within functional regions. The goals of surgery are to establish the correct diagnosis and cytoreduction. The decision to offer surgical resection versus biopsy depends on tumor location and size, patient age, and performance status. Over the past 20 years, a number of studies have enhanced our understanding of the impact of tumor resection on progression-free overall survival in patients with intrinsic brain tumors.[21] Gross total resection affects the natural history of gliomas including progression-free survival and time to malignant transformation. For this reason, maximal safe resection is preferred over biopsy.[22] In a large population-based series of Norwegian patients, early maximal resection was superior to biopsy and watchful waiting with respective 5-year survival rates of 74 and 60%, illustrating the advantage of resection over watchful waiting.[23] Furthermore, 90% extent of resection in low-grade gliomas delays and reduces malignant transformation and improves survival. In the era of glioma molecular subclassification, there has been a new focus directed toward understanding the impact of extent of resection across low- and high-risk subgroups.[24,25,26] This area of investigation is currently incomplete. However, taken together, published reports highlight the fact that clinical outcomes differ independently based on extent of glioma resection and molecular subtype.

11.4.2 Awake Craniotomy for Speech and Language Mapping

Direct cortical stimulation mapping allows for the identification of cortical and subcortical sites critical for language during surgery for removal of intrinsic brain tumors.[17] Intraoperative mapping is critical because individual variability and language pathway distortion from intrinsic brain tumors makes functional neuronavigation using DTI and fMRI less reliable. In addition, critical functions, such as speech arrest, anomia, and alexia, which are classically thought to be located within the anatomical confines of the pars triangularis and opercularis, can be located far outside the anatomic boundaries of Broca area.[27] Direct stimulation mapping is, therefore, the gold standard for identification and preservation of functional areas.

Cortical stimulation is thought to work via depolarization of a focal region of brain, which excites local neurons via diffusion of current using both orthodromic and antidromic propagation. Bipolar stimulation using a 2-mm tip with 5 mm of separation allows for local diffusion and more precise mapping.[27,28] Specialized neuroanesthesia is critical for completion of intraoperative speech mapping[29] during which clear communication between neurosurgeon, anesthesiologist, speech pathologist, neuropsychologist, and other members of the mapping team ensures accuracy and patient safety. Surgery commences with the application of patient monitors and premedicating with midazolam, fentanyl, or dexmedetomidine prior to positioning.[17] Anesthesia during speech mapping is achieved with propofol (up to 100 µg/kg/minute) or dexmedetomidine (up to 1 µg/kg/minute) and remifentanil (0.07–2.0 µg/kg/hour).[30,31,32] Following initiation of drugs, a Foley catheter is inserted and patient is placed in a Mayfield head holder. A scalp block using a mixture of 1% lidocaine with 1:100,000 epinephrine, 0.5% bupivacaine, plus 8.4% sodium bicarbonate is applied by the neurosurgeon. The optimal head positioning allows for ease of operation, patient comfort, and airways access. It is critical that a dedicated intravenous line is filled with a 1 mg/kg bolus of propofol, if needed for suppression of an intraoperative stimulation-induced seizure. In addition, topical ice-cold Ringer's lactate solution is available on the surgical field at all times for seizure suppression.

Administration of speech and language tasks during intraoperative mapping varies in a site-specific manner based on tumor location and baseline performance. However, commonly used tasks include picture naming, text reading, auditory repetition, and syntax comprehension.[17,33] Mapping begins with a stimulation current of 2 mA and increases to a maximum of 6 mA as determined by intraoperative electrocorticography. A constant current generator delivers 1.25 millisecond biphasic square waves in 4-second trains at 60 Hz. Numerical markers are placed on the surgical field spaced 1 cm apart (▶ Fig. 11.3). Continuous electrocorticography is used to improve mapping accuracy, monitor for subclinical seizure activity, and detect after-discharge potentials. The goal for speech mapping is that the patient performs the given language task through the stimulation (or through the after-discharge potential). All language testing is repeated at least three times per cortical site, and a positive site is defined as the inability to count, name objects, or read words during stimulation at least 66% of times.[17,34] Cortical language mapping seeks to identify sites responsible for speech arrest, anomia, and alexia with stimulation testing. Subcortical language mapping applies the same direct stimulation approach and stimulation site relies on the surgeon's understanding of subcortical white matter neuroanatomy. Speech arrest is defined as discontinuation in number

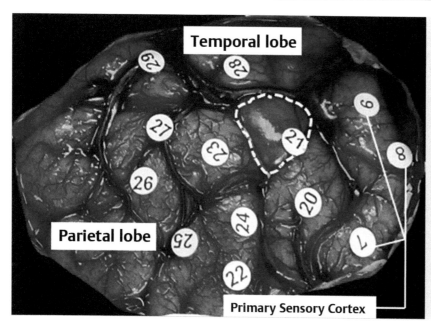

Fig. 11.3 Direct cortical stimulation mapping is the gold standard for identification of functional language and sensorimotor areas. This illustrative case of a left parietal World Health Organization grade III astrocytoma comes to the cortical surface focally (*hashed outline*) but extends under language and sensory motor cortex subcortically. Cortical mapping uses numbered markers placed at 1-cm intervals to mark primary sensory cortex (7, sensory tongue; 8, 9, sensory face) and language areas (20–29). All language sites mapped negative after administration of picture naming, text reading, four syllable repetition, auditory naming, and syntax production.

counting without simultaneous motor response. Dysarthria from motor pharynx stimulation can be distinguished from speech arrest by an absence of involuntary muscle contractions affecting speech.[27] Using this approach, one can administer non-language cognitive tasks in the intraoperative setting including selective attention, calculation, and line bisection.[35,36]

11.5 Complication Avoidance

In the immediate postoperative period, patients are observed closely in the setting of an intensive care unit, where serial neurological examinations are carried out.[19] Depending on tumor location and extent of resection, corticosteroids may be tapered over the days following the surgery. Anticonvulsants are continued in patients who have a history of seizures and for tumors in areas known to have a propensity to cause seizures. The long-term use of seizure medications for prophylaxis remains controversial. Given the prognostic significance of extent of resection for glioma patients and the difficulty in detecting residual tumor during surgery, it is becoming standard practice for surgeons to obtain postoperative MRIs with contrast to evaluate for residual tumor within 24 hours of resection.

Functional performance is the driving force behind maintaining a maximal health-related QOL (HRQOL) and these measures go beyond Karnofsky Performance Status. Preservation of QOL is critically important and is thought to have an impact on survival. Long-term language outcomes following direct cortical and subcortical stimulation mapping of dominant hemisphere gliomas has been evaluated by a number of large clinical series (WHO grades II–IV).[27,37,38] During the immediate postoperative period, language temporarily worsens in 14 to 50% of patients.[27,38,39] One month following surgery, 78 to 100% of patients have return of language to baseline preoperative function.[27,38] However, after 3 to 6 months, only 0 to 2.4% of patients have worsened language function and by and large many patients are satisfied with their functional outcomes.[27,38] Following surgery, 55% of patients had at least transient cognitive

impairments primarily involving speech, executive function, memory, and selective attention.[40,41,42,43] The extent to which functional impairments influence survival has been understudied in adult glioma patients.

11.6 Conclusion

Gliomas are a major cause of morbidity in the United States. This is largely due to the fact that they pose both oncological as well as neurological challenges. It has been established that maximal extent of resection improves both overall and progression-free survival; however, surgical goals must be balanced with preservation of language, motor, and neurocognitive networks. A solid understanding of neuroanatomy safety and surgical goals must be balanced with preservation of language, motor, and neurocognitive networks. Techniques such as intraoperative brain mapping, functional neuronavigation, intraoperative MRI, laser interstitial thermal therapy, and fluorescence-guided surgery have expanded our ability to remove maximal amounts of tumor while preserving these essential functions.

References

[1] Ribas EC, Yagmurlu K, Wen HT, Rhoton AL, Jr. Microsurgical anatomy of the inferior limiting insular sulcus and the temporal stem. J Neurosurg. 2015; 122(6):1263–1273

[2] Chang EF, Raygor KP, Berger MS. Contemporary model of language organization: an overview for neurosurgeons. J Neurosurg. 2015; 122(2):250–261

[3] Deng X, Zhang Y, Xu L, et al. Comparison of language cortex reorganization patterns between cerebral arteriovenous malformations and gliomas: a functional MRI study. J Neurosurg. 2015; 122(5):996–1003

[4] Ille S, Sollmann N, Hauck T, et al. Combined noninvasive language mapping by navigated transcranial magnetic stimulation and functional MRI and its comparison with direct cortical stimulation. J Neurosurg. 2015; 123(1):212–225

[5] Morshed RA, Young JS, Han SJ, Hervey-Jumper SL, Berger MS. The transcortical equatorial approach for gliomas of the mesial temporal lobe: techniques and functional outcomes. J Neurosurg. 201 9; 130(3):822–830

[6] Bogomolny DL, Petrovich NM, Hou BL, Peck KK, Kim MJ, Holodny AI. Functional MRI in the brain tumor patient. Top Magn Reson Imaging. 2004; 15(5): 325–335

[7] Nimsky C, Ganslandt O, Von Keller B, Romstöck J, Fahlbusch R. Intraoperative high-field-strength MR imaging: implementation and experience in 200 patients. Radiology. 2004; 233(1):67–78

[8] Alexander AL, Lee JE, Lazar M, Field AS. Diffusion tensor imaging of the brain. Neurotherapeutics. 2007; 4(3):316–329

[9] Bello L, Gambini A, Castellano A, et al. Motor and language DTI Fiber Tracking combined with intraoperative subcortical mapping for surgical removal of gliomas. Neuroimage. 2008; 39(1):369–382

[10] Berman JI, Berger MS, Chung SW, Nagarajan SS, Henry RG. Accuracy of diffusion tensor magnetic resonance imaging tractography assessed using intraoperative subcortical stimulation mapping and magnetic source imaging. J Neurosurg. 2007; 107(3):488–494

[11] Trinh VT, Fahim DK, Maldaun MV, et al. Impact of preoperative functional magnetic resonance imaging during awake craniotomy procedures for intraoperative guidance and complication avoidance. Stereotact Funct Neurosurg. 2014; 92(5):315–322

[12] Duffau H. New concepts in surgery of WHO grade II gliomas: functional brain mapping, connectionism and plasticity—a review. J Neurooncol. 2006; 79(1): 77–115

[13] Thiel A, Herholz K, Koyuncu A, et al. Plasticity of language networks in patients with brain tumors: a positron emission tomography activation study. Ann Neurol. 2001; 50(5):620–629

[14] Bizzi A, Blasi V, Falini A, et al. Presurgical functional MR imaging of language and motor functions: validation with intraoperative electrocortical mapping. Radiology. 2008; 248(2):579–589

[15] Guggisberg AG, Honma SM, Findlay AM, et al. Mapping functional connectivity in patients with brain lesions. Ann Neurol. 2008; 63(2):193–203

[16] Sarubbo S, De Benedictis A, Merler S, et al. Towards a functional atlas of human white matter. Hum Brain Mapp. 2015; 36(8):3117–3136

[17] Hervey-Jumper SL, Li J, Lau D, et al. Awake craniotomy to maximize glioma resection: methods and technical nuances over a 27-year period. J Neurosurg. 2015; 123(2):325–339

[18] Chang EF, Potts MB, Keles GE, et al. Seizure characteristics and control following resection in 332 patients with low-grade gliomas. J Neurosurg. 2008; 108 (2):227–235

[19] Chang SM, Parney IF, Huang W, et al. Glioma Outcomes Project Investigators. Patterns of care for adults with newly diagnosed malignant glioma. JAMA. 2005; 293(5):557–564

[20] Lima GL, Duffau H. Is there a risk of seizures in "preventive" awake surgery for incidental diffuse low-grade gliomas? J Neurosurg. 2015; 122(6):1397–1405

[21] Hervey-Jumper SL, Berger MS. Role of surgical resection in low- and high-grade gliomas. Curr Treat Options Neurol. 2014; 16(4):284

[22] Smith JS, Chang EF, Lamborn KR, et al. Role of extent of resection in the long-term outcome of low-grade hemispheric gliomas. J Clin Oncol. 2008; 26(8): 1338–1345

[23] Jakola AS, Myrmel KS, Kloster R, et al. Comparison of a strategy favoring early surgical resection vs a strategy favoring watchful waiting in low-grade gliomas. JAMA. 2012; 308(18):1881–1888

[24] Kawaguchi T, Sonoda Y, Shibahara I, et al. Impact of gross total resection in patients with WHO grade III glioma harboring the IDH 1/2 mutation without the 1p/19q co-deletion. J Neurooncol. 2016; 129(3):505–514

[25] Cahill DP, Beiko J, Suki D, et al. IDH1 status and survival benefit from surgical resection of enhancing and nonenhancing tumor in malignant astrocytomas. J Clin Oncol. 2012; 30:2019–2019

[26] Wijnenga MMJ, French PJ, Dubbink HJ, et al. The impact of surgery in molecularly defined low-grade glioma: an integrated clinical, radiological, and molecular analysis. Neuro-oncol. 2018; 20(1):103–112

[27] Sanai N, Mirzadeh Z, Berger MS. Functional outcome after language mapping for glioma resection. N Engl J Med. 2008; 358(1):18–27

[28] Nathan SS, Sinha SR, Gordon B, Lesser RP, Thakor NV. Determination of current density distributions generated by electrical stimulation of the human cerebral cortex. Electroencephalogr Clin Neurophysiol. 1993; 86(3):183–192

[29] Taylor MD, Bernstein M. Awake craniotomy with brain mapping as the routine surgical approach to treating patients with supratentorial intraaxial tumors: a prospective trial of 200 cases. J Neurosurg. 1999; 90(1):35–41

[30] Bekker AY, Kaufman B, Samir H, Doyle W. The use of dexmedetomidine infusion for awake craniotomy. Anesth Analg. 2001; 92(5):1251–1253

[31] Herrick IA, Craen RA, Gelb AW, et al. Propofol sedation during awake craniotomy for seizures: patient-controlled administration versus neurolept analgesia. Anesth Analg. 1997; 84(6):1285–1291

[32] Olsen KS. The asleep-awake technique using propofol-remifentanil anaesthesia for awake craniotomy for cerebral tumours. Eur J Anaesthesiol. 2008; 25 (8):662–669

[33] Fernández Coello A, Moritz-Gasser S, Martino J, Martinoni M, Matsuda R, Duffau H. Selection of intraoperative tasks for awake mapping based on relationships between tumor location and functional networks. J Neurosurg. 2013; 119(6):1380–1394

[34] Sanai N, Berger MS. Glioma extent of resection and its impact on patient outcome. Neurosurgery. 2008; 62(4):753–764, discussion 264–266

[35] Charras P, Herbet G, Deverdun J, et al. Functional reorganization of the attentional networks in low-grade glioma patients: a longitudinal study. Cortex. 2015; 63:27–41

[36] De Witte E, Satoer D, Colle H, Robert E, Visch-Brink E, Mariën P. Subcortical language and non-language mapping in awake brain surgery: the use of multimodal tests. Acta Neurochir (Wien). 2015; 157(4):577–588

[37] Duffau H, Capelle L, Denvil D, et al. Functional recovery after surgical resection of low grade gliomas in eloquent brain: hypothesis of brain compensation. J Neurol Neurosurg Psychiatry. 2003; 74(7):901–907

[38] Duffau H, Moritz-Gasser S, Gatignol P. Functional outcome after language mapping for insular World Health Organization grade II gliomas in the dominant hemisphere: experience with 24 patients. Neurosurg Focus. 2009; 27 (2):E7

[39] Wilson SM, Lam D, Babiak MC, et al. Transient aphasias after left hemisphere resective surgery. J Neurosurg. 2015; 123(3):581–593

[40] Racine CA, Li J, Molinaro AM, Butowski N, Berger MS. Neurocognitive function in newly diagnosed low-grade glioma patients undergoing surgical resection with awake mapping techniques. Neurosurgery. 2015; 77(3):371–379, discussion 379

[41] Douw L, Klein M, Fagel SS, et al. Cognitive and radiological effects of radiotherapy in patients with low-grade glioma: long-term follow-up. Lancet Neurol. 2009; 8(9):810–818

[42] Taphoorn MJ, Klein M. Cognitive deficits in adult patients with brain tumours. Lancet Neurol. 2004; 3(3):159–168

[43] Ahmadi R, Dictus C, Hartmann C, et al. Long-term outcome and survival of surgically treated supratentorial low-grade glioma in adult patients. Acta Neurochir (Wien). 2009; 151(11):1359–1365

12 Motor Mapping (Rolandic, Pre-Rolandic, and Insular Cortex)

N. U. Farrukh Hameed, Wang Peng, Geng Xu, Jie Zhang, and Jinsong Wu

Abstract

This chapter discusses brain parenchymal motor mapping in the perioperative period with glioma as the representative type of tumor. We discuss multimodal techniques for preoperative motor function localization such as comprehensive neuropsychological evaluation and functional brain imaging; neurophysiological methods for intraoperative motor cortex and subcortical motor pathway localization and monitoring; motor mapping-related neuroanesthesia techniques, and advantages and disadvantages of asleep and awake intraoperative mapping; and a typical case illustrating motor mapping.

Keywords: motor, mapping, pre-rolandic, rolandic, insula, cortex

12.1 Introduction

The extent of resection of gliomas has been shown to be most important in the treatment of low- and high-grade gliomas. Since gliomas infiltrate beyond boundaries shown by magnetic resonance imaging (MRI), it has been proposed that true tumor resection encompasses excision beyond tumor boundaries shown by MRI. By excising beyond the traditional fluid-attenuated inversion recovery "true" lesion range, cancer progression is delayed. After defining the benefits of surgery, the primary objective of glioma surgery at present is maximal safe tumor resection to reduce tumor cell burden, thus improving the response rate and efficacy of subsequent adjuvant therapy. In our division, we studied more than 800 patients who underwent surgery for glioma with or without intraoperative neurophysiological monitoring (IONM). Direct electrical stimulation of the brain in functional areas was found to not only reduce the severity of nerve injuries, but also expand the extent of the resection.[1] This explains why intraoperative brain mapping has

become the "golden standard" for tumor resection in functional areas of brain. Depending on individualized cortical and subcortical functional boundaries, true maximum safe resection is aimed with the goal of providing patients with balanced oncological and functional benefits.

The motor cortex is located anterior to the central sulcus (rolandic fissure) and can be divided into the rolandic (primary motor and sensory) cortex, pre-rolandic cortex (premotor cortex), and the supplementary motor area (SMA, ▶ Fig. 12.1). The rolandic cortex, also called the central lobe, consists of the precentral and postcentral gyri.[2] Primary motor cortex is the Brodmann area 4 that consists of most parts of precentral gyrus and the anterior part of paracentral lobule in the medial aspect of frontal lobe. Premotor cortex generally corresponds to Brodmann area 6 and consists of inferior portion of precentral gyrus, posterior parts of superior and middle frontal gyri, and part of medial aspect of superior frontal gyrus. The pre-rolandic cortex and SMA comprise the secondary motor cortex. The insular cortex lies deep within the lateral sulcus like an island and is covered by the insular opercula and is surrounded by critical neural pathways.

12.2 Preoperative Brain Function Localization

12.2.1 Neuropsychological Assessment

In the preoperative work-up of glioma patients, neuropsychological evaluation is very important. The commonly used neuropsychological assessment scales are Edinburgh Handedness Inventory, Karnofsky Performance Score (KPS), Mini Mental State Examination (MMSE), Boston Naming Test (BNT), and the Aphasia Battery test. All patients must undergo neuropsychological

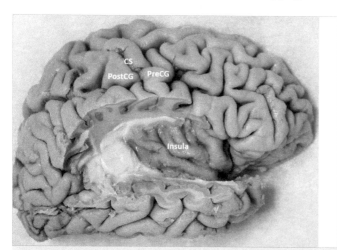
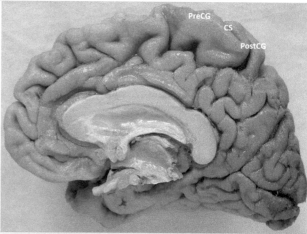

Fig. 12.1 Brain anatomy showing the Rolandic and pre-Rolandic cortices, and the insula. CS, Central sulcus; PreCG, Precentral gyrus; PostCG, Postcentral gyrus.

assessment before and after surgery, since a comprehensive understanding of all types of dominant or recessive neurological dysfunctions before surgery allows surgeons to provide individualized treatment, predict possible temporary postoperative deficits, develop postoperative rehabilitation program, and provide a baseline for continuous assessment of postoperative neurological function.

12.2.2 Functional Magnetic Resonance Imaging

Functional MRI (fMRI) is the most common functional neuroimaging technique. When neurons are excited, the neurovascular coupling mechanism leads to a local increase in the ratio of oxyhemoglobin (antimagnetic) to deoxyhemoglobin (paramagnetic), which can be detected by echo-planner imaging, a fast MRI imaging technique. Although fMRI is fairly accurate in localizing primary motor[3] and sensory cortices, it is less sensitive in localizing language.[4] There are some important considerations underlying fMRI usage in brain tumor surgery. First, fMRI only shows areas of increased cortical blood flow which is an indirect measure of neuronal activity, and is susceptible to errors in the peritumoral brain. Furthermore, there is a temporal delay between neuronal activity and changes in blood flow; therefore, the transient activation of brain regions cannot be detected. In essence, fMRI best reveals areas of the gray matter involved in a particular task but does not indicate areas that are functionally necessary. Therefore, relying on fMRI[3,4] to guide surgery may result in excision of critical functional cortical regions (false negative) or hinder neurosurgeons from removing noncritical cortical regions (false positive) that patients can actually compensate for. More appropriate uses of fMRI include[1] preoperative surgical planning and rehearsal[2]; screening for functional brain regions that need to be verified by intraoperative direct electrical stimulation; or[3] providing cortical motor network information, such as SMA, for patients unable to undergo awake craniotomy.

12.2.3 Transcranial Magnetic Stimulation

This is a newer noninvasive preoperative cortical function mapping technique that involves altering the action potential of cortical neurons through a time-varying magnetic field and combines with navigation technology to accurately localize functional cortical areas. Recent studies have shown that transcranial magnetic stimulation (TMS) localization of cortical motor areas concurs with results of intraoperative direct electrical stimulation.[5,6] TMS can be used in healthy subjects and patients with brain lesions. It can also be used to study cortical function remodeling due to its ability of regulating cortical excitability.

12.2.4 Diffusion Tensor Imaging

This technique is based on anisotropic imaging of the diffusion of water molecules in white matter fibers and can be used to form three-dimensional models of subcortical neural conduction pathways. Tracking imaging (tractography) shows the morphology, structure, and projection of these pathways. In addition to diffusion tensor imaging (DTI) tractography being important for research and teaching, it provides information about virtual structure rather than real function. Brain tumors are often accompanied by edema resulting in distortion and erosion of DTI white matter tracts. Results from our division's clinical trial demonstrated that DTI tractography is clinically effective but not completely reliable in delineating descending motor pathways (corticospinal tract) and must be integrated with direct cortical stimulation for functional glioma surgery (▶ Fig. 12.2).[7] Despite the utility of fMRI and DTI in localizing

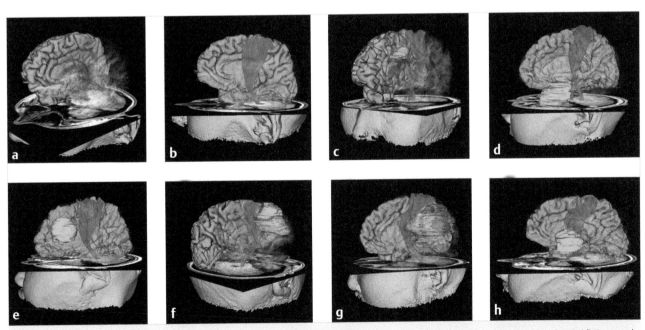

Fig. 12.2 (a) Whole-brain diffusion tensor imaging. (b) Corticospinal tract (CST) of a normal subject. (c) Cingulate gyrus glioma and CST. (d) Temporal lobe glioma and CST. (e) Middle frontal gyrus glioma (pre-rolandic) and CST. (f) Superior frontal gyrus glioma (pre-rolandic) and CST. (g) superior parietal lobe glioma and CST. (h) Insular lobe glioma and CST.

functional cortical areas and subcortical neural pathways, respectively, a multimodal imaging approach comprising IONM is essential to ensure the accuracy and reliability of intraoperative functional brain mapping.

12.3 Intraoperative Neurophysiological Monitoring

Preoperatively, anesthesiologists, electrophysiologists, and surgeons discuss the anesthesia method, monitoring mode, and monitoring parameters for intraoperative cortical and subcortical neural pathways according to the surgical plan. IONM comprises four parts: somatosensory evoked potentials (SSEP) to locate the central sulcus, motor evoked potentials (MEP) to monitor motor pathway integrity, direct cortical electrical stimulation (DCS) in combination with electromyography (EMG) recording to map the primary motor cortex, and direct subcortical electrical stimulation (DsCS) to delineate the subcortical motor pathway (corticospinal tract). In a recent study, we divided primary glioma patients into two groups based on whether or not IONM was applied intraoperatively. The proportion of tumors located in the dominant hemisphere and the eloquent cortex was higher in the IONM versus the non-IONM group. We found the rate of postoperative hospital stay, long-term language deficit, and overall neurological dysfunction to be significantly lower in the IONM group compared to the non-IONM group, suggesting that IONM could reduce the rate of postoperative neurological dysfunction.[1] However, questions still remain on how IONM precisely influences extent of resection in glioma surgery and overall survival.

12.3.1 Somatosensory Evoked Potential

SSEP involves the stimulation of action potentials in peripheral nerves that are recorded in the cerebral cortex which, to some extent, reflect the afferent pathways of specific somatic sensations, the reticular structure of the brainstem, and the functional state of the cerebral cortex. SSEP recording is characterized by continuity, repeatability, and identifiable waveforms, and is advantageous in terms of anatomical monitoring and technique. The stimulation technique involves repetitive stimuli of intensity 15 to 25 mA and duration 0.10 to 0.30 ms at a rate of 2.10 to 4.70 Hz.

An important initial step in sensorimotor function mapping is identifying the central sulcus by SSEP phase reversal technique (▶ Fig. 12.3). A strip electrode with multiple contacts is placed perpendicularly on the surface of the presumed central sulcus to record SSEP by stimulating the median nerve (▶ Fig. 12.4). The strip electrode is moved until it demonstrates polarity reversal.[8] From this, the surgeon and neurophysiologist can estimate the position of the central sulcus which lies between the contacts where polarity reversal occurs. Although it is possible to identify the central sulcus by analyzing anatomical landmarks on neuroimaging,[9] anatomical and neurophysiological discrepancies resulting from large rolandic and prerolandic brain lesions can significantly impact the reliability of direct visual identification of the central sulcus.

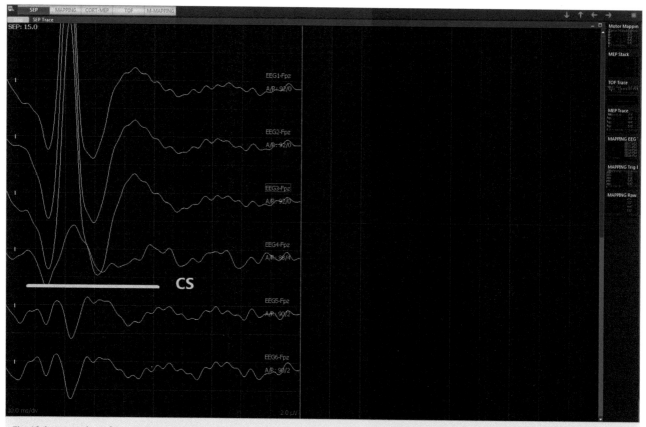

Fig. 12.3 A snapshot of somatosensory evoked potential recording showing identification of central sulcus by phase reversal technique.

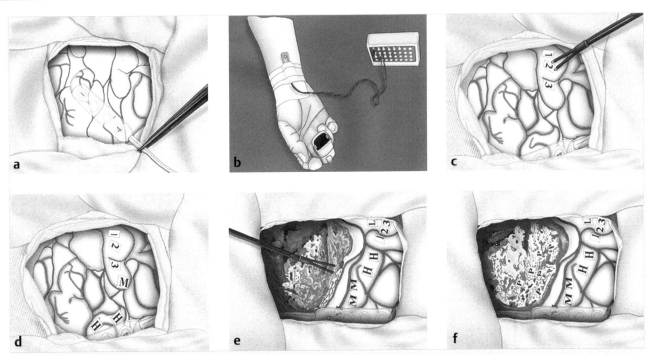

Fig. 12.4 (**a**) Placement of subdural strip electrodes on the central sulcus for continuous detection of somatosensory evoked potentials (SSEP). (**b**) Electrical stimulation of the median nerve to evoke SSEP. (**c**) Language and motor function mapping. (**d**) Labeling of functional cortical areas with sterile tags (1, 2, 3, speech arrest; M, mouth motor area; H, hand movement) and covering with thin film for both visualization and protection. (**e**) Following tumor debulking, subcortical stimulation is performed to ensure there is no residual injury to language and motor tracts. (**f**) Tagging of positive subcortical areas, P, to guide surgeon to safely resect tumor around these regions. (Illustration by Tongxiong Chen).

12.3.2 Motor Evoked Potential

Intraoperative MEP monitoring involves electrical or magnetic stimulation of the motor cortex to produce a downstream electrical response through the corticospinal tract, and ultimately, a measurable electrophysiological signal in the form of a compound muscle action potential (CMAP; ▶ Fig. 12.5). Clinically, the latency and amplitude of CMAP are often used as monitoring indicators. However, it must be noted that sometimes, transcranial MEP is not suitable for intracranial tumors because current from scalp stimulation can penetrate deeper brain tissues and activate corticospinal fibers. This poses problems in identifying more superficial lesions and yields false-negative results. Continuous transcortical MEPs are widely used for tumor surgeries of the rolandic, pre-rolandic, or insular cortex to monitor the integrity of motor pathways to achieve maximum resection of lesions while preserving motor function (▶ Fig. 12.5). Also, prior to closing the dura, transcortical MEPs are assessed one last time to assess the integrity of distal motor activity and subsequent postoperative motor deficits are considered transient. The stimulation consists of a train of five pulses (rate 250 pulse/second), at a stimulation intensity of 20 to 100 V by 5V for a duration of 75 μs and rate 1 Hz. MEP is also used for monitoring cortical and subcortical ischemia during carotid endarterectomy or intracranial aneurysm surgery.

12.3.3 Direct Cortical Stimulation and Direct Subcortical Stimulation

Intraoperative direct electrical stimulation for both cortical and subcortical functional mapping and monitoring of neural pathways is currently the "gold standard" technique for functional brain mapping (▶ Fig. 12.4c, e). This technique decreases long-term neurological deficits while maximizing overall tumor resection, and is suitable for intra-axial glioma surgeries of the rolandic, pre-rolandic, or insular cortex. DCS mapped motor pathways are often used to determine the edges of lesions after resection, white matter area, internal capsule, corona radiation, boundaries of the corticospinal tract, relationship between tumor and the corticospinal tract, and the extent of resection (▶ Fig. 12.4).

Identification of the central sulcus by SSEP is followed by DCS to trigger muscle MEP in the contralateral muscles of an awake or anesthetized patient. The DCS technique involves repetitive stimuli of intensity 1.5 to 6 mA in increments of 0.5 mA and duration 1 ms at a rate of 60 Hz. EMG records are more sensitive than muscle contractions and are monitored to reduce stimulation threshold and risk of intraoperative epilepsy (▶ Fig. 12.6). The primary motor cortex is identified by electrical responses triggered at the lowest current amplitude, and it is continuously monitored intraoperatively together with the corticospinal tract via continuous stimulation of the motor strip. For this, the primary motor cortex is stimulated by either a handheld electrode or the same strip electrode that was initially used for locating SSEP polarity reversal by repositioning it parallel to the central sulcus on the precentral gyrus. The handheld electrodes are of two kinds: monopolar or bipolar electrodes. Bipolar electrodes have separated ball tips and are advantageous over monopolar electrodes because an additional return electrode is not required. However, the presence of two electrodes creates ambiguity in stimulation and limits the spatial resolution because it is difficult to identify which of the two electrodes

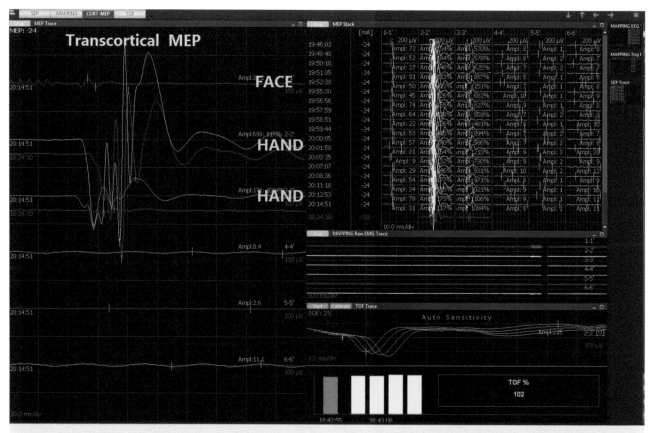

Fig. 12.5 Intraoperative motor evoked potential monitoring involves measurement of downstream electrophysiological signals in the form of compound muscle action potential.

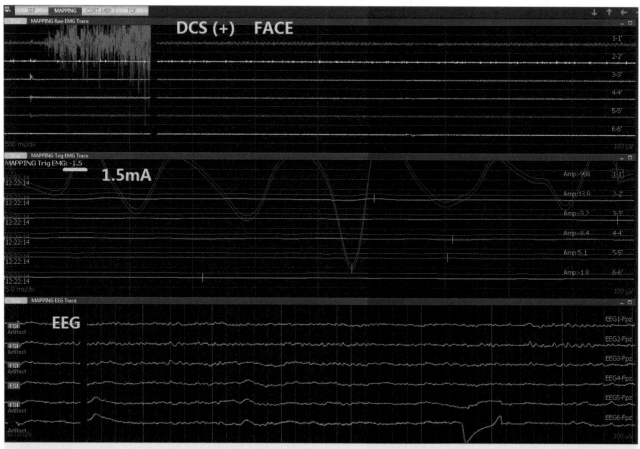

Fig. 12.6 Snapshot of direct cortical stimulation recording.

was the effective site of stimulation. Consequently, when precise demarcation of the motor homunculus is needed, monopolar stimulation is favored. Monopolar stimulation is preferred for initial mapping of functional brain regions because the number of trials needed corresponds to the number of electrodes, all of which act as anodes connected to the same cathode. In bipolar stimulation, the possibilities are much more with each contact possibly being an anode, cathode, or both. This is not practical in a real-life scenario since surgeons will have to take extended breaks during brain mapping. However, bipolar stimulation is preferred for prolonged monitoring during tumor surgeries due to the higher spatial resolution of DCS in comparison to transcranial stimulation. Each bipolar electrical stimulation is approximately 5 mm apart, such that when resecting subcortical regions near the functional area, the stimulation should be repeated frequently (2 mm per resected tumor).

The use of these stimulation methods extends beyond cortical stimulation, and is also applied for subcortical stimulation for identifying and localizing the corticospinal tract. Bipolar electrodes can map both subcortical motor and language pathways, whereas monopolar electrodes detect only motor pathways. The DsCS technique by bipolar electrodes involves repetitive stimuli of intensity 2 to 16 mA in increments of 1 mA and duration 1 ms at a rate of 60 Hz (▶ Fig. 12.7). For monopolar electrodes, the stimulus intensity is 5 mA with adjustments of 1 mA, duration of 0.5 second at a rate of 1 Hz, and train of five pulses (rate 250 pulse/second). The adjustment of 1 mA translates to a distance of approximately 1 mm during resection,

making the monopolar electrodes more suitable for subcortical stimulation.

The identified functional cortical areas, as well as the subcortical functional margin, are marked with sterile tags and recorded in MRI navigation. Following this, surgical incisions are performed to reach deep lesions. When excising close to the corticospinal tract (corticospinal tract [deep, rolandic and pre-rolandic lesions], internal capsule [insular lesions], cerebral peduncle [mesial temporal and insular lesions]), the DsCS stimulation parameters used are similar to that of DCS. DsCS also allows us to distinguish somatosensory pathways in the thalamic cortex that blunt patients' sensation during resection of intra-axial lesions. In addition to transient sensory disorders, stimulation of the central and posterior deep white matter can also cause motor control disorders. This may result from disruption of its connection with the primary motor function of the rolandic cortex.

12.4 Neuroanesthesia

An awake brain surgery is conducted without the use of general anesthesia and avoids the use of endotracheal intubation. Together with DCS, awake intraoperative mapping allows surgeons to elicit transient dysfunction of functional areas allowing their localization and preservation during tumor resection.[10,11,12] Awake DCS and DsCS has many advantages over brain function localization under general anesthesia. Awake mapping allows for (1) testing of more neurological

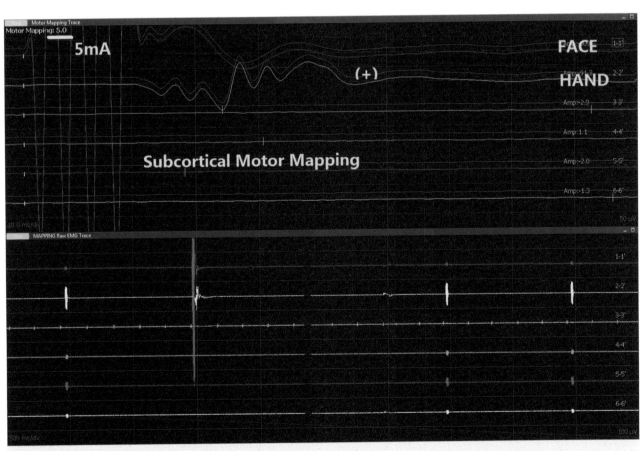

Fig. 12.7 Snapshot of direct subcortical electrical stimulation recording.

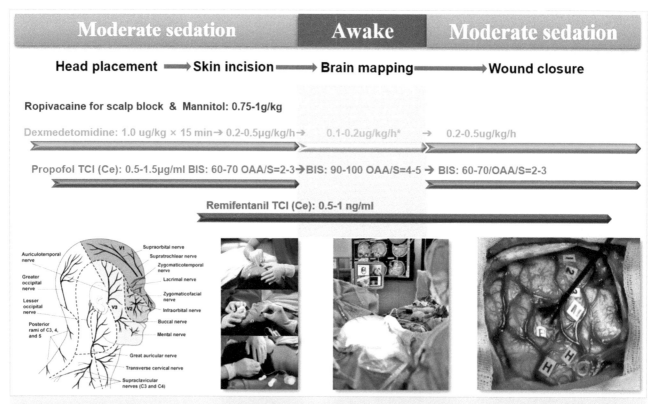

Fig. 12.8 Monitored anesthesia care approach for awake intraoperative mapping.

functions such as language, sensory, visual, and spatial awareness that require patients to be awake; (2) lower stimulating current intensity compared to general anesthesia, reducing the risk of intraoperative seizures and improving accuracy; (3) localizing functional auxiliary motor regions in the SMA and parietal cortex that can be tested when awake; and (4) monitoring advanced cognitive functions such as attention, judgment, computational power, and mental state.

The indications for awake mapping include age ≥ 14 years, dominant-sided and eloquent tumors, good patient communication, tolerance, and cooperation. Pediatric brain language networks are immature and plastic, and hence, awake brain stimulation is not recommended. Other contraindications include unstable mental status (anxiety), high intracranial pressure, sleep apnea syndrome, difficult airway, morbid obesity, and claustrophobia. For awake intraoperative mapping, a monitored anesthesia care (MAC) approach is used (▶ Fig. 12.8). The process and anesthetic regimen of MAC includes lidocaine/ropivacaine for scalp block, mannitol for brain relaxation/protection, controlled infusion of dexmedetomidine and propofol for sedation, and remifentanil for analgesia. The effects of different anesthetic drugs on MAC are summarized in ▶ Table 12.1.

12.5 Illustrative Case

We present the case of a 55-year-old man who came with sudden onset numbness for 4 months in his right limbs. Preoperative MRI revealed a nonenhancing lesion in the left insular lobe. Following craniotomy and dural opening, intraoperative awake

Table 12.1 Effect of inhaled and intravenous anesthetics on motor evoked potential

Anesthetic	MEP latency	MEP volatility
Desflurane	↑	↓
Enflurane	↑	↓
Halothane	↑	↓
Isoflurane	↑	↓
Sevoflurane	↑	↓
Laughing	↑ ↑	↓
Barbiturates	↑	N
Benzodiazepines	↑	↓
Opioids	↑	↓
Etomidate	N	↓
Propofol	N	↓
Ketamine	↑	↑
Dexmedetomidine	N	↓

Abbreviations: MEP, motor evoked potential; N, no detectable effect.

DCS was used to map motor and language areas. After identification of functional cortical areas, transcortical incisions were made in noneloquent cortical regions to access the underlying tumor through which the tumor was then carefully debulked. The first branch of the lenticulostriate artery marked the medial plane of dissection. Subcortical mapping combined with DTI tractography-based navigation was also performed to localize and preserve motor pathway. Intraoperative MRI evaluation showed residual tumor which was reinspected and resected. Pathological studies revealed grade II IDH-mutant astrocytoma. Gross total tumor resection was achieved, and the patient recovered without language or motor deficits (see **Video 12.1**).

For an additional case where a similar strategy was used, the paper *"Awake Brain Mapping in Dominant Side Insular Glioma Surgery: 2-Dimensional Operative Video"*[13] can be studied.

12.6 Conclusion

The critical location and need for maximal resection of cerebral gliomas, especially in the dominant hemisphere, rolandic, pre-rolandic, or insular cortex, pose a significant risk of irreversible postoperative motor and critical functional deficits. From our experience in complex glioma surgery and evidence in literature, awake brain mapping combined with a multimodal image-guided surgical approach offers best motor outcomes in neuro-oncological surgery.

References

[1] Zhang N, Yu Z, Hameed NUF, et al. *Long-term functional and oncological outcomes of glioma surgery with and without intraoperative neurophysiological monitoring: a retrospective cohort study in a single center. World Neurosurg. 2018; 119:e94–e105

[2] Delev D, Send K, Wagner J, et al. Epilepsy surgery of the Rolandic and immediate perirolandic cortex: surgical outcome and prognostic factors. Epilepsia. 2014; 55(10):1585–1593

[3] Qiu TM, Yan CG, Tang WJ, et al. Localizing hand motor area using resting-state fMRI: validated with direct cortical stimulation. Acta Neurochir (Wien). 2014; 156(12):2295–2302

[4] Qiu T-M, Gong FY, Gong X, et al. Real-time motor cortex mapping for the safe resection of glioma: an intraoperative resting-state fMRI study. AJNR Am J Neuroradiol. 2017; 38(11):2146–2152

[5] Lehtinen H, Mäkelä JP, Mäkelä T, et al. Language mapping with navigated transcranial magnetic stimulation in pediatric and adult patients undergoing epilepsy surgery: comparison with extraoperative direct cortical stimulation. Epilepsia Open. 2018; 3(2):224–235

[6] Garcia-Cossio E, Witkowski M, Robinson SE, Cohen LG, Birbaumer N, Soekadar SR. Simultaneous transcranial direct current stimulation (tDCS) and whole-head magnetoencephalography (MEG): assessing the impact of tDCS on slow cortical magnetic fields. Neuroimage. 2016; 140:33–40

[7] Zhu F-P, Wu JS, Song YY, et al. Clinical application of motor pathway mapping using diffusion tensor imaging tractography and intraoperative direct subcortical stimulation in cerebral glioma surgery: a prospective cohort study. Neurosurgery. 2012; 71(6):1170–1183, discussion 1183–1184

[8] Wood CC, Spencer DD, Allison T, McCarthy G, Williamson PD, Goff WR. Localization of human sensorimotor cortex during surgery by cortical surface recording of somatosensory evoked potentials. J Neurosurg. 1988; 68(1):99–111

[9] Bittar RG, Olivier A, Sadikot AF, Andermann F, Reutens DC. Cortical motor and somatosensory representation: effect of cerebral lesions. J Neurosurg. 2000; 92(2):242–248

[10] De Witt Hamer PC, Robles SG, Zwinderman AH, Duffau H, Berger MS. Impact of intraoperative stimulation brain mapping on glioma surgery outcome: a meta-analysis. J Clin Oncol. 2012; 30(20):2559–2565

[11] Duffau H, Capelle L, Sichez N, et al. Intraoperative mapping of the subcortical language pathways using direct stimulations. An anatomo-functional study. Brain. 2002; 125(Pt 1):199–214

[12] Sanai N, Martino J, Berger MS. Morbidity profile following aggressive resection of parietal lobe gliomas. J Neurosurg. 2012; 116(6):1182–1186

[13] Hameed NUF, Zhu Y, Qiu T, Wu J. Awake brain mapping in dominant side insular glioma surgery: 2-dimensional operative video. Oper Neurosurg (Hagerstown) 2018;15(4):477

13 Awake Subcortical Mapping of the Ventral and Dorsal Streams for Language

Hugues Duffau

Abstract

The aim of surgery for cerebral lesions is to optimize the extent of resection while preserving neural networks. In tumors within language structures, awake surgery with electrostimulation mapping and cognitive monitoring must be achieved with the goal to identify not only cortical epicenters but also white matter pathways critical for this complex function. This original concept consists of the exploration of the individual organization of language subnetworks mediating articulation, phonology, and semantics as well as their dynamic interaction in real time throughout the resection in awake patients. Such a paradigmatic shift, from classical image-based resection to function-based resection, has led to an increase of surgical indications for lesions involving language structures with a significant decrease in the rate of persistent aphasias and an optimization of the extent of resection. These results can be obtained only in a connectomal view of language processing that breaks with the traditional Broca–Wernicke's model. Surgical technique should be adapted to a dual-stream distribution of language, with a dorsal phonological route working in parallel with a ventral semantic route. The role of the so-called right nondominant hemisphere should be looked at again. Neurosurgeons have to better understand the networking organization of language and its interaction with nonverbal functions, opening the door to a huge potential of neuroplasticity, which makes large resections of lesions that were deemed inoperable feasible with an improvement in both functional and oncological outcomes. Nonetheless, this is possible only if one adopts the condition to preserve subcortical white matter pathways and deep gray nuclei underpinning the language connectome.

Keywords: awake surgery, direct electrical stimulation, language mapping, white matter tracts, extent of resection, function-based resection, quality of life

13.1 Introduction

The goal of brain lesion surgery is to maximize the extent of resection while preserving the quality of life. This is particularly true in neuro-oncology, since a greater extent of tumor removal is associated with a significant increase in overall survival for low-grade gliomas,[1,2] high-grade gliomas,[3,4] and/or metastases.[5] It has been proposed to achieve supratotal resection, that is, to take a margin around the signal abnormality visible on magnetic resonance imaging (MRI), both in diffuse low-grade glioma[6] and glioblastoma,[7] in order to improve the oncological outcomes.

To optimize the oncofunctional balance, the principle is to switch from a traditional image-guided resection to a mapping-based resection performed up to the individual functional boundaries, both at cortical and subcortical levels. When the lesion is located near or within eloquent structures, such as

structures critical for language, awake surgery is mandatory to identify and preserve not only the cortical hubs but also the white matter tracts underpinning neural networks. Intraoperative direct electrical stimulation (DES) mapping combined with real-time cognitive monitoring throughout the resection is the sole method for allowing the detection of the subcortical pathways essential for brain functions.[8]

Here, the purpose is to detail how cortical and axonal DES participated in improving our knowledge regarding the subnetworks mediating language as well as their dynamic interactions: such a better understanding of language connectome resulted in an improvement of the benefit-to-risk ratio of surgery for lesions involving this complex circuitry, on the condition to adapt the surgical technique accordingly.

13.2 Illustrative Case

This case is about a 25-year-old right-handed man who experienced seizures. The neurological examination was normal, but the neurocognitive assessment revealed slight disorders of verbal working memory. The MRI demonstrated an imaging typical for a diffuse low-grade glioma (despite a small enhancement in the middle of the tumor) invading the posterior part of the left inferior frontal gyrus and the lateral part of the Rolandic operculum (▶ Fig. 13.1). Awake surgery was performed with intraoperative DES mapping. Cortically, the ventral premotor cortex (inducing speech arrest when stimulated) and the primary cortex of the face (eliciting involuntary face movement with dysarthria during stimulation) were identified and preserved as the posterior limit of the resection. Of note, the so-called Broca area did not generate any disturbances when stimulated. Glioma removal was achieved according to functional boundaries, as well as at the subcortical level. Indeed, axonal DES at the end of resection allowed the detection of the anterior part of the dorsal route (causing articulatory troubles) as well as the frontal part of the ventral route (inducing semantic paraphasias). A complete resection was achieved, as shown by the postoperative MRI, and the patient improved his neuropsychological scores after surgery in comparison with the preoperative scores, especially concerning verbal working memory, thanks to postsurgical cognitive rehabilitation.

13.3 Evidence-based Clinical Decisions

A recent review of the literature confirmed that maximal safe resection is the first therapeutic option in glioma patients,[9] as already recommended by the current guidelines.[10]

Beyond the oncological considerations, preoperative functional neuroimaging is not reliable enough at the individual level for language mapping. While allowing a noninvasive mapping of the entire brain, functional MRI (fMRI) and diffusion

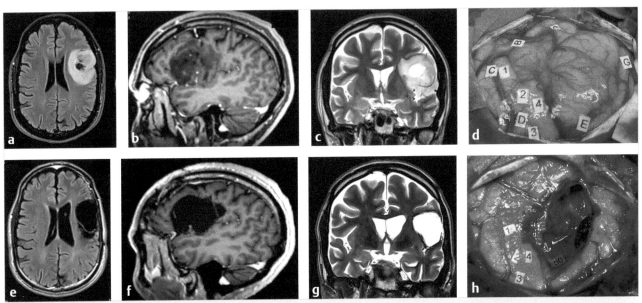

Fig. 13.1 Preoperative axial fluid-attenuated inversion recovery (FLAIR)-weighted (**a**), sagittal enhanced T1-weighted (**b**) and coronal T2-weighted (**c**) magnetic resonance imaging (MRI) in a 25-year-old right-handed man who presented with partial seizures, revealing a left frontoinsular low-grade glioma involving the so-called Broca area. The neurological exam was normal but the neurocognitive assessment found deficits in verbal working memory. Intraoperative view before resection in this awake patient (**d**). The anterior part of the left hemisphere is on the right and its posterior part is on the left. Letter tags correspond to the tumor limits identified using ultrasonography. Number tags show zones of positive DES mapping as follows: 1 and 2, ventral premotor cortex (evoking speech arrest); 3 and 4, primary motor cortex of the face. Preoperative axial FLAIR-weighted (**e**), sagittal enhanced T1-weighted (**f**), and coronal T2-weighted (**g**) MRI demonstrating a complete resection, including the Broca area. Intraoperative view after resection (**h**). At the cortical level, the eloquent sites detected before resection have been preserved. Moreover, DES of white matter tracts allowed the detection of the anterior part of the superior longitudinal fasciculus (eliciting articulatory disorders, tag 9) and of the ventral stream subserved by the inferior fronto-occipital fasciculus (eliciting semantic paraphasias, tag 50). Therefore, surgical resection was achieved according to functional boundaries (language pathways) and not on the basis of the preoperative MRI. The patient resumed a normal familial, social, and professional life within 3 months following surgery, with no functional deficits (no neurological, no seizures), and even had an improvement in his neuropsychological assessment after postsurgical cognitive rehabilitation.

tensor imaging cannot be used in clinical practice for surgical selection and planning, because they do not provide a direct reflection of the real neural functions but only a very indirect approximation of brain processing based upon biomathematic reconstructions. At the cortical level, correlation between preoperative language fMRI and intraoperative DES revealed that fMRI sensitivity and specificity were only 37.1 and 83.4%, respectively.[11] An open international tractography challenge including 20 research groups demonstrated that algorithms produce tractograms which contain many more invalid than valid bundles, and that half of these invalid bundles occur systematically across research groups.[12]

By contrast, a meta-analysis of the literature examining over 8,000 patients who underwent excision for low-grade or high-grade gliomas evidenced that the use of intraoperative DES led to a significant decrease of postoperative permanent worsening, while the rate of surgical selection for tumors involving eloquent structures, especially language, increased. The extent of resection was also improved.[13] This is in agreement with a large series using awake mapping that reported less than 2% risk of severe persistent deficit.[14,15]

In summary, the current literature supports early and radical resection under the guidance of intraoperative DES mapping for brain tumors.

13.4 Surgical Technique

Even if anatomical landmarks are important for brain surgery, they are not sufficient. DES is nowadays the sole technique that permits the detection and preservation of the corticosubcortical circuits critical for neural functions, especially for language, executive functions, and emotion.[8] The goal is to perform real-time structural-functional correlations in an awake patient by means of DES which mimics a focal and transitory virtual lesion, in order to obtain an individual mapping of the cortex and white matter tracts. This enables one to check if a cerebral structure infiltrated by a tumor is still functionally essential—what is frequently observed in diffuse glioma, particularly in the peripheral and deep part of the neoplasm. The principle is that DES of eloquent structures causes a transient disruption of the tasks performed by the patient with normalization of function as soon as the stimulation is stopped and that this area (which is only a part of a more complex neural circuit) must be preserved. DES is an easy, reliable, reproducible, safe and inexpensive method of brain mapping.[12,14,16]

From a technical point of view, a positive cortical mapping has to be obtained prior to the resection in order to tailor it according to the organization of the neural networks, in this given patient at this moment.[17] In studies which advocate for negative mapping, up to 9% of new permanent language worsening have been generated, illustrating that such negative mapping paradigms cannot guarantee the lack of critical structures and cannot prevent persistent deteriorations in all cases.[15,18,19] A wider bone flap is thus recommended in order to elicit functional responses in a systematic manner before starting the tumor removal: this is possible by exposing at least the ventral premotor cortex which induces articulatory disturbances in all cases when stimulated, including in the right hemisphere.[20] In other words, "minimal invasive neurosurgery" does not mean "minimal bone flap size," it means "minimal morbidity."

A bipolar electrode with a 5-mm space between the tips and delivering a biphasic current (pulse frequency 60 Hz, single pulse phase duration 1 millisecond) is directly applied to the brain. When using low intensity of electrical current (e.g., 1.5 to 3 mA), electrocorticography is not mandatory to obtain a positive mapping and to decrease the risk of intrasurgical seizures: this risk is less than 3% in a prospective series without electrocorticography based upon 374 supratentorial brain lesions, with no aborted awake surgeries.[14] The duration of each stimulation is 1 to 4 seconds. No site is stimulated twice in succession to avoid seizures. Each cortical site (size 5 × 5 mm, due to the spatial resolution of the probe) of the entire cortex exposed by the bone flap should be tested three times. Indeed, three trials are sufficient to assure if a cortical site is functionally critical. The patient is never informed when the brain is stimulated. Furthermore, since the subcortical connectivity is the main limitation of the neuroplastic potential,[21] it is crucial to spare the white matter fibers to avoid persistent neurological deteriorations. In order to map and preserve these pathways that underly the brain connectome, such tracts must be detected using subcortical DES throughout the resection.[8] The stimulation parameters are the same as those used at the cortical level.

Beyond DES mapping, real-time cognitive monitoring also needs to be achieved in awake patients, regardless of the hemisphere, to confirm that no neurological and/or neuropsychological disturbances are generated by the resection.[20,22] A strong collaboration is critical between the patient, neurosurgeon, and speech therapist/neuropsychologist in the operating theater. Of note, the current dogma is to perform awake surgery to map and monitor language in the "left dominant" hemisphere, but to achieve resection under general anesthesia (possibly with motor mapping) in the "right nondominant" hemisphere. Nonetheless, when accurate neuropsychological examinations are performed, they often reveal cognitive and behavioral disturbances after surgery, even in the right hemisphere. Consequently, to preserve an optimal quality of life, awake surgery with cortical and axonal DES mapping should also be considered more systematically for removal of right-sided tumors. Right hemisphere plays a key role in movement execution and control, visual processes and spatial cognition, language and nonverbal semantic processing, executive functions (e.g., attention or working memory), and social cognition (mentalizing and emotion recognition).[20] In all cases, objective neurocognitive assessment must be performed before and after each surgery.

To sum up, the original concept is to disconnect the part of the brain infiltrated by the tumor according to functional boundaries detected from the beginning of the resection, and not to debulk the neoplasm from inside to outside. Since eloquent areas may be located within the glioma, the traditional surgical principle of debulking tumor from inside is not safe, especially in diffuse low-grade gliomas. Moreover, if one comes closer to the functional structures (especially the subcortical bundles) only at the end of the resection, the patient will be less cooperative. By contrast, once the invaded parenchyma has been disconnected up to eloquent limits provided by the individual mapping, it can be excised under general anesthesia during the last stage of the surgical procedure, since the real-time feedback of the patient is not needed anymore.[17]

13.5 Complication Avoidance

To prevent postoperative persistent deficits, neurosurgeons should evolve toward a "connectomal surgery," based on the mapping of the eloquent subnetworks and their dynamic interactions, as well as on the use of the individual neuroplastic potential.[16] Because tumors often involve language pathways, the neural basis underlying this complex function must be better understood, especially thanks to original data issues from DES. Schematically, the language connectome is mediated by a dual route, including a ventral semantic pathway devoted to mapping visual information to meaning (the "what" stream), and a dorsal phonological pathway involved in mapping visual information to articulation through visuophonological conversion.[23] From an anatomic perspective, the ventral route is subserved by a direct subcircuit represented by the inferior fronto-occipital fasciculus (IFOF), and by a parallel indirect subpathway itself constituted by the anterior part of the inferior longitudinal fasciculus, which links the posterior occipitotemporal region and the temporal pole, then relayed by the uncinate fasciculus which connects the temporal pole to the orbitofrontal regions. Similarly, the dorsal route is underpinned by two parallel subpathways: the arcuate fascicle and, more laterally, the lateral part of the superior longitudinal fasciculus (SLF). From a functional point of view, DES of the IFOF generates semantic paraphasia, while stimulation of the indirect ventral pathway causes lexical access disorders (such as anomia). DES of the arcuate fasciculus elicited conduction aphasia (i.e., phonemic paraphasia and repetition disturbances), while stimulation of the lateral SLF results in articulatory deficits. In addition, preservation of the deep gray nuclei (eliciting perseveration or anarthria when stimulating the head of the caudate or the lentiform nucleus, respectively) is crucial. Therefore, these new data resulted in a reexamination of language organization, from the traditional Broca–Wernicke localizationist model to a connectomal account based upon multiple direct and indirect cortico-subcortical interconnected subcircuits implied in phonological, articulatory, and semantic processes.[23]

However, language mapping is not enough to avoid complications. As already mentioned, DES should also be used throughout the resection to detect and spare the connectivity sustaining sensorimotor functions, visuospatial processing (to prevent the onset of visual field deficit or hemineglect), executive functions, and emotional processing. Moreover, the integration of those subfunctions is necessary to allow a normal behavior, based on the preservation of multimodal semantic processes as well as different levels of consciousness (especially self-awareness and consciousness of environment).[8]

In conclusion, although the brain has a considerable potential of neuroplasticity, partly generated by the tumor itself (especially in slow-growing lesion such as low-grade glioma), there are also limitations that should be taken in consideration to avoid postsurgical deterioration. These limitations are mainly represented by the input (as the visual cortex), the output (as the primary motor cortex), and the subcortical structures, which must be surgically preserved. Thus, when a resection cannot be completed for functional reasons, it is also possible to facilitate neural reorganization, thanks to postoperative rehabilitation, and to consider a subsequent surgery after remapping that may enable an increase in the extent of resection while preserving quality of life.[24]

Finally, beyond functional mapping, another cornerstone in glioma surgery is to preserve the entire vascularization (both arteries and veins) by performing subpial dissection and minimizing the use of coagulation.[17]

13.6 Conclusion

DES mapping has contributed in challenging the traditional fixed and modular model of the central nervous system, by revealing a dynamic organization based on parallel and interactive large-scale subnetworks. Such better understanding of the cerebral connectivity has resulted in redefining the surgical anatomy of the brain, which is particularly helpful for tumor removal. Resecting a part of the parenchyma invaded by diffuse glioma cells until functional boundaries have been encountered in an awake patient allows the emergence of a "connectomal neurosurgery." This original concept permits an improvement of the oncofunctional balance in brain tumor patients, with a longer survival and a better quality of life.

References

[1] Jakola AS, Myrmel KS, Kloster R, et al. Comparison of a strategy favoring early surgical resection vs a strategy favoring watchful waiting in low-grade gliomas. JAMA. 2012; 308(18):1881–1888

[2] Capelle L, Fontaine D, Mandonnet E, et al. Spontaneous and therapeutic prognostic factors in adult hemispheric WHO grade II gliomas: a series of 1097 cases. J Neurosurg. 2013; 118:1157–1168

[3] Sanai N, Polley MY, McDermott MW, Parsa AT, Berger MS. An extent of resection threshold for newly diagnosed glioblastomas. J Neurosurg. 2011; 115(1): 3–8

[4] Chaichana KL, Jusue-Torres I, Navarro-Ramirez R, et al. Establishing percent resection and residual volume thresholds affecting survival and recurrence for patients with newly diagnosed intracranial glioblastoma. Neuro-oncol. 2014; 16(1):113–122

[5] Kamp MA, Rapp M, Slotty PJ, et al. Incidence of local in-brain progression after supramarginal resection of cerebral metastases. Acta Neurochir (Wien). 2015; 157(6):905–910, discussion 910–911

[6] Duffau H. Long-term outcomes after supratotal resection of diffuse low-grade gliomas: a consecutive series with 11-year follow-up. Acta Neurochir (Wien). 2016; 158(1):51–58

[7] Li YM, Suki D, Hess K, Sawaya R. The influence of maximum safe resection of glioblastoma on survival in 1229 patients: Can we do better than gross-total resection? J Neurosurg. 2016; 124(4):977–988

[8] Duffau H. Stimulation mapping of white matter tracts to study brain functional connectivity. Nat Rev Neurol. 2015; 11(5):255–265

[9] Sanai N, Berger MS. Surgical oncology for gliomas: the state of the art. Nat Rev Clin Oncol. 2018; 15(2):112–125

[10] Weller M, van den Bent M, Tonn JC, et al. European Association for Neuro-Oncology (EANO) Task Force on Gliomas. European Association for Neuro-Oncology (EANO) guideline on the diagnosis and treatment of adult astrocytic and oligodendroglial gliomas. Lancet Oncol. 2017; 18(6):e315–e329

[11] Kuchcinski G, Mellerio C, Pallud J, et al. Three-tesla functional MR language mapping: comparison with direct cortical stimulation in gliomas. Neurology. 2015; 84(6):560–568

[12] Maier-Hein KH, Neher PF, Houde JC, et al. The challenge of mapping the human connectome based on diffusion tractography. Nat Commun. 2017; 8 (1):1349

[13] De Witt Hamer PC, Robles SG, Zwinderman AH, Duffau H, Berger MS. Impact of intraoperative stimulation brain mapping on glioma surgery outcome: a meta-analysis. J Clin Oncol. 2012; 30(20):2559–2565

[14] Boetto J, Bertram L, Moulinié G, Herbet G, Moritz-Gasser S, Duffau H. Low rate of intraoperative seizures during awake craniotomy in a prospective cohort with 374 supratentorial brain lesions: electrocorticography is not mandatory. World Neurosurg. 2015; 84(6):1838–1844

[15] Sanai N, Mirzadeh Z, Berger MS. Functional outcome after language mapping for glioma resection. N Engl J Med. 2008; 358(1):18–27

[16] Duffau H. Mapping the connectome in awake surgery for gliomas: an update. J Neurosurg Sci. 2017; 61(6):612–630

[17] Duffau H. A new concept of diffuse (low-grade) glioma surgery. Adv Tech Stand Neurosurg. 2012; 38:3–27

[18] Serletis D, Bernstein M. Prospective study of awake craniotomy used routinely and nonselectively for supratentorial tumors. J Neurosurg. 2007; 107 (1):1–6

[19] Kim SS, McCutcheon IE, Suki D, et al. Awake craniotomy for brain tumors near eloquent cortex: correlation of intraoperative cortical mapping with neurological outcomes in 309 consecutive patients. Neurosurgery. 2009; 64(5): 836–845, discussion 345–346

[20] Vilasboas T, Herbet G, Duffau H. Challenging the myth of right "non-dominant" hemisphere: lessons from cortico-subcortical stimulation mapping in awake surgery and surgical implications. World Neurosurg. 2017; 103:449–456

[21] Herbet G, Maheu M, Costi E, Lafargue G, Duffau H. Mapping neuroplastic potential in brain-damaged patients. Brain. 2016; 139(Pt 3):829–844

[22] Fernández Coello A, Moritz-Gasser S, Martino J, Martinoni M, Matsuda R, Duffau H. Selection of intraoperative tasks for awake mapping based on relationships between tumor location and functional networks. J Neurosurg. 2013; 119(6):1380–1394

[23] Duffau H, Moritz-Gasser S, Mandonnet E. A re-examination of neural basis of language processing: proposal of a dynamic hodotopical model from data provided by brain stimulation mapping during picture naming. Brain Lang. 2014; 131:1–10

[24] Picart T, Herbet G, Moritz-Gasser S, Duffau H. Iterative surgical resections of diffuse glioma with awake mapping: how to deal with cortical plasticity and connectomal constraints? Neurosurgery. 201 9; 85(1):105–116

14 Surgery Around the Command and Control Axis: The Default Mode, Control, and Frontal Aslant Systems

Michael E. Sughrue

Abstract

The initiation axis is a novel concept in neurosurgical anatomy which is based on the idea that some part of the brain needs to give the "start" signal for goal-directed action to occur. This chapter describes this anatomy and discusses methods for avoiding injury to the initiation axis during brain surgery.

Keywords: default mode network, salience network, abulia, frontal aslant tract

14.1 Introduction

For a long time, the frontal lobe has been a synonym for "safe" in neurosurgery. In most surgical management schemes, the "eloquent areas" are principally the motor strip, the language areas, and perhaps the supplementary motor area (SMA). The term "eloquent" is a principal term in the neurosurgical community that refers to areas of the brain which when transgressed cause a visible observable deficit, usually one that can easily be described by a nonexpert, for example, the inability to talk or move one's arm. In this paradigm, our only mandate is to avoid destroying these areas, and we theoretically have carte blanche to do whatever with the rest of the largest lobe in the human brain.

Of late, this paradigm is being challenged by a growing voice, as it is unlikely that the lobe evolved to absorb cerebrospinal fluid, and all parts of the brain are doing something. Certainly, we know this from neuropsychology, as frontal lobe syndromes are reproducible, roughly localizable to gross areas of the frontal lobe, and debilitating, and the functional imaging community has been arguing this for some time. In this paradigm, we should respect all parts of the brain as if they were the motor cortex.

I will argue that uncritically applying either strategy is ridiculous and deprives patients of an ideal approach. While neither deficit is ideal, reducing an adult patient to a child is hardly better than paralyzing the hand, and in many ways, it leaves a less functional patient: some people with motor deficits can hold jobs as compared to patients with severely impaired judgment. At the same time, conventional wisdom is not entirely baseless, and the frontal lobe clearly has more redundancy, bilaterality, and plasticity than the primary motor cortex in many people, and approaching malignant cancers in the frontal lobe overly cautiously to "save function" frequently ends in saving neither the function nor the patient. A key problem in balancing our goals is very limited knowledge we have about how the frontal lobe works and how to do rational surgery there.

It is beyond any question that the medial frontal lobe can punish an unwary neurosurgeon, often in ways which are hard to nail down using 5-point scales, but which damage the patient's quality of life in profound ways. Again, a patient who can talk, but rarely speaks or initiates any activities is almost certainly less functional than the one who struggles to find words. A patient with a paralyzed arm is easier to rehabilitate than one who merely stares blankly into space.

This chapter addresses the command and control axis of the frontal lobe which summarizes the parts of the lobe that initiate behaviors and transmit intentions to areas that can act on them. This axis comprises several interconnected large-scale functional networks that have been found to play key roles in these processes and, which I am increasingly convinced, underlie many of the clinical syndromes we see with surgery or around in the medial frontal lobe; these syndromes can often be overlooked if you limit your assessments to "moving all four extremities," but families do notice these as such syndromes have often more profound implications. Knowing the exact anatomy of these areas can and should alter your surgical plan, as it is probable that many syndromes which we have long accepted as inevitable consequences of certain operations can be avoided in many people with better knowledge of anatomy, especially connectomics.

14.2 The Command and Control Axis Defined

We take it as a given that there is a system of places in the brain that makes the decisions, such as one is thirsty, and translates them into a series of actions starting from reaching for a glass of water and putting it to the mouth to drink it. While hypothalamic, motor planning, visual, somatosensory, attention, and executive systems all are part of this series of events, it is self-evident that some part of the brain needs to say "Go," or in other words, needs to tell to stop one task and start another. Given that a large percentage of problems with initiation and motivation occur, in clinical neurology, due to medial frontal damage, it also seems self-evident that at least some of the key machinery for initiation and motivation is located in the medial frontal lobe. Given that much of the experience with akinetic and abulic problems have come from stroke, trauma, and surgical manipulation, such as with the anterior interhemispheric approaches which are for imprecise lesions, we have long had a poor understanding of this problem and how to avoid it.

This is not entirely understood by anyone at present, but a large body of evidence supports the idea that a coordinated interplay of three large-scale cerebral networks—the default mode network (DMN), the central executive or control network (CTRL), and the salience network—is strongly linked with the process of transitioning from internal to external mental states, and several related behaviors such as goal-directed behavior versus mind wandering. The proximity of these networks to the SMA and specific clinical observations related to the nature of syndromes from these areas raise the possibility that this is an axis needed to get actions going, and that the consequences for disrupting this axis are some form of failure to start an action or the lack of motivation to do so. In some ways, this is an axis similar to the visual pathway where lesions in different places lead to different variants on the same basic issue, though obviously initiation is a subtler problem which is harder to definitively identify than a field cut. The subsequent text provides some summary about what is known about these networks, our work defining the anatomy of these networks as precisely as possible which will provide some ideas of how they exactly interconnect with each other, and eventually insights into how to make good decisions regarding appropriate surgery for gliomas in these parts of the brain. We will start with the key large-scale functional networks and then segue into a discussion about the frontal aslant tract (FAT) which contains the SMA and salience network interconnections.

14.3 The Large-Scale Functional Networks

The DMN was first noted by Marcus Raichle and colleagues in 2001, when they noted areas in the anteromedial frontal lobe, the posterior cingulate cortex (PCC), and the lateral parietal lobe that were activated only in the task-negative state. Since then, thousands of reports confirm these areas to activate on correlated time courses (thus forming a functional network), and to anticorrelate with several other networks involved in performing externally directed goals, notably the CTRL network. The DMN is probably the most consistently identifiable network in the brain that is involved in numerous complex cognitive abilities, such as speech, theory of mind, and memory, among others.

▶ Fig. 14.1 provides a simple schematic of DMN–CTRL interactions. The salience network is a third network which appears to be the key in this transition. Failure to alternate these networks has been found in minimally conscious and vegetative patients, and it has been shown to be impaired in schizophrenics with severe negative symptoms. Thus, it seems reasonable to hypothesize that disruption of this system might impair patients' ability to organize their thoughts, create a plan, and transition toward executing the plan, though obviously this is a complex process.

14.3.1 Network Anatomy

The Human Connectome Project (HCP) recently published their scheme for parcellating the human neocortex based on functional connectivity and physical characteristics. ▶ Fig. 14.2 provides an example of the scheme which we have heavily utilized to describe brain connectivity in ways which can be compared, reproduced, and utilized by surgeons. Next we describe the anatomy of the large-scale functional networks in HCP parcellation format, based on coordinate based meta-analysis, combined with diffusion spectrum tractography to provide the best possible anatomic model for these networks, given existing technology. There is extreme interindividual variability in the human cortex, and gliomas can cause functional reorganization, so these models are merely the starting point in the discussion, but a key starting point compared to a previous lack of knowledge of these areas.

14.3.2 Default Mode Network

The DMN is classically a three-part system with hubs anteromedial frontal lobe, PCC, and angular gyrus. Careful study shows this is not entirely adequate, as parts of the middle temporal gyrus, the thalamus, and the hippocampus also strongly correlate with these regions in many datasets. ▶ Fig. 14.3 shows our model of the DMN. The anterior frontal regions include areas a24, s32, p32, and 10r. PCC areas include areas 31a, 31pd, 31pv, d23ab, v23ab, 7m, POS1, POS2, and the retrosplenial cortex (RSC). The lateral parietal regions include PFm, PGs, and PGi. The anterior frontal and PCC areas are clearly joined by the cingulum. We have found no evidence of direct white matter connection of the lateral parietal regions and the medial regions, and this suggests that the network is functionally constructed by the thalamocortical rhythms or by interplay with other neighboring areas (see below).

14.3.3 Central Executive Network

The CTRL is basically a frontopolar and parietal network (▶ Fig. 14.4). At present, we think this likely involves connections between HCP areas, prefrontal areas 9a, 9p, 9–46d, a9–46v,

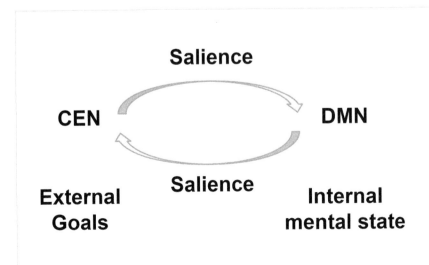

Fig. 14.1 A schematic diagram demonstrating the interactions between the default mode, salience, and central executive networks.

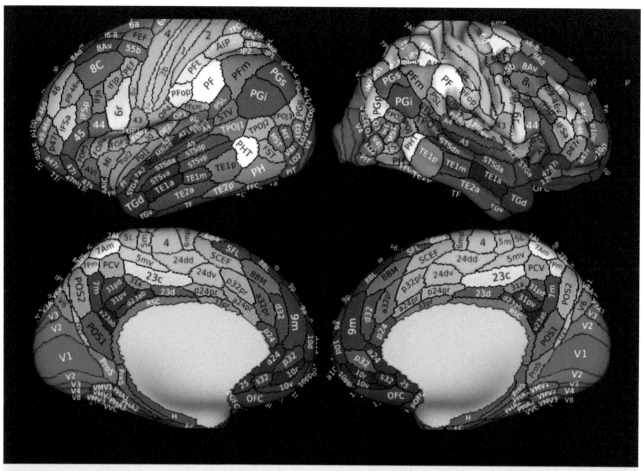

Fig. 14.2 Image demonstrating the cortical parcellation scheme based on data from the Human Connectome Project.

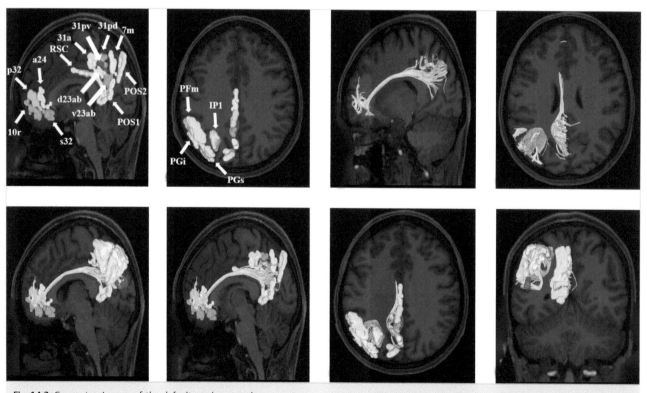

Fig. 14.3 Connectomic map of the default mode network.

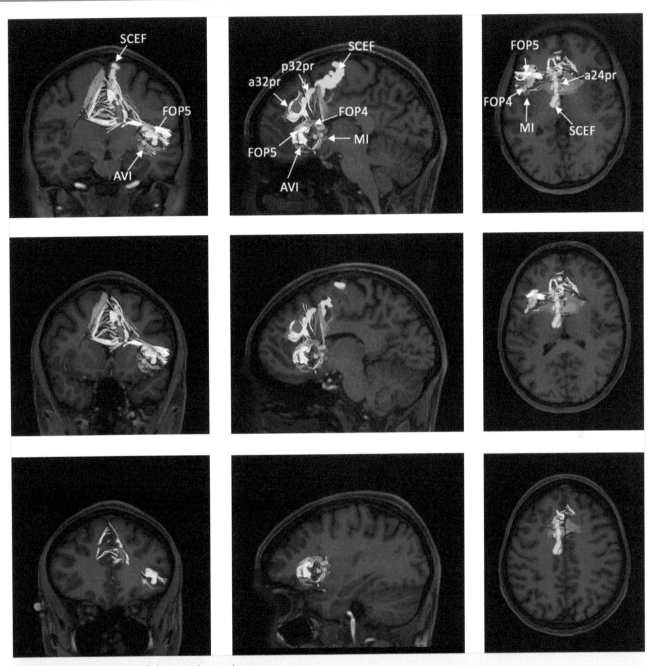

Fig. 14.4 Connectomic map of the control network.

46, polar areas a10p, p10p, and inferior frontal sulcus areas IFSa, and IFSp with the parietal areas Pft and PF, opercular area OP4, and intraparietal sulcus areas AIP, IP1, and IP2. These areas are probably linked by the superior longitudinal fasciculus (SLF).

14.3.4 Salience Network

The salience network (▶ Fig. 14.5) is a middle cingulate and anterior insula network. Its middle cingulate structure includes areas a32prime, p32prime, and supplementary and cingulate eye field (SCEF) and its insular regions include anterior ventral insula (AVI), middle insula (MI), and the frontal opercular areas FOP4 and FOP5. These are linked via the FAT. Most interestingly, the SCEF is also a part of the SMA complex, providing a critical

link between the large-scale networks and the motor planning system.

14.3.5 Supplementary Motor Area

These areas in the medial bank of the posterior superior frontal gyrus (SFG) include areas 6ma, 6mp, SCEF, and superior frontal language (SFL) area (▶ Fig. 14.6). In addition to its immediate neighbors, the SMA connects to the contralateral SMA via the corpus callosum, the ipsilateral premotor, opercular, and insular areas via the FAT, the contralateral premotor areas via the crossed FAT which runs in the middle callosum, as well as contributing to fibers entering the basal ganglia and corticospinal tract. Interestingly, direct connections to the primary motor

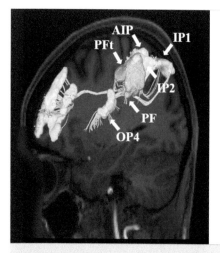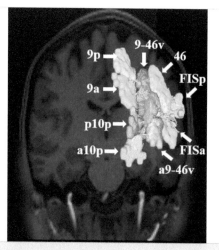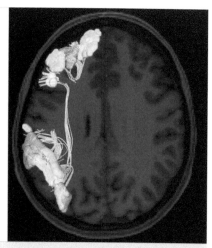

Fig. 14.5 Connectomic map of the salience network.

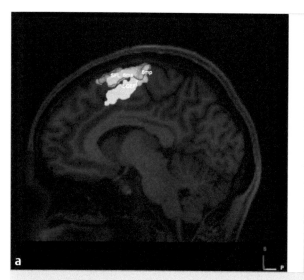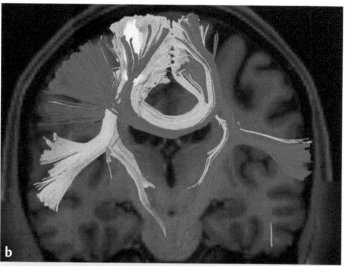

Fig. 14.6 (a) Connectomic map of the supplementary motor area (SMA), (b) tractography of the SMA region showing the connections of each SMA in different colors. Note that recovery from SMA syndrome probably requires these bilateral connections.

cortex are surprisingly sparse. The fact that the SMA contains a connection between the SFL area and the canonical Broca regions, such as area 44, is a likely mechanism behind the mutism component of SMA syndrome.

14.4 How to Operate Around the Command and Control System

Whatever illusions you have about your ability to "stay within the tumor," during glioma surgery, you are cutting neurons somewhere or you are severely subtotally resecting the tumor, if for no other reason than the infiltrative nature of the boundary of gliomas. Thus, I have found that it is best to think of resecting a glioma in terms of a set of disconnections, with the goal being to minimize unnecessary destruction of salvageable networks (note that not all networks are salvageable especially with high-grade gliomas). Intraoperative use of tractography,

while not accurate enough to follow blindly, is extremely helpful for structuring your plan about how to cut around the brain networks—without it, there are no landmarks to structure your maneuvers in the subcortical white matter.

14.4.1 The Fundamental Division Cuts of the Posteromedial Frontal Lobe

The Motor System and FAT

The motor system is best considered as having semblance to a bouquet of flowers: somewhat conical and widening near the top of the branching (▶ Fig. 14.7). Most of our cuts in previous chapters addressed protecting this system by cutting parallel to these fibers with cuts in the coronal plane paralleling the precentral or postcentral sulci, which maintain the cortical motor networks and their connections with the cerebellum, basal ganglia, thalamus, and spinal cord.

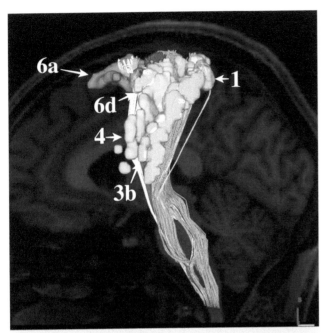

Fig. 14.7 Tractography map of the sensorimotor and motor planning system. Note that it is has a bouquet shape, and safe cuts are usually in the coronal plane.

Preservation of the FAT, in my experience, has largely eliminated the SMA syndrome from my glioma practice. Again, this is not surprising given what it is connecting. This generally involves a coronal cut also, similar to the motor cortex. I have found that a coronal cut beginning from the opercular areas and ending in the frontal horn can be safely made, provided that the FAT is respected.

If you think about all maneuvers in the posterior frontal lobe as respecting a coronal plane including the FAT and the head of caudate, you will seldom cause unexpected motor deficits.

Moreover, in my experience if you transgress both the mid-callosum and the SMA region, the SMA syndrome does not recover. Consider the crossed FAT in your surgical planning (▶ Fig. 14.8).

Cuts with the Cingulate

The callosal fibers make a bend around the cingulum bundle as they connect mostly analogous parts of the parasagittal brain, that is, SFG to SFG, paracentral lobule to paracentral lobule, etc. This important fact suggests that it is possible to preserve the cingulate system while removing the corpus callosum. This should not be surprising given that we have been safely cutting this for years and have been entering the frontal horn transcortically (which cuts the forceps minor).

It is important to note that anterior callosum tumors are really frontal tumors which involve the callosum and should be taken out through the middle frontal gyrus, which both addresses the tumor and avoids the DMN and salience systems. This means you usually find the cingulate from its deep surface. In addition to using the cingulate sulcus as a key landmark, intraoperative mapping tells you when you need to deviate laterally to avoid cutting the cingulum bundle on your way to the

ventricle. Thus, the cut with the cingulum is a sagittal cut and the deviations needed to avoid it are movements of this sagittal plane in response to changes in the patient.

14.5 How Do You Test the "Command and Control" System in Surgery?

One reason this system is poorly understood in neurosurgery is that it is relatively hard to access it. The medial frontal lobe is not usually very easy to visualize and you are working on it from the white matter side, at least in our surgeries. More importantly, it lacks an easy sign which can be elicited by direct electrical stimulation telling you that this is the place.

Intraoperative testing in these tumors is basically continuous monitoring of alertness and concentration. This is challenging testing which requires a dedicated and experienced intraoperative tester, as the problems can be subtle; the patients frequently have some impairment at baseline, and almost everyone has worse concentration with their brain open and some anesthetic in their blood.

The ideal testing paradigm is some combination of multimodality test requiring focus. We have had patients sew, assemble auto parts, play musical instruments, etc. If nothing unique is available, placing pegs in and out of a grooved pegboard is usually possible (see **Video 14.1**). More impaired patients may have to merely perform a simple task which tells us we are not making them worse. Ideally, they will name objects at the same time, but usually only high-functioning patients can do this.

The video demonstrates two forms of failures that we usually see as we approach the cingulate. One is freezing which often involves dropping the object. The other is a lack of attention to task. In both cases, the best thing to do is to stop and let the patient recover and then deviate your resection laterally.

14.6 Specific Techniques and Strategies for Tumors Near the Command and Control Axis

14.6.1 Medial Frontal Tumors

Medial frontal tumors threaten function on their posterior edge which abuts the motor planning system and FAT, and medially where they abut the DMN and salience networks as well as their connections to the SMA.

It is helpful to view surgery in this region as making an "L"-shaped cut that separates the tumor from the motor system and SMA/FAT network posteriorly, the SLF and parts of inferior fronto-occipital fasciculus laterally, eventually ending in the frontal horn of the lateral ventricle.

The lateral limb of this cut is always done first, typically with an arm/naming double task. This is because the posterior cut can lead to abulia or mutism which can prevent you from monitoring other areas like language networks or cingulate areas.

The posterior cut often involves a switch to motor-based tasks, especially ones which require concentration as these can be used to protect the SMA/FAT and the medial networks such

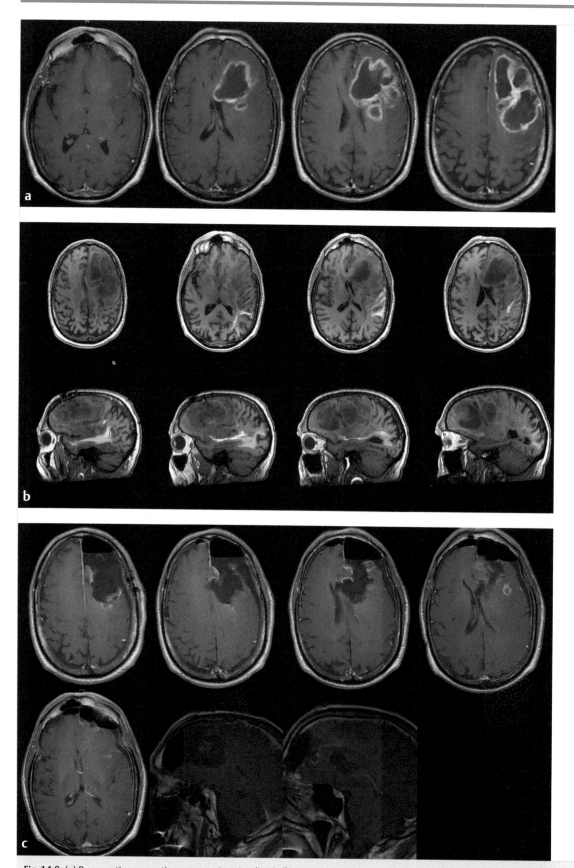

Fig. 14.8 (**a**) Preoperative magnetic resonance imaging (MRI), (**b**) preoperative diffusion tensor imaging tractography, and (**c**) postoperative MRI from a medial frontal glioma case described in the text.

as the DMN. I start by finding the midline and continue the cut down to the falx. This allows me to find the cingulate sulcus, which is where I expect to find the attention networks. The rest of the cut follows the direction of the sulci as superior to inferior as possible, the goal being not to drift into the FAT or the descending communications with the basal ganglia/thalamus in the subcortex.

14.6.2 Medial Frontal Cases

▶ Fig. 14.8 demonstrates a large frontal resection of a glioblastoma which spares the orbitofrontal cortex. The patient was mostly mute and had severe abulia preoperatively; however, we mapped as much as possible given his poor function to permit our cuts with the SLF and FAT systems.

1. This is a large tumor which fills most of the superior frontal lobe. The cingulate gyrus is compressed but not involved and the orbitofrontal cortex is uninvolved as the tumor is not especially close to it.

2. The diffusion tensor imaging shows us the nature of his mutism: the FAT is compressed by the tumor. This is a challenging case as we do not have much information from mapping.

3. Our resection spared the orbitofrontal cortex and cingulum, and this patient made an excellent recovery to nearly normal. This case highlights the importance of preserving the anatomic continuity of the FAT.

▶ Fig. 14.9 demonstrates an interesting case where the tumor lies between the FAT (in red) and the motor system (in blue). We were able to remove it without motor deficit by working between these two tracts, suggesting that direct connections between the SMA and motor strip are not necessary to maintain function.

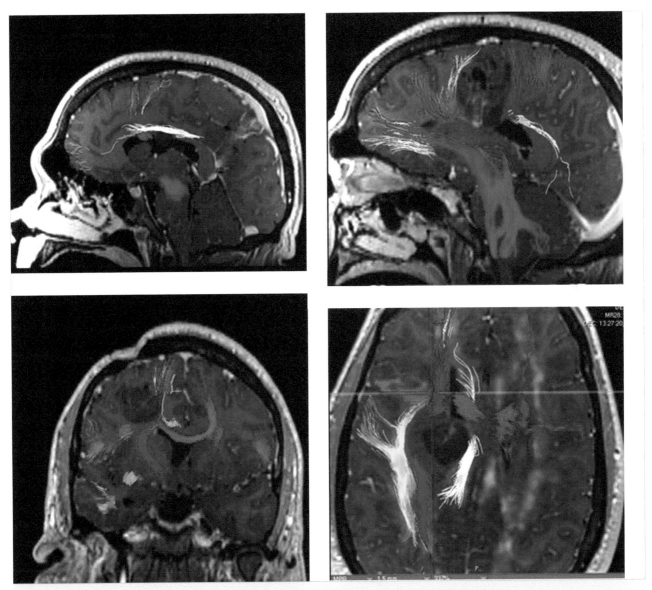

Fig. 14.9 Preoperative diffusion tensor imaging tractography from a medial frontal glioma case described in the text.

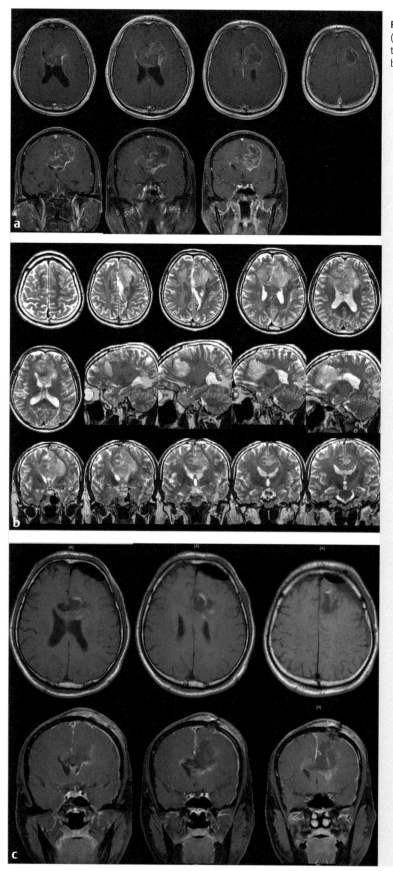

Fig. 14.10 (a) Preoperative magnetic resonance imaging (MRI), (b) preoperative diffusion tensor imaging tractography, and (c) postoperative MRI from an anterior butterfly glioma case described in the text.

14.6.3 Anterior Butterfly Gliomas

It is an essential observation that the corpus callosum and its fibers wrap around the cingulate gyrus and thus the tumor can surround it on all sides. Protecting the cingulate gyrus is paramount and this can be achieved by defining the cingulate and callosal sulci as early as possible, and staying lateral to their deepest extent. Awake mapping studying attention to complex tasks can also guide you to stay out of the cingulum, which you can drift into from the lateral side as there is no pial bank, as there is on the other surfaces, to protect you. The cingulum and corpus callosum can be separated in the lab, and this is often possible in patients with careful patient dissection.

You should always be aware that these tumors are mainly in the frontal lobe and not in the callosum most of the time. If you spend your time fixating on the corpus callosum (it is unique to this case), you will not deal with the actual bulk of the tumor.

Removing a butterfly glioma means opening biventricularly. There is no way to avoid this and shunts are often unavoidable. I prepare the patient for this. The tumor is approached by a transcortical middle frontal gyrus approach. The trajectory you need is dictated by a balance between your desire to have a lateral trajectory which looks down the long axis of the callosum fibers and the reality that the SLF and FAT may force you to deviate more medially. At the angle you approach the tumor, removing the corpus callosum generally involves working down the long axis of the corpus callosum until you have widely removed the front wall of both frontal horns. The callosal sulcus and the anterior cerebral artery (ACA) complex are key landmarks for remaining out of the cingulum and basal forebrain. When working in the rostrum and genu, remember that the forceps minor has a superior and inferior radiation into the frontal lobe. Note that the inferior radiations form a pyramid as they exit the rostrum and enter the bilateral inferior frontal lobes. If you transgress these pyramids and head inferiorly, you have entered the subcallosal cingulate structures and/or the septal nuclei/basal forebrain. This should be avoided.

In short, the steps of this surgery are as follows (see **Video 14.1**):

1. Separate the tumor from the cingulum medially, the SLF laterally, and the motor system posteriorly.
2. Enter the ventricle and identify the boundaries of the caudate head. Clear the tumor from the anterior border of the caudate based on the landmarks in the ventricular wall and based on the gross appearance of the caudate tissue.
3. Remove the frontal lobe tumor on the ipsilateral side.

4. Identify the callosal sulcus and/or ACA and orient yourself to the ventricular anatomy and ventricular walls. This shows you where the corpus callosum is.
5. Define the parts of the corpus callosum which need to be removed. Follow this to the body and the rostrum to get a game plan.
6. Remove the corpus callosum until you have widely opened into both ventricles. Separate the tumor from the septum pellucidum.
7. Follow the forceps minor until you have cleared the other side or functional considerations force you to stop. Take care to stay above the pyramid overlying the septal nuclei and subcallosal areas.

▶ Fig. 14.10 demonstrates a mostly unilateral butterfly glioma which was aggressively removed using awake mapping techniques.

1. This patient presented with mild abulia and this is likely due to the proximity of these tumors to the cingulate gyrus. Note that the tumor almost exclusively follows the corpus callosum fibers as shown in several figures in this book, and has only minor association with the cingulate.
2. The cingulum is not well visualized in this case on either side, likely due to edema, and this requires that we preserve the anatomic structure of the cingulate gyrus, using anatomic landmarks and functional mapping.
3. The tumor is mostly removed. At minimum, it is quite hard to get the caudate head to stop bleeding without packing it off which leads to some of the blood in the cavity. The cingulate gyrus is mostly anatomically preserved, but thin in places. He recovered well from this surgery.

14.6.4 Middle Callosum Butterfly Gliomas

These are bad tumors because they threaten the SMA, and command and control axes on both sides, making it possible to cause deficits which cannot be compensated for the other side. In my practice, the best way to achieve optimum outcomes with these cases involves focusing on the corpus callosum only and removing it through an interhemispheric transcallosal approach. It is important to have reasonable goals in such cases, as the mutism and weakness can become permanent, which defeats the goals of surgery.

15 Mapping and Surgery of Insular Tumors

Matthew A. Kirkman, D. Ceri Davies, and George Samandouras

Abstract

Resection of insular tumors remains one of the most challenging areas of neuro-oncological surgery. This chapter examines the incidence and unique characteristics of insular tumors, and the evidence behind attempts to maximize extent of resection. Subsequently, key elements of the complex surgical anatomy of the insula are described, including surface and relational topographic anatomy, arterial networks, and eloquent cortical parcels and subcortical segments along with proposed mapping paradigms based on our current understanding of function. The focus is then placed on classification schemes, surgical principles, and step-by-step paradigms, along with nuances and caveats in achieving maximum safe resection.

Keywords: awake craniotomy, brain mapping, cortical mapping, insular gliomas, insular surgery, white matter tracts

15.1 Introduction

The surgical management of insular gliomas remains a formidable challenge as the insula is covered by eloquent cortical parcels; is encased by complex arterial and venous networks; has disputed function; is surrounded by white matter tracts; and superimposes the basal ganglia nuclei. Therefore, the surgeon embarking upon maximum safe resection of insular tumors should have a clear understanding of its surgical and physiological anatomy; be familiar with cortical and subcortical direct electrical stimulation (DES) techniques predicated on thorough working knowledge of functional significance of cortical parcels and subcortical segments; and work with the support of wider teams, including specialists from the fields of advanced functional neuroimaging, neuroanesthesia, neuropsychology, and cognitive neuroscience.

15.2 Epidemiology

Gliomas are the commonest primary intraparenchymal tumors of the brain in adults, with an incidence rate of 4.7 to 5.7 per 100,000 population. The insula is a common location for gliomas, with studies reporting approximately 25 and 10% incidence of low- and high-grade gliomas, respectively. It remains unclear as to why the insular location is relatively overrepresented in glioma epidemiology, although several explanations have been proposed.[1]

Insular gliomas are considered to have worse outcomes than gliomas in other locations, with a higher frequency of the astrocytic phenotype and, consequently, reduced incidence of the better prognostic profile of oligodendrogliomas. In one study of World Health Organization (WHO) grade II gliomas involving the insula, no patients had complete 1p and 19q deletions and only 25% had partial deletions.[2] Indeed, it has been shown in a large Chinese sample of 1,210 high- and low-grade glioma (LGG) samples that lesions in the insular lobe were more likely to be IDH-mutant astrocytomas (29.6%).[3] However, other authors have suggested insular gliomas follow a more indolent course than gliomas elsewhere.[4] Although other types of tumors, including dysembryonic neuroepithelial tumors and gangliogliomas, have been described in the insular region, the focus of this chapter is on mapping of gliomas which are by far the commonest tumors encountered in the insula.

15.3 Clinical Presentation

Insular gliomas tend to present differently than gliomas located elsewhere. Although some have argued that they present with a protracted and slowly progressive clinical course,[5] others have proposed that populations of patients with insular gliomas have a high proportion of patients with intractable seizures.[6] Indeed, epilepsy is commonly the only presenting symptom of insular gliomas.[5,7,8] Other presentation symptoms and signs may include expressive dysphasia with or without paresis of the facial muscles.[9] Cognitive dysfunction is also common in patients with insular glioma, potentially due to infiltration of white matter tracts and in particular the inferior fronto-occipital fasciculus (IFOF) which is involved in supramodal semantic processing.[10] This necessitates a comprehensive preoperative neuropsychological and cognitive assessment prior to surgical intervention.

15.4 Evidence on Extent of Resection

15.4.1 Low-Grade Gliomas

Maximum safe resection of LGGs as initial therapeutic option, regardless of topographical location, is strongly supported by current literature.[11,12,13,14,15] Progression-free survival (PFS), overall survival (OS), and rates of malignant transformation are statistically improved with greater extent of resections (EOR), although discrepancy exists in the current literature with regard to the percentage of residual tumor volume and absolute residual tumor volume (cm^3) required to produce a statistically significant survival benefit. More specifically, Smith et al reported that a minimum EOR of > 90% of original volume is required to produce survival benefit and, more recently, absolute residual tumor volumes stratified between 0, 0.1 to 5.0, and > 5.0 cm^3 were associated with consecutively decreasing survival benefit for each group.[11] Also, in a "near-randomized" trial, Roelz et al reported that survival benefit was recorded in patients with absolute residual tumor volume of < 15 cm^3 and patients, in their series, where this threshold was not reached fared similar to the biopsy-only group.[12] Finally, also accounting for molecular subtyping, a recent large retrospective study showed that any residual postoperative volume affected negatively the OS regardless of the tumor's molecular profile, even if the residual volume was only 0.1 to 5.0 cm^3.[15]

15.4.2 Insular Low-Grade Gliomas

EOR has been shown to strongly influence OS and PFS, among additional factors such as age, performance status, tumor volume, and histological grade and molecular profile.[16,17,18,19,20] Multiple studies have shown that a greater EOR in low- and high-grade insular gliomas is associated with improved OS and PFS,[5,21,22] as well as seizure control.[17,23,24] Transient immediate postoperative worsening of functional status is not uncommon in some of the reported series (14.4–59%),[5,7,23,25] but permanent neurological deficits in more recent series are low (0–6%).[5,7,23,25,26]

One research group has proposed four factors as indicators to select the candidates that are most likely to have reduced risks and improved outcomes following radical resection of insular gliomas: patients with clear tumor boundaries, no enhancement, lack of involvement of the lenticulostriate arteries, and preservation of the superior extremity of the central insular sulcus.[27] Another group found that preoperative identification of the IFOF on diffusion tensor imaging (DTI) was associated with a high probability of achieving a resection of > 80%.[28]

In a consecutive series of 115 patients with insular gliomas, 70 low-grade (WHO grade I and II) and 45 high-grade (WHO grade III and IV), a 16% increase in 5-year OS in the low-grade group was noted when EOR was 90% or more; a 16% increase in the 2-year OS was noted in the high-grade group also with an EOR of 90% or more.[5] Crucially, EOR ≥ 90% was associated with an increased malignant-progression-free survival by 17%.[5] In one German study of 72 patients undergoing intraoperative continuous motor mapping for insular gliomas, intraoperative motor evoked potentials (MEPs) remained stable in 40 (56%) cases.[29] In the remainder, a deterioration was observed that was reversible in 21 (29%) cases, with no new permanent deficit in 9 (13%) of these cases. Furthermore, a higher rate of permanent motor deficit occurred in those where no useful MEP monitoring was obtained compared to those where irreversible MEP loss was associated with permanent paresis (18 vs. 4%).

A single-surgeon series of 51 consecutive WHO grade II insular gliomas operated on with DES (some awake) found that although there was an immediate postoperative deficit in over half of the patients (59%), the condition in all but two returned to baseline or actually improved over baseline status during follow-up.[7] The same study also found that 78% of patients, with chronic epilepsy preoperatively, had relief of seizures following surgery.[7] A study from the same author focusing on 24 patients with WHO grade II insular gliomas who underwent awake craniotomy with intraoperative language mapping involving DES, found similar results: exactly 50% of patients had immediate postoperative language worsening, but all recovered within 3 months, and six patients improved their preoperative neurological deficits following surgery.[26]

A retrospective review from a single center of 22 patients with insular gliomas operated via a transopercular approach found that the majority (91%) of patients were seizure free and only 1 had persisting neurological deficit after a mean follow-up of 33.4 months. In this series, 73% of patients had an EOR ≥ 90%, and the remainder had macroscopic gross total resection. Finally, a recent retrospective series of patients with insular gliomas who were reoperated on for recurrence has shown that such operations can be undertaken safely with an acceptable degree of resection, irrespective of insular zone and pathology.[30]

15.4.3 Anatomical Basis of Insular Mapping and Surgery

Using a modified Klinger technique, the authors used formalin-fixed cadaveric brains which were subsequently frozen at −10 to −15 °C for 10 to 14 days and then thawed under running water in a technique described extensively in the literature. The brains were dissected by the authors, under a Zeiss operating microscope (Zeiss, Oberkochen, Germany) with use of microinstruments and wooden spatulas. The anatomical structures were observed. Institutional permission for dissections obtained and photographs were taken from identifiable and electronically tagged specimens, according to Human Tissue Act, 2004, Human Anatomy Unit best practice guidelines and the Data Protection Act, 1998. Authorization was obtained from the Human Anatomy Unit, Division of Surgery, Imperial College London, London, UK. Structures were sequentially identified and are described below, with accompanying photographs.

15.4.4 Cortical Insular Anatomy

The pyramid-like, three-dimensional body of the insula lies in the depth of the Sylvian fissure and is covered by the opercula of frontal, parietal, and temporal lobes. The insula consists of paralimbic mesocortex which is phylogenetically between iso- (or neo-) cortex and allocortex. Other paralimbic structures include the caudal orbitofrontal cortex, the temporal pole, and the parahippocampal and cingulate gyri.

The insula is demarcated by the triangular limiting, rather than circular, sulcus of the insula and its three parts—the anterior, superior, and inferior limiting sulci; there is no posterior limiting sulcus. The surface projections of the limiting sulci are the anterior part of the pars triangularis for the *anterior limiting sulcus (ALS)*; the inferior frontal gyrus anteriorly and the supramarginal gyrus (SMG) posteriorly for the *superior limiting sulcus (SLS)*; and the depth of the superior temporal sulcus for the *inferior limiting sulcus (ILS)* of the insula (▶ Fig. 15.1).[31] The ALS and SLS are straight sulci but the ILS is curved and divided into an anterior and a posterior part with the junction of the two parts lying medial to the anterior part of the Heschl gyrus.[32]

The surface of the insula is divided by the central sulcus of the insula, which lies in the same plane to the central sulcus of the ipsilateral hemisphere, into an anterior and posterior part. The anterior insula has five gyri, the anterior, middle, and posterior short gyri, and also the transverse and the accessory gyrus, placed most anteriorly and concealed by the pars orbitalis. All five gyri converge to the apex of the insula, the most prominent part of the insular surface. The posterior short insular gyrus is considered to be the Dronkers territory, involved in articulatory planning of speech (▶ Fig. 15.1).[33]

The anterior Sylvian point, a visible expansion of the subarachnoid space of the Sylvian fissure at the bottom of pars triangularis, corresponds to the apex of the insula, allowing the surgeon to mentally reconstruct the projection of the insula into the lateral aspect of the brain. The posterior insula displays two long gyri, anterior and posterior, separated by the postcentral sulcus.

The *limen insula* is a hook-like structure consisting of a narrow strip of olfactory cortex[34] that creates a gap between the ALS and ILS. It is readily seen when the Sylvian fissure is split[32]

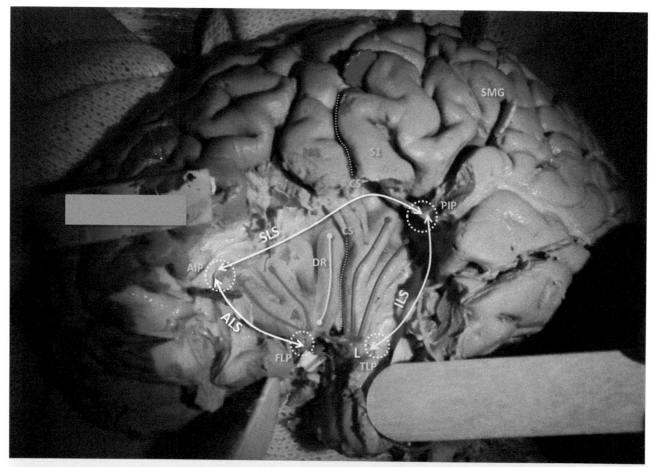

Fig. 15.1 Overview of the left insular anatomy after removal of the frontal, parietal, and temporal opercula and separation of the orbitofrontal and temporopolar parts with wooden spatulas. The insula is limited circumferentially by the anterior (ALS), superior (SLS), and inferior (ILS) limiting sulci. The short gyri, in *light red* and *yellow*, converge to the insular apex (**a**). The short precentral gyrus, in *yellow*, is the seat of the Dronker region (DR) and lies anterior to the central sulcus of the insula (CS) which lies in the same plane with the central sulcus of the cerebral cortex, between the primary motor (M1) and somatosensory (S1) cortices. AIP, anterior insular point; FLP, frontal limen point; ICA, internal carotid artery; L, limen insula; M1 (superior, in larger font), primary motor cortex; M1 (inferior, in smaller font), first segment of the middle cerebral artery; PIP, posterior insular point; SMG, supramarginal gyrus, long gyri in *dark red*; TLP, temporal limen point.

and represents the lateral limit of the anterior perforating substance.[35] The limen insula, which covers part of the uncinate fasciculus (UF), lies just inferior to the insula apex having the temporal incisura anteroinferiorly (temporal connection) and the posteromedial orbital lobule superoanteriorly (frontal connection).

Four superficial insular points have topographical importance: (1) the *anterior insular point*, at the junction of the ALS and SLS; (2) the *posterior insular point*, at the junction of the SLS and ILS; (3) the *frontal limen point*, at the junction of the ALS and limen insula; and (4) the *temporal limen point*, at the junction of the ILS and limen insula (▶ Fig. 15.1).[31]

15.4.5 Vascular Anatomy of the Insular Region

Although the focus of this chapter remains on mapping, surgery for insular tumors is obstructed by the dense, complex arterial system of the insular region. Arterial injury of critical branches may result in permanent neurological deficits, rendering

mapping irrelevant; therefore, vessel identification and preservation is essential and prerequisite for successful mapping. The insular region is characterized by the presence of approximately 100 (range: 77–112), mostly submillimeter caliber (range: 0.1–0.8 mm), arteries.[35] In addition, the complex arterial anatomy of the normal insula is complicated even further by the presence of gliomas that often encase and distort the expected topography of sphenoidal (M1) and insular (M2) arteries.[36]

For the surgeon, it is essential to conceptually and topographically group the arteries of the insular region into three groups:

- A superficial group of arteries that supply mainly the insular cortex, extreme capsule, and claustrum.
- An intermediate group that, in addition, occasionally may supply the external capsule, putamen, globus pallidus, and rarely, can even reach the internal capsule, mainly in the posterior insula.
- The lateral lenticulostriate arteries (LLAs) which do not supply the insular structures but supply the putamen, globus pallidus, and internal capsule. Despite their proximity, the insular arteries and LLAs are separate arterial systems with no direct communication.

All three arterial groups originate from the middle cerebral artery (MCA) and its main segments. The M1 segment of the MCA extends in the posterior continuation of the internal carotid artery (ICA), starting at the branching of the much smaller anterior cerebral artery and extending up to the branching of M1 into, most commonly, two (superior and inferior) segments constituting the M2 segment, covering with multiple branches the insular cortex; the bifurcation is located at the limen insula. The opercular (M3) segment extends from the limiting sulci to the cortex; due to the sharp angulation in the transition, the M3 branches are called candelabra arteries.[35] The para-Sylvian (M4) and terminal (M5) segments are cortical only, with the M5 being visible without parting the Sylvian fissure.

The M1 segment gives rise to three arterial groups:

- Seven to eight (range: 1–15), straight, slim (< 0.5 mm), parallel to each other LLAs arising from the inferomedial aspect of the M1 which do not supply the insula or adjacent superficial structures, but instead, after penetrating the anterior perforating substance, supply the putamen, anterior commissure, substantia innominata, globus pallidus, caudate nucleus, and internal capsule.
- Frontal branch.
- Temporal branch.

This bifurcation, called by Yasargil "false," is observed before the bifurcation of the M1 into superior and inferior trunks. The frontal and temporal branch of M1 should be distinguished from the superior and inferior trunk of the M2, although their course may be parallel. A number of branching variations exist; most commonly a temporal branch only is observed (> 50%) and the second most common variation is the presence of both frontal and temporal branches (35%).[35]

The insular cortex is supplied by the M2 segment with a few branches occasionally coming from M1 or, more rarely, M3 segments. The superior and inferior trunks of the M2 give rise to approximately 10 branches (range: 8–12), and most consistently, from anterior to posterior, the prefrontal, precentral, central, anterior and posterior parietal, and angular arteries. The temporal branch of M1 often gives rise to middle and posterior temporal arteries.

The M1 (*proximal or sphenoidal*) segment of the MCA results from the bifurcation of the ICA in the region of the anterior perforating substance and extends to the region of the limen insula where it branches to a number of patterns, including the most commonly observed bifurcation to a superior and inferior trunk, trifurcation, quadfurcation, or no branching. The M2 segment most commonly includes the superior and inferior trunks and gives off 9 to 12 arterial branches mostly from its superior

trunk before transitioning with acute angles (candle tree arteries) at the level of the SLS to M3 segment.[35]

15.5 Classification Schemes of Insular Tumors

A number of surgical classification schemes of insular tumors have been proposed, aiming to better understand the extent of anatomical involvement,[36,37] resectability, and surgical morbidity.[5]

15.5.1 Yasargil Classification System

In 1992, in a thoughtful article, Yasargil reviewed 177 cases of tumors affecting the mesocortical limbic system (*insula, temporal pole, parahippocampal and cingulate gyri*) and the phylogenetically older allocortical paralimbic system (*amygdala, hippocampus, septal region, substantia innominata, and piriform cortex*), and observed a propensity for tumors to prefer expansion within meso- or allocortical regions. He grouped these tumors into mediobasal temporal, insular, and orbitofrontal-insular-temporal pole tumors.[36] Yasargil's classification is an anatomical/developmental classification model (► Table 15.1): **Type 3** tumors involve all, or part, of the insula (**3A**) or may involve adjacent opercula (**3B**); **type 5** tumors may involve either or both of the orbitofrontal and temporopolar (paralimbic) regions (**5A**) and may involve the limbic system (**5B**).[38]

15.5.2 Berger–Sanai Zone Classification System (2010)

Using two planes, one along the Sylvian fissure, and one across the foramina of Monro, the insular region is divided into four quadrants: clockwise starting from the frontal operculum I and II superiorly, and III and IV inferiorly to the Sylvian plane (► Table 15.2). Consequently, quadrants I and IV are anterior, and quadrants II and III are posterior to the plane of Monro (► Table 15.2). As insular tumors do not respect arbitrary planes, the grading depends on the location of the majority of tumor volume. Berger–Sanai model is a surgical planning/surgical morbidity prediction model. It has been shown that this classification can reliably predict EOR[5,21] and morbidity due to insular gliomas.[21] Due to its relevance to topographic anatomy and surgical planning, the Berger–Sanai classification system will be used in the remaining of the chapter.

15.5.3 The Putamen Classification (2017)

This classification is based on the work of a Chinese group that studied 211 consecutively treated patients with insular glioma

Table 15.1 Yasargil classification of tumors of the limbic and paralimbic systems (1992)

Type 3A	Involves the insula only
Type 3B	Extends to adjacent opercula
Type 5A	Extends to +/– orbitofrontal +/– temporopolar structures (paralimbic system)
Type 5B	Extends to mesiotemporal structures (limbic system)

Source: From (Yasargil et al 1992).[36]

Table 15.2 Berger–Sanai classification of the insular tumors (2010)

Type I	Anterior-superior quadrant
Type II	Posterior-superior quadrant
Type III	Posterior-inferior quadrant
Type IV	Anterior-inferior quadrant

Source: From (Sanai et al 2010).[5]

and classified them accordingly to whether or not there was putaminal involvement.[37] It was proposed that the putamen, which is parallel to a large surface of the opposing insula, can stop or delay medial extension of gliomas. In contrast with the claustrum, putamen can easily be identified in high-resolution magnetic resonance imaging (MRI). In the studied group, 47% of patients were found to have putaminal involvement; these tumors were significantly larger, less likely to be associated with seizures, more likely to be IDH1 wild type, and less likely to be removed totally at surgery. In addition, the putamen classification was found to independently predict survival outcome. The binary putaminal classification scheme is survival predictor based on the singular fact of putaminal involvement. However, it should be noted that insular tumors involving the putamen have higher tumor volumes and tend to proportionally involve other adjacent structures and are also less likely to be resected.

15.6 Surgical Anatomy and Mapping Paradigms of Cortical Parcels/Subcortical Segments in Insular Surgery

15.6.1 Opercula

In insular surgery, three parcels of the frontal operculum are relevant and mapped according to their precise anatomical location. There is no consensus in the literature with regard to function and testing of specific cortical parcels and subcortical segments, and variations in practice are considerable among different institutions and teams.[39] The discussion below is based on the senior author's practice supported by his multidisciplinary team and also a critical review of the literature. Parts of function and testing described below do not apply universally, as many of these functions are still a matter of controversy.[39]

The **pars orbitalis (Brodmann area 47)** is the most prominent part of the inferior frontal gyrus connected anteriorly to the lateral orbital gyrus, and posteriorly it is separated from the pars triangularis by the anterior horizontal ramus of the Sylvian fissure.[40]

The function of the pars orbitalis is disputed. Most evidence supports the role of the dominant pars orbitalis in semantic processing,[41] but it has also been shown to have a role in phonological processing.[42,43] It is therefore likely to have a role in both the processes, and recent evidence also suggests that the pars orbitalis plays a role in converging semantic and emotional aspects of communication.[44] The semantic function of pars orbitalis can be tested with semantic association tasks and word retrieval using the Boston Naming Test, and the phonological function by word generation tasks, such as asking patients to generate words beginning with a specific letter.

The **pars triangularis (Brodmann area 45)** is defined between the anterior horizontal (anteriorly) and anterior ascending (posteriorly) rami of the Sylvian fissure,[40,45] and points to the anterior Sylvian point and the insular apex. The dominant pars triangularis is involved in syntactic processing and grammar and can be tested with sentence completion and negation tasks. Some semantic functions have also been

attributed to pars triangularis and can be tested with word retrieval using the Boston Naming Test.

The **pars opercularis (Brodmann area 44)** lies posterior to pars triangularis, and the two cortical parcels are separated by the anterior ascending ramus of the Sylvian fissure. The pars opercularis continues with a "U" connection to the inferior part of the precentral gyrus.

The dominant pars opercularis is involved in phonological processing and word generation and can be tested asking patients to generate words beginning with a specific letter. The nondominant pars triangularis and opercularis are involved in emotional intonation (*I can't believe this!*) and semantic metaphorical meanings (*I have butterflies in my stomach*). However, these functions are not routinely tested in nondominant insular mapping. It appears that the posterior part of pars opercularis is particularly involved in speech production.[46,47]

The inferior part of the obliquely arranged **precentral gyrus** (primary motor cortex or M1; Brodmann area 4) is connected at its base to the inferior part of the postcentral gyrus with another "U," the subcentral gyrus, which lies over the transverse gyrus of Heschl of the temporal lobe.[40] Resection of gyrus of Heschl, usually required for type III insular gliomas, is not expected to result in auditory deficits.[46] The inferior part of M1, the facial motor cortex, can be resected producing a usually temporary unilateral, central facial paralysis.[38,46] For insular gliomas type II, resection of the inferior part of S1 may result in somatosensory deficits of the contralateral face.[46]

15.6.2 Insular Cortex

In 1996, Nina Dronkers described a group of 25 patients with stroke in a discrete area involving the left insular posterior short gyrus with disorders in motor (articulatory) planning of speech resulting in apraxia of speech (AOS; ▶ Fig. 15.1). Patients with AOS inconsistently and effortfully misarticulate words and attempt multiple times to self-correct.[33] The muscles involved in speech are not weak and this differentiates AOS from dysarthria.

Dronkers territory can be tested by asking patients to repeat five times polysyllabic (> three syllables) words with an initial cluster of consonants (gravity; spaghetti).[33,48]

However, it should be noted that other groups have subsequently used functional MRI (fMRI) studies to suggest different findings,[49] indicating that any such association is perhaps due to a high base rate of ischemic damage and fMRI activation in this region,[50] as well as proximity to regions that more directly support speech articulation, such as the precentral gyrus or posterior aspects of the inferior frontal gyrus.[51] More recently, a meta-analysis of 42 fMRI studies of healthy adults has shown speech perception tasks to preferentially activate the left dorsal mid-insula, and expressive language tasks activated the left ventral mid-insula suggesting that distinct regions of the mid-insula play different roles in speech and language processing.[52] Interestingly, all tasks result in activation of insula regions bilaterally.

The anterior ventral insula (▶ Fig. 15.2) is involved in social and emotional awareness and empathy.[53,54] This aspect is often recorded in preoperative neuropsychological testing but is challenging to test intraoperatively, although emotional mapping has been reported in awake brain mapping.

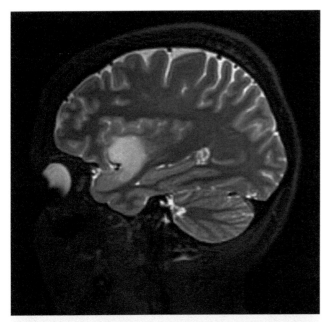

Fig. 15.2 Sagittal T2-weighted magnetic resonance imaging showing a hyperintense lesion involving the ventral anterior insula of a 33-year-old patient presenting with seizures. The preoperative neuropsychology report recorded "Performance was intact on a task of theory of mind (Reading the Mind in the Eyes Test, 48th percentile). Subjectively, although she has not noticed a change in her ability to understand the intentions and emotions of others, she now feels less empathy."

15.6.3 Extreme Capsule

The extreme capsule (▶ Fig. 15.3) is revealed upon removal of the insular cortex and consists of short association fibers connecting the adjacent insular gyri, but it also contains long association fibers connecting the inferior frontal area, the superior temporal gyrus, and the inferior parietal lobule suggesting a role in semantic processing of language.[39,55] It is postulated that the extreme capsule contains fibers of the IFOF and UF.[56,57] The extreme capsule is not routinely tested by DES.

15.6.4 External Capsule

Removal of the extreme capsule reveals two systems of white matter fibers—one traveling from superior to inferior, and the other traveling from anterior to posterior. These are the dorsal and ventral external capsule, respectively (▶ Fig. 15.4). An island of gray matter lies between the two fiber systems, known as the claustrum, which has two components: (1) a distinct, compact, larger dorsal claustrum posterosuperiorly, and (2) a much less well-defined, fragmented, ventral claustrum, anteroinferiorly, imbedded between the white matter tracts of the IFOF and UF (▶ Fig. 15.4).

The dorsal external capsule originates from the dorsal claustrum like sun rays and contributes to the corona radiata as the claustrocortical projection fibers. The ventral external capsule is formed by the UF and IFOF association fibers (▶ Fig. 15.4). The function of the dorsal external capsule has been proposed to involve integration of multiple sensory modalities (visual-audio-tactile). More recent studies suggest that due to an extensive connectivity of the claustrum to the prefrontal cortex,

it might be involved in detection of novel sensory stimuli and directing attention.[58]

Electrical stimulation of the dorsal external capsule (claustrum and the dorsal claustrocortical fibers) is hindered by its thin consistency and uncertainty of its functional properties, and at present it cannot be practically mapped. For mapping of the ventral external capsule, please see IFOF and UF.

15.6.5 Uncinate Fasciculus

The UF, a short, hook-like frontotemporal association fiber system, forms part of both the extreme and external capsules arching over the stem of M1 where it is covered by the gray matter of limen insula, and in this area, is placed inferiorly and slightly medially to the IFOF (▶ Fig. 15.4). It connects, mostly bidirectionally, with the uncus and the amygdala via the lateral orbitofrontal cortex, and with the medial orbitofrontal cortex and septal areas via its dorsolateral and ventromedial components, respectively.[31,59,60]

The UF has been associated with numerous psychiatric disorders and two neurological disorders—epilepsy and frontotemporal dementia. Putative functions attributed to UF, linked to its topographic relation to the limbic system, include episodic memory including reward/punishment-based learning, famous face naming, and social/emotional processing.[59,61]

The UF can be tested with DES using famous faces naming, verbal fluency, object naming, and semantic testing, although any deficits can be compensated.[62,63]

15.6.6 Inferior Fronto-occipital Fasciculus

Similar to the UF, the IFOF forms part of both the extreme and external capsules (▶ Fig. 15.4); however, unlike to the UF, it has a long, protracted, anteroposterior course, measuring approximately > 80 mm, connecting the dorsolateral prefrontal cortex of the middle frontal gyrus, the pars orbitalis and triangularis to the temporal, posterior parietal and occipital lobes. In the frontal lobe it is covered by the superior longitudinal fasciculus (SLF) II, SLF III, and arcuate fasciculus (AF), but covers the optic radiation in the posterior temporal and occipital lobes.[31]

First described by Curran in 1909, the IFOF is currently thought to be part of the ventral semantic stream. In 2007, Hickock and Poeppel introduced a dual stream language model, consisting of a largely bilateral, ventral, semantic stream involved in comprehension and a dorsal, phonological stream involved in articulation which is strongly left-hemisphere dominant.[64] The SLF and AF are involved in the dorsal, phonological stream and DES produces dysarthria and other phonological disorders.[65] The IFOF and UF are believed to participate in the ventral, semantic stream, although the latter appears to be compensated.[63,65] DES of the IFOF induces semantic paraphasias,[65,66] although nonverbal semantic disorders in the nondominant hemisphere are possible.[67,68]

15.6.7 Superior Longitudinal Fasciculus III

There still remains controversy in the literature and numerous anatomical and neurosurgical atlases with regard to the SLF and

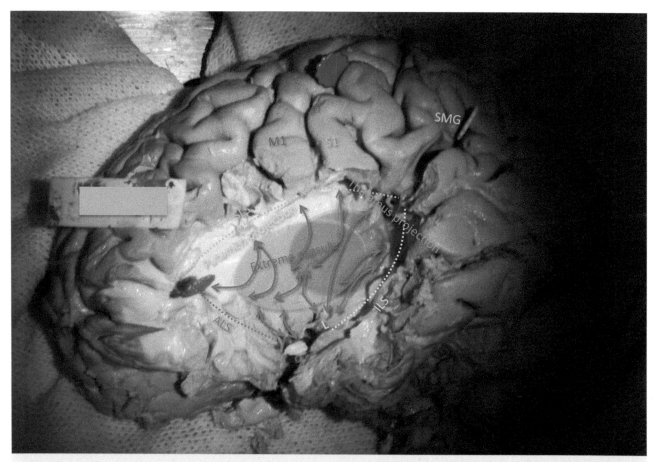

Fig. 15.3 Following removal of the insular short and long gyri, the short association fibers of the extreme capsule are demonstrated in the form of white matter folds (*orange arrows*). It should be noted that the extreme capsule also contains the long association fibers of the inferior fronto-occipital fasciculus and uncinate fasciculus. Please note the surface projection of the extreme capsule (anteriorly) and the thalamus (posteriorly). ALS, anterior limiting sulcus; ILS, inferior limiting sulcus; L, limen insula; M1, primary motor cortex; S1, somatosensory cortex; SLS, superior limiting sulcus; SMG, supramarginal gyrus.

AF perisylvian systems. Some researches use these terms interchangeably or consider the AF as part of the SLF.[56] It should be noted that the SLF is a parietotemporal fasciculus while the AF is a temporofrontal fasciculus. SLF I, II, and III are located in the superior (F1), middle (F2), and inferior (F3) frontal gyri, respectively (▶ Fig. 15.5). The SLF III connects posterior-inferior prefrontal and ventral premotor cortices with the SMG and intraparietal sulcus.[69] One hypothesis is that the SLF III is right-lateralized, in contrast with the AF which is left-lateralized.[70,71] On the dominant side, SLF is involved with phonological and articulatory function; DES can produce dysarthria or anarthria.

15.6.8 Ventral Arcuate Fasciculus

There is substantial controversy in the literature with regard to the anatomy, components, and function of the AF with produced models differing considerably between research groups, using different or even similar methodologies. The authors would currently agree to an anatomical model, as this is in concordance with their own anatomical dissection using the Klinger technique, describing a ventral (vAF) and a dorsal (dAF) component of the AF (▶ Fig. 15.5). The vAF connects the T1 and

T2 with the F3, passing through the SMG; the dAF connects the T2 and T3 with the F2 and F3, passing through the angular gyrus. The vAF is placed medially to SLF III at the frontal operculum; the dAF is placed ventrally to SLF II (▶ Fig. 15.5).

On the dominant side, vAF is involved in phonological function and DES can produce hesitation, dysarthria, and typically, repetition disorders; in the latter case, the patient is asked to repeat a phrase he or she just heard, for example *"no ifs, ands, or buts."* During positive DES, the patient, either cannot repeat the phrase or hesitates significantly.

15.6.9 Internal Capsule

The corona radiata transitions to internal capsule at the level of the SLS of the insula and superior aspect of the putamen (▶ Fig. 15.6).[72] The corticospinal fibers are found at the posterior limb of the internal capsule, covered with the globus pallidus laterally. However, the internal capsule remains unprotected from the putamen and globus pallidus at the level of the SLS (▶ Fig. 15.6).[33] DES at the depth of the middle of the SLS can identify movement arrest and localize the corticospinal tract (CST).

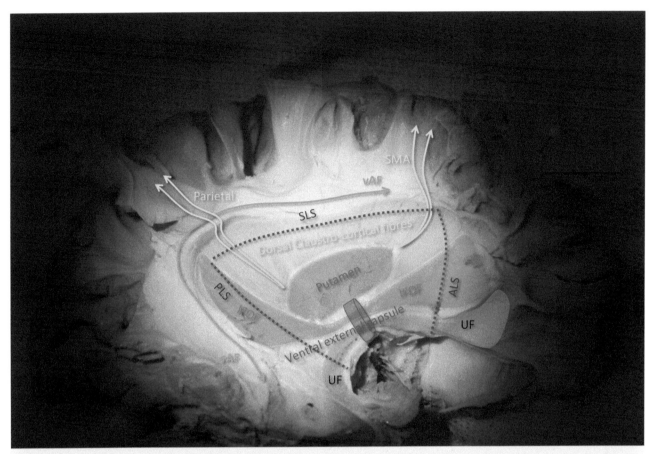

Fig. 15.4 Following removal of the extreme capsule, the dorsal and ventral parts of the external capsule are revealed. Please note the relationship of the inferior fronto-occipital fasciculus (IFOF) and uncinate fasciculus (UF), especially at their convergence at the level of the limen insula. Two main dorsal claustrocortical fiber groups terminate at the SMA, anteriorly, and the parietal lobes, posteriorly. ALS, anterior limiting sulcus; SLS, superior limiting sulcus; SMA, supplementary motor area; vAF, ventral arcuate fasciculus.

15.7 Illustrative Case

A 40-year-old patient presented with history of sensory seizures affecting the face and mouth. An MRI scan showed a left-sided intrinsic lesion involving the superior part of the long insular gyri. There was faint enhancement. The lesion was considered inoperable at a different department and was referred to our service. The patient underwent perfusion MRI, fMRI, DTI, and transcranial magnetic stimulation (TMS; ▶ Fig. 15.7).

After presenting the management options to the patient and family, they elected to have maximum safe resection with awake brain mapping. The case was performed with intraoperative MRI (iMRI). Volumetric structural MRI, fMRI, DTI, and navigated TMS were uploaded in the neuronavigation software and images were fused. Mapping was performed using Boston Naming Test, sentence repetition task, and phonological tasks. Distinct positive cortical areas were identified at 4 mA, and a functionally silent and safe entry point was identified. The tumor was removed completely macroscopically. Postoperatively, the patient developed a transient phonological deficit which resolved within days. The iMRI images at the end of the operation showed no obvious residual tumor (▶ Fig. 15.8).

15.8 Surgical Techniques

Insular gliomas approached with the intent of maximum safe resection remain challenging tumors due to complex three-dimensional anatomy, eloquent cortical parcels and subcortical segments, and the presence of multiple arteries. Two main approaches are traditionally employed: a trans-Sylvian (TS) approach and a transopercular/transcortical (TC) approach.

15.8.1 Trans-Sylvian Approach

Initially introduced by Yasargil, the TS approach is considered an effective alternative to the TC approach in anterior insular tumors (zones I and IV).[36,46] There are three potential disadvantages with the TS approach relating to the need for opercular retraction, arterial injury or spasm, and need for venous sacrifice, particularly in posterior insular lesions (types II and III).[46,73]

Although in theory, the TS approach does not involve sacrificing eloquent opercular tissue unless directly infiltrated by tumor, it appears that a minimum of 2 to 2.5 cm of opercular retraction is required to expose the insula.[46,73] The distance between the insular apex to the SLS of the insula is 19.1 mm

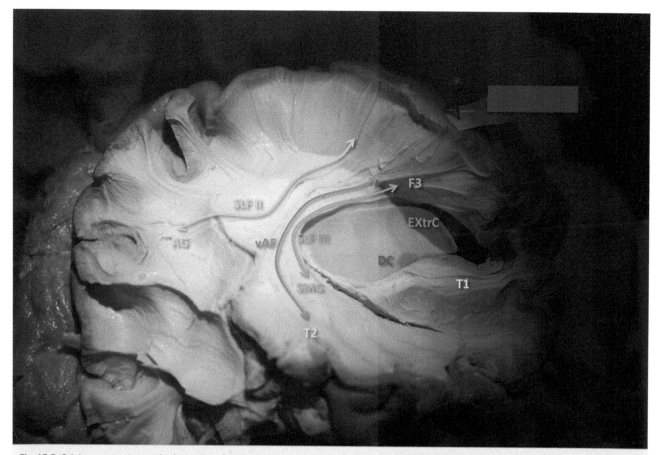

Fig. 15.5 Origin, termination, and relationship of the ventral arcuate fasciculus between the superior longitudinal fasciculus (SLF) II and SLF III. AG, angular gyrus; DC, dorsal claustrum; EXtrC, extreme capsule; F3, T1, T2, inferior frontal, superior and middle temporal gyri; SMG, supramarginal gyrus.

(range: 17–23 mm), although gliomas expand this distance further.[34,73] This retraction can bruise the pars triangularis and opercularis in anterior insular tumors (types I and IV) or bruise the SMG in posterior insular tumors (type II and III), and can also produce ischemia to M3 branches.[73] Yasargil recommended cotton balls rather than metal retractors.[36]

In the TS approach, although the short and intermediate insular vessels can be theoretically sacrificed as they do not reach the corona radiata or putamen/globus pallidus, vessel tearing from tumor manipulation can also avulse their origin from M2 superior or inferior trunk.[35,73] In addition, the surgeon has no knowledge whether a perforating artery is short, intermediate, or long, or supplying part of the corona radiata, except the theoretical notion that long perforators are more likely to be present in the posterior insula.[35]

The principle of Yasargil's description of the trans-Sylvian approach was to initially find out whether the tumor was located in the anterior or posterior part of the Sylvian fissure and usually open the Sylvian fissure along its entire length allowing control to the M1 to M3 segments. Yasargil emphasized meticulous microsurgical technique and preservation of the Sylvian veins.[74] Part of this technique was to devascularize the tumor from small feeding arteries and decompress the tumor internally. He also suggested using soft sponges to allow retraction of the opercula rather than retractors and also frequent use of papaverine to prevent vasospasm.[74]

The Bonn group, in one of the original large series of insular gliomas, employed the TS approach for insular tumors restricted to the insula but added the transopercular route for opercular tumor extensions without using awake craniotomies or intraoperative brain mapping.[75] In their series of 101 operations, they performed this technique on 94 patients and achieved EOR > 90% in 42% of cases and EOR > 70% in 51% of cases. They did not find a relationship between EOR and surgical approach, or, interestingly, dominant versus nondominant location.[75]

A potential disadvantage of the TS approach is the venous clustering around the area of pars triangularis, opercularis, and M1 observed in > 50% of cases in a cadaveric study, obstructing the corridor in insular gliomas anterior to the foramen of Monro, types I and IV, and vital venous drainage in insular gliomas posterior to the foramen of Monro, types II and III, that may result in venous infarctions in 30% of cases.[46] It is unclear whether the insula is drained by the deep venous system, but cadaveric studies have shown numerous anastomoses from the superficial system,[76] emphasizing the importance of the Sylvian bridging veins. Sacrificing the bridging veins may be necessary during the TS approach for posteriorly placed insular tumors thus increasing the risk of venous infarction in patients with poor collateral outflow through the vein of Labbé or superior sagittal sinus.[46]

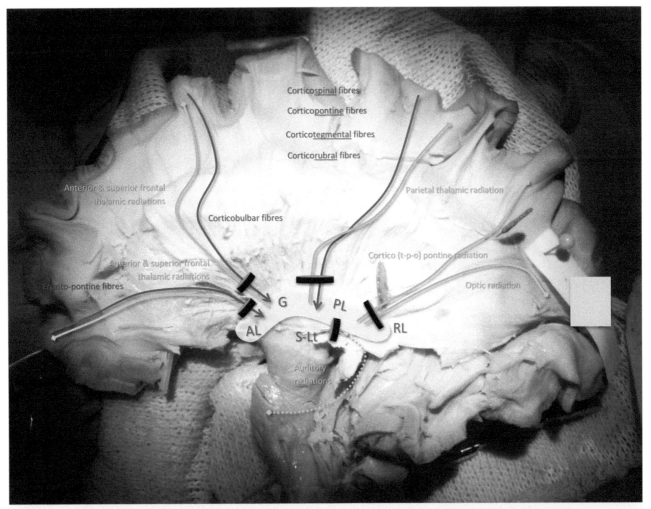

Fig. 15.6 Diagrammatic depiction of the complex fiber arrangements of the internal capsule (IC) as they converge through the five segments of the projected IC: anterior limb (AL); genu (G); posterior limb (PL); and retro- (RL) and sub-lenticular (S-Lt) segments. Please note the extensive fiber network of thalamic radiations (*dark yellow*) including the optic radiation. The corticospinal fibers constitute a very small part of the IC.

15.8.2 Transopercular/Transcortical Approach

Although insular surgery has been traditionally performed under general anesthesia, it can be inferred from more recent studies and the initial series of Yasargil[36,73] that the TC approach, especially in the left insula, required awake brain mapping. There are numerous studies showing that brain mapping for insular tumors can help maximize the extent of tumor resection while preventing adverse neurological outcomes.[77] In a meta-analysis of over 8,000 glioma patients, DES was shown to be safe, well tolerated, and permitted a greater EOR and lower rate of permanent neurological deficits.[78] Tumors on the nondominant side can, in theory, be resected under general anesthesia with motor mapping of the face area, whereas tumors in the dominant hemisphere require awake speech mapping. However, some surgeons perform all insular glioma resections awake irrespective of the laterality of the tumor. In the senior author's practice, most nondominant insular tumors

are also removed with awake brain mapping, mainly to monitor and protect motor function.

The TS approach does not require opening of the Sylvian fissure but creating entries through one, or more, opercular windows, thereby requiring cortical mapping to identify safe entry points. The exact description of the technique remains sparse in the literature. The aim is to develop a surgical trajectory medially to superior and inferior trunks of M2 and branches of M3, avoiding the risk of manipulating arterial trunks or sacrificing Sylvian bridging veins, especially in the case of posteriorly placed insular tumors. The senior author employs awake brain mapping in both left and right insular gliomas, with mapping paradigms depending on the exact anatomical location. Although the TC approach can be used for all insular tumors, it may be particularly useful for posterior insular (zone 2 and 3 in the Sanai–Berger classification) lesions where the trans-Sylvian approach is limited by the narrow Sylvian cistern. The technique is described in detail in subsequent text.

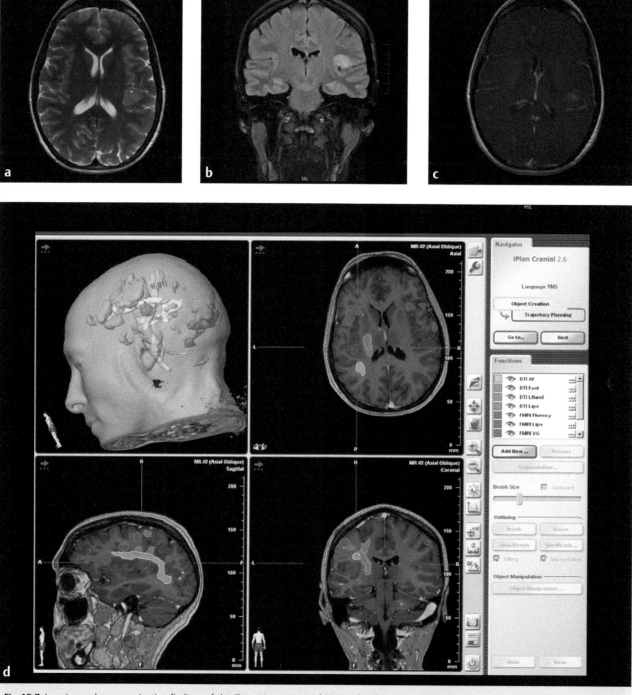

Fig. 15.7 Imaging and neuronavigation findings of the illustrative case. Axial T2-weighted magnetic resonance imaging (**a**), coronal fluid-attenuated inversion recovery scan (**b**), and axial T1 after administration with gadolinium (**c**) showing a lesion of the posterior/superior insula with faint enhancement. (**d**) Functional imaging uploaded to the neuronavigation shows the lesion (*magenta*) adjacent to the arcuate fasciculus (*yellow*), corticospinal tract (*green*), and verbal fluency (*orange*). Positive, navigated transcranial magnetic stimulation (nTMS) sites are depicted as *magenta dots*.

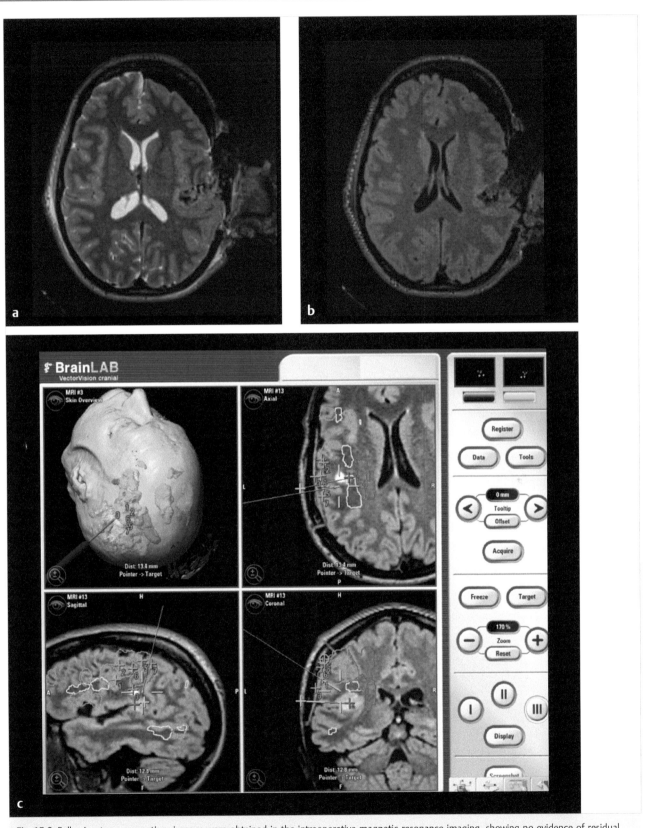

Fig. 15.8 Following tumor resection, images were obtained in the intraoperative magnetic resonance imaging, showing no evidence of residual disease on axial T2 (**a**) and axial T1 fluid-attenuated inversion recovery (**b**) sequences. A screen shot of the neuronavigation monitor (**c**) demonstrates the arcuate fasciculus (*yellow*); verbal fluency (*orange*); and corticospinal tract (*red*). Positive navigated transcranial magnetic stimulation sites are depicted as *cyan dots*. The numbers correspond to the positive direct electrical stimulation points during mapping. Although advanced technologies can be useful, they are not prerequisite to successful operations and cannot replace surgical knowledge and skill.

15.9 Step-by-Step Surgical and Mapping Paradigms in Insular Surgery

15.9.1 Preoperative Assessment

All patients with insular tumors, similar to all brain tumor cases, are discussed at the neuro-oncology multidisciplinary meeting (MDT), which is equivalent to a tumor board meeting, where a range of neuro-oncology specialists review individual cases. Patients are seen at a neuro-oncology MDT clinic where the options of conservative management, biopsy with potential adjuvant treatment and maximum safe resection, usually with awake brain mapping, are discussed extensively with the patients and their families. The patients are also provided with written information specifically addressing difficult points in the decision-making. It is the senior author's experience that the vast majority of patients with LGGs, including those in eloquent locations such as the insula, elect to proceed with maximum safe resection. Part of the authors' preoperative work-up for insular gliomas include structural MRI along with perfusion MRI, MR spectroscopy, fMRI, and DTI of CST and perisylvian pathways. Dopamine positron emission tomography is requested for identification of potential higher-grade foci within the tumor volume. The authors do not perform preoperative computed tomography angiography or digital subtraction angiography to study the location of the LLAs of the M2 and M3 segments, as despite displacement from tumor volume, the arterial anatomy tends to be consistent. The patient also undergoes routine preoperative neuropsychological assessment.

In addition, the authors present cases at a specialized, weekly *Brain Mapping MDT*, where each case is discussed for a minimum of 30 to 40 minutes with a group of neuropsychologists, cognitive neuroscientists, speech and language therapists, specialized neuroradiologists, other neurosurgeons, and, in selected cases, neuro-ophthalmologists and motor neurophysiologists. Following this meeting, where functional imaging, imaging anatomy, neuropsychology, and cognitive neurology aspects are reviewed by the team, a mapping plan is formulated based on individual patient anatomy, presumed function, and patient's preoperative testing parameters. Then, the neuropsychologist and speech and language therapist rehearse the testing well before the operation, so the patient is prepared and familiar with all components of intraoperative testing.

15.9.2 Surgical Technique

All patients are coached before and during surgery. A circumferential scalp block with equal parts of lidocaine 1% with epinephrine (1:200,000) and bupivacaine 0.25% are used while the patient is under a small amount of target-controlled infusion (TCI) of propofol and remifentanil aiming to a target blood concentration of 0.8 to 1.2 µg/mL and 1 to 2 ng/mL, respectively. Infusion rates are typically 15 to 50 µg/kg/minute for propofol and 0.003 to 0.008 µg/kg/minute for remifentanil. This method allows rapid titration of level of sedation and rapid offset to ensure quick recovery, so the patient can comply with intraoperative testing. During this time, the patient is fully conscious with his or her eyes open and interacting normally. We found

that even slightly higher than necessary sedation at this stage may render the patient disinhibited, so strict control of sedation is essential. No intubation or laryngeal mask are used. Once the Mayfield Clamp is applied, all sedation is stopped.

The senior author employs a modified TC approach. The patient is positioned supine with his or her head turned to the contralateral side. Patients adjust the position themselves for maximum comfort with support of the shoulders and back of the neck. The patients should look and feel comfortable with no stretching of neck or unnatural head positioning; this is important for achieving patient tolerance during the operation for many hours. The surgeon sits on the side of the craniotomy looking at the brain laterally, and not upside down, as depicted in many diagrams.

A frontotemporal craniotomy is performed, with the exact extent and placement depending on the size and anatomical predilection of the tumor. The senior author employs the TC approach but elects to open the Sylvian fissure before the transcortical entry to visualize the superior and inferior trunks of the M2. All tumor removal is achieved through a TC/transopercular approach; the subpial resection is generally a safe way to avoid vascular injury but the pia mater can easily be violated, not only with the ultrasonic aspirator but also with the suction or microinstruments. Having sound anatomical information on the position of the superior and inferior trunks of the M2 provides security and minimizes the risk of vascular injury through the subpial route. In addition, the senior author avoids coagulating any arteries or veins, regardless of size, to avoid small vascular infarcts; any small hemorrhages are usually readily controlled with hemostatic agents (e.g., Surgiflo, Ethicon, Somerville, NJ).

After splitting the Sylvian fissure under the operating microscope, from a proximal to distal direction, and identifying M1 and superior and inferior trunks of M2, cortical mapping is performed. For 6 years, the senior author was using the 5 mm hand-held bipolar probe attached to the Ojemann Cortical Stimulator, model OCS2 (Integra, Plainsboro, NJ), with stimulation parameters including pulse duration 0.5 millisecond, pulse rate 50 Hz, and current output 2.0 to 6.0 mA, maintaining contact with the neural tissue for 3 seconds at a time. However, it appears that Ojemann stimulation production has ceased and the stimulation is now performed with the C2 Xtend nerve monitor (Inomed, Emmendingen, Germany) with high-frequency, train of five, monopolar stimulation for motor system testing and low-frequency bipolar stimulation for language testing. Electrocorticography is used for recording after-discharge potentials with a six-contact electrode strip (Brain Quick EEG System, Micromed, Treviso, Italy). Ice-cold saline is used to irrigate the brain between stimulation discharges; this also can be used in the rare event of intraoperative seizures. Sterile tickets with numbers are used to mark positive mapping sites. Overlays of DTI and fMRI are fused with the volumetric fluid-attenuated inversion recovery sequences for neuronavigation, which is performed with the StealthStation S8 (Medtronic, Minneapolis, MN) unless the case is being performed in iMRI, as this suite is equipped with BrainLab (Munich, Germany). It is important to emphasize that anatomy is more important than neuronavigation, and that iMRI is a useful addition to the surgeon's armamentarium but is not essential.

The location and number of cortical windows depends on the location and size of insular tumors. Based on the anatomical, cortical, and subcortical mapping principles described in detail above, and provided that no deficits are recorded on DES, entry at the frontal operculum is usually achieved through the pars orbitalis and anterior half of parts triangularis. For tumors involving the anterior/superior insula, creating a frontal window may be sufficient; for larger tumors involving the superior and inferior anterior insula, a temporal window, at the superior temporal gyrus, after mapping, can also be created. For more posteriorly placed tumors, the face motor area and the SMG are mapped. The nondominant face motor area can be resected, as it has bilateral representation and recovers within months;[79] however, care should be taken to avoid the motor hand area.

After successfully mapping and creating transopercular entries to the insula, the aim is to perform a subpial resection, utilizing one, or more, windows, and aiming to join the frontal and temporal trajectories, behind the superior and inferior trunks of M2. Cortical and subcortical mapping is particularly important during the TC approach to the posterior zones (II and III), as the facial and somatosensory functions (zone II) and language areas (zone III) may be involved.[46] Subcortical mapping is performed at times adjacent to critical white matter tracts, as described above. The tumor is removed with a combination of suction and ultrasonic aspirator, preferably with low cavitation and medium/high tissue select settings, to minimize the risk of vascular injury.

Two additional caveats should be emphasized: First, at the level above the SLS, the internal capsule is not protected by the putamen and globus pallidus.[73] Subcortical DES deep to the level of SLS can produce movement arrest.[73] This is particularly relevant to zone II tumors; although the pyramidal tract can be monitored during general anesthesia,[80] awake mapping is more sensitive to identify the somatosensory thalamocortical tracts that lie more lateral than the motor pathways in the posterior limb of the internal capsule.[7,26]

Second, it should be noted that despite the subpial resection technique, the LLAs are still exposed and vulnerable, and the optimal method to avoid their injury is a sound anatomical knowledge of their exact location—branching medially to the UF and anteriorly to the anterior commissure, and fanning out ascending toward the putamen, globus pallidus, and internal capsule.

15.10 Pearls

- Understanding the complex anatomy and, partially solved, physiology of the insula remains the key in successful insular surgery.
- The anterior Sylvian point indicates the insular apex, and therefore provides the surgeon an accurate surface projection of the insula before starting any dissection.
- The limen insula indicates the inferior limit of dissection and the origin of LLAs.
- At the depths of the middle of the SLS of the insula lies the internal capsule, and therefore risk of motor deficit, if resection proceeds to a deeper level.
- The ultrasonic aspirator should be avoided where possible—it can cause vascular injury[81]; the safest setting close to arteries is with tissue select high and medium/low amplitude. The ultrasonic aspirator has good and precise aspirational

capacity and can be used as a very effective, advanced suction, without any cavitation effect.

15.11 Conclusion

Maximum safe resection of insular tumors remains a formidable challenge. This chapter attempts to provide specific and practical advice, based on the senior author's experience. A number of technical nuances and caveats were provided. Surgeons are encouraged to perform their own cadaveric dissections, as the complex anatomy of neural surfaces, arteries, and deep white matter tracts in and around the insula are difficult to conceptualize. Mapping remains challenging due to lack of consistency in assigned functions to cortical parcels and subcortical segments. However, efforts to deeply understand surgical anatomy and relevant cognitive neuroscience may lead to robust results in achieving maximum safe resections.

References

[1] Duffau H, Capelle L. Preferential brain locations of low-grade gliomas. Cancer. 2004; 100(12):2622–2626

[2] Gozé C, Rigau V, Gibert L, Maudelonde T, Duffau H. Lack of complete 1p19q deletion in a consecutive series of 12 WHO grade II gliomas involving the insula: a marker of worse prognosis? J Neurooncol. 2009; 91(1):1–5

[3] Jiang H, Cui Y, Wang J, Lin S. Impact of epidemiological characteristics of supratentorial gliomas in adults brought about by the 2016 world health organization classification of tumors of the central nervous system. Oncotarget. 2017; 8(12):20354–20361

[4] Johannesen TB, Langmark F, Lote K. Progress in long-term survival in adult patients with supratentorial low-grade gliomas: a population-based study of 993 patients in whom tumors were diagnosed between 1970 and 1993. J Neurosurg. 2003; 99(5):854–862

[5] Sanai N, Polley M-Y, Berger MS. Insular glioma resection: assessment of patient morbidity, survival, and tumor progression. J Neurosurg. 2010; 112(1):1–9

[6] Michaud K, Duffau H. Surgery of insular and paralimbic diffuse low-grade gliomas: technical considerations. J Neurooncol. 2016; 130(2):289–298

[7] Duffau H. A personal consecutive series of surgically treated 51 cases of insular WHO Grade II glioma: advances and limitations. J Neurosurg. 2009; 110 (4):696–708

[8] Duffau H, Capelle L, Lopes M, Bitar A, Sichez JP, van Effenterre R. Medically intractable epilepsy from insular low-grade gliomas: improvement after an extended lesionectomy. Acta Neurochir (Wien). 2002; 144(6):563–572, discussion 572–573

[9] Signorelli F, Guyotat J, Elisevich K, Barbagallo GMV. Review of current microsurgical management of insular gliomas. Acta Neurochir (Wien). 2010; 152 (1):19–26

[10] Almairac F, Herbet G, Moritz-Gasser S, de Champfleur NM, Duffau H. The left inferior fronto-occipital fasciculus subserves language semantics: a multilevel lesion study. Brain Struct Funct. 2015; 220(4):1983–1995

[11] Smith JS, Chang EF, Lamborn KR, et al. Role of extent of resection in the long-term outcome of low-grade hemispheric gliomas. J Clin Oncol. 2008; 26(8):1338–1345

[12] Roelz R, Strohmaier D, Jabbarli R, et al. Residual tumor volume as best outcome predictor in low grade glioma—a nine-years near-randomized survey of surgery vs. biopsy. Sci Rep. 2016; 6(1):32286

[13] Jakola AS, Myrmel KS, Kloster R, et al. Comparison of a strategy favoring early surgical resection vs a strategy favoring watchful waiting in low-grade gliomas. JAMA. 2012; 308(18):1881–1888

[14] Jakola AS, Skjulsvik AJ, Myrmel KS, et al. Surgical resection versus watchful waiting in low-grade gliomas. Ann Oncol. 2017; 28(8):1942–1948

[15] Wijnenga MMJ, French PJ, Dubbink HJ, et al. The impact of surgery in molecularly defined low-grade glioma: an integrated clinical, radiological, and molecular analysis. Neuro-oncol. 2018; 20(1):103–112

[16] Capelle L, Fontaine D, Mandonnet E, et al. French Réseau d'Étude des Gliomes. Spontaneous and therapeutic prognostic factors in adult hemispheric World

Health Organization grade II gliomas: a series of 1097 cases: clinical article. J Neurosurg. 2013; 118(6):1157–1168

[17] Pallud J, Audureau E, Blonski M, et al. Epileptic seizures in diffuse low-grade gliomas in adults. Brain. 2014; 137(Pt 2):449–462

[18] Pallud J, Mandonnet E, Duffau H, et al. Prognostic value of initial magnetic resonance imaging growth rates for World Health Organization grade II gliomas. Ann Neurol. 2006; 60(3):380–383

[19] Metellus P, Coulibaly B, Colin C, et al. Absence of IDH mutation identifies a novel radiologic and molecular subtype of WHO grade II gliomas with dismal prognosis. Acta Neuropathol. 2010; 120(6):719–729

[20] Gozé C, Blonski M, Le Maistre G, et al. Imaging growth and isocitrate dehydrogenase 1 mutation are independent predictors for diffuse low-grade gliomas. Neuro-oncol. 2014; 16(8):1100–1109

[21] Hervey-Jumper SL, Li J, Osorio JA, et al. Surgical assessment of the insula. Part 2: validation of the Berger-Sanai zone classification system for predicting extent of glioma resection. J Neurosurg. 2016; 124(2):482–488

[22] Eseonu CI, ReFaey K, Garcia O, Raghuraman G, Quinones-Hinojosa A. Volumetric analysis of extent of resection, survival, and surgical outcomes for insular gliomas. World Neurosurg. 2017; 103:265–274

[23] Ius T, Pauletto G, Isola M, et al. Surgery for insular low-grade glioma: predictors of postoperative seizure outcome. J Neurosurg. 2014; 120(1):12–23

[24] Wang DD, Deng H, Hervey-Jumper SL, Molinaro AA, Chang EF, Berger MS. Seizure outcome after surgical resection of insular glioma. Neurosurgery. 2018; 83(4):709–718

[25] Wu AS, Witgert ME, Lang FF, et al. Neurocognitive function before and after surgery for insular gliomas. J Neurosurg. 2011; 115(6):1115–1125

[26] Duffau H, Moritz-Gasser S, Gatignol P. Functional outcome after language mapping for insular World Health Organization grade II gliomas in the dominant hemisphere: experience with 24 patients. Neurosurg Focus. 2009; 27(2):E7

[27] Kawaguchi T, Kumabe T, Saito R, et al. Practical surgical indicators to identify candidates for radical resection of insulo-opercular gliomas. J Neurosurg. 2014; 121(5):1124–1132

[28] Martino J, Mato D, Marco de Lucas E, et al. Subcortical anatomy as an anatomical and functional landmark in insulo-opercular gliomas: implications for surgical approach to the insular region. J Neurosurg. 2015; 123(4):1081–1092

[29] Neuloh G, Pechstein U, Schramm J. Motor tract monitoring during insular glioma surgery. J Neurosurg. 2007; 106(4):582–592

[30] Morshed RA, Young JS, Han SJ, Hervey-Jumper SL, Berger MS. Perioperative outcomes following reoperation for recurrent insular gliomas. J Neurosurg. 2018; 151(18):1–7

[31] Yagmurlu K, Vlasak AL, Rhoton AL, Jr. Three-dimensional topographic fiber tract anatomy of the cerebrum. Neurosurgery. 2015; 11 Suppl 2:274–305, discussion 305

[32] Ribas EC, Yağmurlu K, de Oliveira E, Ribas GC, Rhoton A. Microsurgical anatomy of the central core of the brain. J Neurosurg. 2018; 129(3):752–769

[33] Dronkers NF. A new brain region for coordinating speech articulation. Nature. 1996; 384(6605):159–161

[34] Türe U, Yaşargil DC, Al-Mefty O, Yaşargil MG. Topographic anatomy of the insular region. J Neurosurg. 1999; 90(4):720–733

[35] Türe U, Yaşargil MG, Al-Mefty O, Yaşargil DC. Arteries of the insula. J Neurosurg. 2000; 92(4):676–687

[36] Yaşargil MG, von Ammon K, Cavazos E, Doczi T, Reeves JD, Roth P. Tumours of the limbic and paralimbic systems. Acta Neurochir (Wien). 1992; 118(1–2):40–52

[37] Wang Y, Wang Y, Fan X, et al. Putamen involvement and survival outcomes in patients with insular low-grade gliomas. J Neurosurg. 2017; 126(6):1788–1794

[38] Duffau H, Capelle L, Lopes M, Faillot T, Sichez JP, Fohanno D. The insular lobe: physiopathological and surgical considerations. Neurosurgery. 2000; 47(4):801–810, discussion 810–811

[39] Dick AS, Tremblay P. Beyond the arcuate fasciculus: consensus and controversy in the connectional anatomy of language. Brain. 2012; 135(Pt 12):3529–3550

[40] Ribas GC. The cerebral sulci and gyri. Neurosurg Focus. 2010; 28(2):E2

[41] Devlin JT, Matthews PM, Rushworth MFS. Semantic processing in the left inferior prefrontal cortex: a combined functional magnetic resonance imaging and transcranial magnetic stimulation study. J Cogn Neurosci. 2003; 15(1):71–84

[42] Leff AP, Schofield TM, Stephan KE, Crinion JT, Friston KJ, Price CJ. The cortical dynamics of intelligible speech. J Neurosci. 2008; 28(49):13209–13215

[43] Hope TMH, Prejawa S, Parker Jones, et al. Dissecting the functional anatomy of auditory word repetition. Front Hum Neurosci. 2014; 8(787):246

[44] Belyk M, Brown S, Lim J, Kotz SA. Convergence of semantics and emotional expression within the IFG pars orbitalis. Neuroimage. 2017; 156:240–248

[45] Naidich TP, Hof PR, Gannon PJ, Yousry TA, Yousry I. Anatomic substrates of language: emphasizing speech. Neuroimaging Clin N Am. 2001; 11(2):305–341, ix

[46] Benet A, Hervey-Jumper SL, Sánchez JJG, Lawton MT, Berger MS. Surgical assessment of the insula. Part 1: surgical anatomy and morphometric analysis of the transsylvian and transcortical approaches to the insula. J Neurosurg. 2016; 124(2):469–481

[47] Rolston JD, Englot DJ, Benet A, Li J, Cha S, Berger MS. Frontal operculum gliomas: language outcome following resection. J Neurosurg. 2015; 122(4):725–734

[48] Baldo JV, Wilkins DP, Ogar J, Willock S, Dronkers NF. Role of the precentral gyrus of the insula in complex articulation. Cortex. 2011; 47(7):800–807

[49] Fedorenko E, Fillmore P, Smith K, Bonilha L, Fridriksson J. The superior precentral gyrus of the insula does not appear to be functionally specialized for articulation. J Neurophysiol. 2015; 113(7):2376–2382

[50] Yarkoni T, Poldrack RA, Nichols TE, Van Essen DC, Wager TD. Large-scale automated synthesis of human functional neuroimaging data. Nat Methods. 2011; 8(8):665–670

[51] Richardson JD, Fillmore P, Rorden C, Lapointe LL, Fridriksson J. Re-establishing Broca's initial findings. Brain Lang. 2012; 123(2):125–130

[52] Oh A, Duerden EG, Pang EW. The role of the insula in speech and language processing. Brain Lang. 2014; 135:96–103

[53] Chang LJ, Yarkoni T, Khaw MW, Sanfey AG. Decoding the role of the insula in human cognition: functional parcellation and large-scale reverse inference. Cereb Cortex. 2013; 23(3):739–749

[54] Uddin LQ, Kinnison J, Pessoa L, Anderson ML. Beyond the tripartite cognition-emotion-interoception model of the human insular cortex. J Cogn Neurosci. 2014; 26(1):16–27

[55] Makris N, Pandya DN. The extreme capsule in humans and rethinking of the language circuitry. Brain Struct Funct. 2009; 213(3):343–358

[56] Fernández-Miranda JC, Rhoton AL, Jr, Alvarez-Linera J, Kakizawa Y, Choi C, de Oliveira EP. Three-dimensional microsurgical and tractographic anatomy of the white matter of the human brain. Neurosurgery. 2008; 62(6) Suppl 3:989–1026, discussion 1026–1028

[57] Kier EL, Staib LH, Davis LM, Bronen RA. MR imaging of the temporal stem: anatomic dissection tractography of the uncinate fasciculus, inferior occipito-frontal fasciculus, and Meyer's loop of the optic radiation. AJNR Am J Neuroradiol. 2004; 25(5):677–691

[58] Brown SP, Mathur BN, Olsen SR, Luppi P-H, Bickford ME, Citri A. New breakthroughs in understanding the role of functional interactions between the neocortex and the claustrum. J Neurosci. 2017; 37(45):10877–10881

[59] Von Der Heide RJ, Skipper LM, Klobusicky E, Olson IR, Heide Von Der RJ. Dissecting the uncinate fasciculus: disorders, controversies and a hypothesis. Brain. 2013; 136(Pt 6):1692–1707

[60] Schmahmann JD, Pandya DN, Wang R, et al. Association fibre pathways of the brain: parallel observations from diffusion spectrum imaging and autoradiography. Brain. 2007; 130(Pt 3):630–653

[61] Papagno C. Naming and the role of the uncinate fasciculus in language function. Curr Neurol Neurosci Rep. 2011; 11(6):553–559

[62] Papagno C, Gallucci M, Casarotti A, et al. Connectivity constraints on cortical reorganization of neural circuits involved in object naming. Neuroimage. 2011; 55(3):1306–1313

[63] Duffau H, Gatignol P, Moritz-Gasser S, Mandonnet E. Is the left uncinate fasciculus essential for language? A cerebral stimulation study. J Neurol. 2009; 256(3):382–389

[64] Hickok G, Poeppel D. The cortical organization of speech processing. Nat Rev Neurosci. 2007; 8(5):393–402

[65] Chang EF, Raygor KP, Berger MS. Contemporary model of language organization: an overview for neurosurgeons. J Neurosurg. 2015; 122(2):250–261

[66] Duffau H, Moritz-Gasser S, Mandonnet E. A re-examination of neural basis of language processing: proposal of a dynamic hodotopical model from data provided by brain stimulation mapping during picture naming. Brain Lang. 2014; 131:1–10

[67] Duffau H. Stimulation mapping of white matter tracts to study brain functional connectivity. Nat Rev Neurol. 2015; 11(5):255–265

[68] Moritz-Gasser S, Herbet G, Duffau H. Mapping the connectivity underlying multimodal (verbal and non-verbal) semantic processing: a brain electrostimulation study. Neuropsychologia. 2013; 51(10):1814–1822

[69] Wang X, Pathak S, Stefaneanu L, Yeh F-C, Li S, Fernández-Miranda JC. Subcomponents and connectivity of the superior longitudinal fasciculus in the human brain. Brain Struct Funct. 2016; 221(4):2075–2092

[70] Thiebaut de Schotten M, Dell'Acqua F, Forkel SJ, et al. A lateralized brain network for visuospatial attention. Nat Neurosci. 2011; 14(10):1245–1246

[71] Glasser MF, Rilling JK. DTI tractography of the human brain's language pathways. Cereb Cortex. 2008; 18(11):2471–2482

[72] Ribas GC. Applied Cranial-Cerebral Anatomy: Brain Architecture and Anatomically Oriented Microneurosurgery. Cambridge: Cambridge University Press; 2018

[73] Lang FF, Olansen NE, DeMonte F, et al. Surgical resection of intrinsic insular tumors: complication avoidance. J Neurosurg. 2001; 95(4):638–650

[74] Yaşargil MG. Microneurosurgery: Operative Treatment of CNS Tumors 4B. Stuttgart: Thieme; 1995

[75] Simon M, Neuloh G, von Lehe M, Meyer B, Schramm J. Insular gliomas: the case for surgical management. J Neurosurg. 2009; 110(4):685–695

[76] Tanriover N, Rhoton AL, Jr, Kawashima M, Ulm AJ, Yasuda A. Microsurgical anatomy of the insula and the sylvian fissure. J Neurosurg. 2004; 100(5):891–922

[77] Alimohamadi M, Shirani M, Shariat Moharari R, et al. Application of awake craniotomy and intraoperative brain mapping for surgical resection of insular gliomas of the dominant hemisphere. World Neurosurg. 2016; 92:151–158

[78] De Witt Hamer PC, Robles SG, Zwinderman AH, Duffau H, Berger MS. Impact of intraoperative stimulation brain mapping on glioma surgery outcome: a meta-analysis. J Clin Oncol. 2012; 30(20):2559–2565

[79] LeRoux PD, Berger MS, Haglund MM, Pilcher WH, Ojemann GA. Resection of intrinsic tumors from nondominant face motor cortex using stimulation mapping: report of two cases. Surg Neurol. 1991; 36(1):44–48

[80] Nossek E, Korn A, Shahar T, et al. Intraoperative mapping and monitoring of the corticospinal tracts with neurophysiological assessment and 3-dimensional ultrasonography-based navigation. Clinical article. J Neurosurg. 2011; 114(3):738–746

[81] Rey-Dios R, Cohen-Gadol AA. Technical nuances for surgery of insular gliomas: lessons learned. Neurosurg Focus. 2013; 34(2):E6

16 Mapping of the Visual Pathway

Lina Marenco-Hillembrand and Kaisorn L. Chaichana

Abstract

Vision is a multistep process that involves several different anatomical regions whereby optical signals begin in the retina and are transmitted throughout various parts of the brain. This process is complex and contributes human ability to perform higher level tasks in addition to just visualizing an object, such as object identification, motion acquisition, recognition, and naming, among others. Lesions, namely gliomas, can reside adjacent to and/or interfere with the function of these visual pathway components. In this chapter, we discuss the anatomical pathways involved in primary vision, the pathways involved in hierarchical visual processing, and brain mapping techniques for identifying optic radiations and hierarchical visual functions. Preserving vision is a key, often overlooked, component of one's quality of life.

Keywords: brain mapping, brain tumors, vision, visual pathway

16.1 Introduction

Vision is a multistep process that involves several different anatomical regions whereby optical signals begin in the retina and are transmitted throughout various parts of the brain.[1,2,3] In order for visual perception to occur, the physiological signal must be identified by the retina, the impulses must be transmitted through the optic nerves to the optic pathways, and then these nerve signals must be processed by various areas of the brain including the occipital, parietal, and temporal lobes and eventually the frontal lobes.[1,2,3] This process is complex and contributes the human ability to perform higher level tasks in addition to just visualizing an object, such as object identification, motion acquisition, recognition, and naming, among others.[1,2,4] Visual functions, including visual fields and visual processing, are critical components of one's daily functioning and intraoperative damage to these pathways can significantly affect one's quality of life.[5] Lesions, namely gliomas, can reside adjacent to and/or interfere with the function of these visual pathway components.[1,2,4] An understanding of these pathways and how to map these pathways intraoperatively can help facilitate extensive resection and complication avoidance.[1,2,4,5] In this chapter, we report how we perform awake brain mapping with direct electrical stimulation for lesions involving the visual pathways.

16.2 Visual Pathway and Cognitive Processing of Vision

Visual perception is the process whereby an object is visualized and cognitively recognized.[1,2,3] This process involves multiple steps, several different anatomical structures, and a connectome that spans the entire sagittal distance of the brain.[6,7,8] Lesions can occur along this entire pathway and lead to different deficits depending on the location and degree of pathway disruption.[6,7,8] Knowledge about the process of visual percep-

tion is in constant evolution as the brain connectome is being better understood with brain imaging and brain mapping techniques.[1,2,3]

Light strikes the retinal ganglion cells and the impulse is conducted through the retinal ganglion cell axons into the optic nerve.[6,7,8] The optic nerve then traverses from the retina through the intraorbital space, followed by the optic canal, and then to the optic chiasm where there is partial crossing of the temporal optic nerve axons.[6,7,8] The postchiasmatic optic nerve or optic tract, which carries axons from both optic nerves, synapses in the lateral geniculate nucleus of the thalamus.[6,7,8] The nerve fibers from the lateral geniculate nucleus form the optic radiations that travel through the white matter adjacent to the lateral ventricles to the primary and late visual cortices in the occipital, temporal, and parietal lobes.[6,7,8]

The occipital lobe is referred to as the primary visual cortex, while the temporal and parietal lobes are the late cortices.[6,7,8] In the primary occipital cortex, the lower bank of the calcarine sulcus represents the upper visual field, while the upper back represents the lower visual field.[6,7,8] Moreover, the right visual field is represented in the left occipital lobe and the left visual field is represented in the right occipital lobe.[6,7,8] The fovea is represented in a large cortical area within the occipital lobe where there are a large number of neurons that enable fine spatial vision.[6,7,8] The ability to visualize an object, therefore, requires the optic pathway from the retina to the primary visual cortex of the occipital lobe to be intact.[1,2,3]

Although visualization is a primary function, there are other hierarchical functions that vision is a component of. These hierarchical systems are involved in a number of tasks including object recognition, object naming, detection of motion, and memory, among others, and require input from other sensory systems and brain regions.[1,2,3] In this hierarchical system, several different networks combine their inputs from lower levels and the information is combined and processed in higher levels that allow for visual analysis.[1,2,3] As with language and hearing, there are ventral and dorsal streams that subserve vision.[9] In this dual-stream model, the ventral stream is involved with object identification and recognition, while the dorsal stream is involved with spatial location.[9] The ventral stream involves the processing of information within the parvocellular layer of the lateral geniculate nucleus of the thalamus and projects this information to the V1 cell layer of the occipital cortex, followed by the V2 and V4 cell layers, and then to the inferior temporal lobe primarily through inferior longitudinal fasciculus (ILF).[9] Damage to this region results in difficulty with object recognition, but mostly recognizing faces and facial expression.[9] The posterior portion of the ILF, especially the temporal-occipital area plays a crucial role in reading.[9] In comparison to the ventral stream, the dorsal stream involves the V1 layer of the primary visual cortex of the occipital lobe and transmits information into the parietal lobe, and plays a role in detecting and analyzing movements and spatial awareness.[9] This spatial awareness is most prominent at the right parieto–temporal junction and the information is transmitted through the second portion of the superior longitudinal fasciculus (SLF II).[9] Damage to this region results in incoordination and poor spatial resolution. In addition to these dual streams, the occipital-callosal fibers of the corpus callosum allow information to be communicated to the bilateral occipital lobes for visual processing.[1,2,3]

16.3 Preoperative Imaging

Preoperative imaging can help identify and delineate components of the optic pathway.[10,11,12,13,14] The optic nerves are typically best visualized with high-resolution T2-weighted magnetic resonance imaging (MRI).[10,11,12,13,14] The differential in intensity between the optic nerves and the cerebrospinal fluid space allows the delineation of the optic nerves from the back of the globe, through the optic canal and to the chiasm.[10,11] In the setting of lesions involving or adjacent to the optic nerves, sequences such as inversion recovery (fast gray and white matter acquisition T1 inversion recovery), contrast-enhanced fast imaging employing steady-state acquisition (FIESTA), and heavily weighted T2 sequences can help better delineate the optic nerve and chiasm especially nearby bony structures.[12,13,14]

The retrochiasmatic optic pathway involving the optic radiations can be visualized with a number of different MRI modalities.[10,11] The most commonly used method is diffusion tensor imaging (DTI; ▶ Fig. 16.1).[10,11] This method is based on the diffusion of water molecules in the extra and intracellular spaces.[10,11] When this diffusion is not random and limited to directional structures such as axons, the diffusion of water follows these axon bundles rather than random path.[10,11] This anisotropic diffusion allows the identification of these white matter tacts.[10,11] In addition to DTI, functional MRI (fMRI) can also help identify components of the optic pathway, namely the primary visual cortex.[10,11] FMRI is based on neurovascular coupling, where neural activity in a specific cortical region will trigger a change in the regional blood flow that is captured on the MRI.[10,11] A component of this fMRI is called retinotopic mapping.[10,11] In retinotopic mapping, visual stimuli are presented to different visual fields that create a wave of specific neural activity within the cortex.[10,11] This allows one to identify the correspondence between the position of the stimuli within the visual field and the cortex to be identified.[10,11] More complex functional mapping involves hierarchical functions such as object perception and recognition of object motion, where cortical areas that are activated during specific tasks are identified.[10,11] For object perception, an object is shown in its entire form or scrambled, while, for motion, an object is shown in motion or stationary.[10,11] The corresponding cortical areas that are activated are then identified for their respective function.[10,11]

These preoperative imaging modalities have significant limitations for intraoperative utilization.[10,11,12,13,14] This is especially true for the optic radiations.[10,11] For DTI, the normal anisotropic diffusion of water can be disrupted by various pathologies.[10,11] Lesions that induce perilesional edema interfere with the normal anisotropic diffusion of water thereby making this imaging modality less precise and subject to false positive and false negative identification intraoperatively.[1,2,4] Moreover, pathologies that destroy and/or infiltrate these white matter tracts can also interfere with the anisotropic diffusion of water within these tracts.[1,2,4] In addition to the limitations associated with DTI, fMRI can be associated with error as this imaging modality requires large-scale neural activation with specific tasks.[10,11]

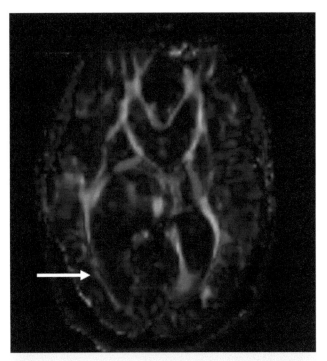

Fig. 16.1 Diffusion tensor imaging of the visual pathway. The nerve impulse after visualizing an object starts in the retina and then is transmitted in the optic nerve through the chiasm and then to the optic pathway. The optic pathway goes from the chiasm to the lateral geniculate nucleus of the thalamus and then forms the optic radiations (*white arrow*) around the ventricles to the primary visual cortex in the occipital lobe. Information from the primary visual cortex is then transmitted to hierarchical areas that control other visual functions through the ventral and dorsal streams (not pictured).

These foci of neural activation can be associated with false positive and false negative localization with intraoperative direct electrical stimulation.[1,2,4] Despite the widespread availability of these imaging modalities and others, the problem remains that they are associated with false positive and false negative identification of eloquent and noneloquent areas.[1,2,4] Most importantly, they do not accurately identify functional from nonfunctional areas and therefore should not be used solely for functional brain area identification and avoidance during surgery.[1,2,4] This is why many advocate a 5 to 10 mm avoidance of these critical cortical and subcortical regions identified on DTI and fMRI during surgery, which can significantly limit extent of resection.[1,2,4]

16.4 Intraoperative Mapping— Visual Evoked Potentials (VEP)

Visual evoked potentials (VEP) are not commonly used for glioma surgery.[15,16,17] VEP records the electrical signal over the occipital lobes at the scalp in response to light stimulus.[15,16] This light stimulus has to be repetitive and time-locked in order to be identified on the electroencephalogram (EEG).[15,16] The VEPs are designed to assess the afferent visual pathway and therefore a decrease or loss in signal signifies damage to any part of the afferent visual pathway.[15,16] On the EEG, the VEP waveforms typically consist of an initial negative peak (N1), followed by a positive peak (P1), a second negative peak (N2), and a second positive peak (P2) in that order.[15,16] The latency of peak onset after the light stimulus and, to a lesser extent, the amplitude of the peak are analyzed to detect vision loss.[15,16] These values are compared to the starting VEP, the contralateral eye, and to each hemisphere to delineate where along the optic pathway an insult has occurred.[15,16]

VEP monitoring, however, has not typically been used for intra-axial surgery since it primarily evaluates central visual function.[15,16,17] In a recent study in awake patients, Shahar and colleagues found no association between the presence of VEP monitoring and presence of visual field deficits.[17] Central visual function in the macula is distributed through a large portion of the occipital cortex and the electrodes in the scalp are not sensitive enough to detect visual field deficits.[15,16] This modality has been used for sellar and suprasellar surgery, but more commonly it is used for detecting deficits in the visual pathway in infants and inarticulate adults and to detect nonorganic disease.[15,16] Since its ability to detect peripheral vision loss is limited, its use in intra-axial surgery is limited and therefore it is not routinely used.[15,16,17]

16.5 Intraoperative Mapping with Awake Brain Surgery and Direct Electrical Stimulation

16.5.1 Importance of Awake Brain Surgery with Direct Electrical Stimulation

It is well established that increasing extent of resection is associated with improved outcomes for both low- and high-grade gliomas as long as iatrogenic deficits are avoided.[18,19,20,21,22,23,24,25,26] In eloquent regions, primarily involving language and motor cortices and their respective subcortical white matter tracts, awake surgery with direct electrical stimulation has been associated with improved outcomes.[27,28,29] In a meta-analysis by DeWitt Hammer et al, 90 published studies between 1990 and 2010 evaluated the effects of direct electrical stimulation mapping and found that late severe neurological deficits were less (3.4 vs. 8.2%), percent of gross total resections were more (75 vs. 58%), and the technique was more commonly used in eloquent locations (99.9 vs. 95.8%).[29] When comparing the awake-asleep-awake versus the monitored anesthesia care for gliomas, the awake-asleep-awake approach was associated with shorter duration of surgery and no differences in intraoperative complications such as seizures, aborted cases, and conversion to monitored anesthesia care.[30] For tumors involving the peri-Rolandic region, awake surgery with brain mapping was associated with higher postoperative Karnofsky Performance Scores (93 vs. 81), increased extent of resection (86.3 vs. 79.6%), more gross total resections (25.9 vs. 6.5%), and shorter hospital stays (4.2 vs. 7.9 days) as compared to general anesthesia.[27] This use of awake surgery has been associated with decreased hospital costs and improved quality of life for patients with low- and high-grade gliomas.[28]

The overwhelming majority of studies on awake surgery with intraoperative mapping typically applies to lesions involving language and/or motor cortical and subcortical white matter.[27,28,29] Studies devoted to mapping the visual cortex, optic pathways, and hierarchical visual functions are limited.[1,2,4,17,31] The retrochiasmatic visual pathway and optic radiations are more difficult to map than language and/or motor function for several reasons. This is because visual field function has not been a primary concern as this function has been considered secondary to "more critical" functions such as language and/or motor.[4] In addition, visual field mapping can be difficult to execute intraoperatively because it requires more intensive patient cooperation and examinations, and cannot be done asleep.[1,2,4,17,31] Moreover, an understanding of higher level visual functions, such as object recognition and movement, and the brain regions responsible for these functions has been limited.[1,2,4,17,31] However, visual field function is a critical component of one's quality of life as it dictates the ability to drive and participate in activities. It is also critical for several occupations and, therefore, attempts at preserving one's visual function is important for many patients.

16.5.2 Visual Field Mapping

Visual function is widely distributed throughout the brain. Visual field mapping, a component of visual function, is only part of the mapping armamentarium, as we typically map language and motor functions concomitantly with visual field function. This is because these areas are in close proximity with each other, these functions subserve one another, and lesions often involve multiple cortical and subcortical areas that control many different critical neurological functions.[2,3,4,31] For visual field mapping, we typically perform these mapping techniques for lesions involving the area of the brain between the posterior part of the temporal lobe and the temporal–occipital–parietal junction on either hemisphere. In addition, we typically only map for visual field function in patients with no or minimal preoperative visual field deficits on formal visual field testing. It is challenging to maintain visual field function in a patient with preexisting visual field deficits because of the difficulty of intraoperative examinations. The typical goal of surgery is to avoid homonymous hemianopia, while quadrantanopia is tolerated since patients can still drive with this deficit.[1,2,4]

Patients are positioned in the lateral position under local anesthesia as previously described.[28,30] The patient is kept asleep until the craniotomy is done, prior to dural opening. The craniotomy typically spans multiple cortical and subcortical functional areas to facilitate positive and negative mapping, and typically includes motor and language functions in addition to visual fields. Once the dura is exposed, the patient is awakened and examinations are done continuously until the tumor is disconnected from eloquent regions and then the patient is put back to sleep. This process typically does not take longer than 30 minutes as patient fatigue interferes with evaluating various neurological functions especially language including semantic and paraphasic evaluations. Direct electrical stimulation is applied to brain and is done with the use of a bipolar electrode with 5-mm spaced tips that delivers a biphasic current with a pulse frequency of 60 Hz, single pulse duration of 1 millisecond, and amplitude that varies from 1 to 6 mA (Nicolet Cortical Stimulator, Natus, Middleton, WI). This amplitude is selected on the basis of positive mapping with sensorimotor or language cortex stimulation whereby transient movement, paresthesias, speech arrest, or picture naming inhibition are elicited with direct electrical stimulation. For lesions involving the nondominant hemisphere, sensorimotor mapping is typically done first because of the close proximity of the visual fields and primary visual cortex to the sensorimotor cortex. Positive mapping in this area is achieved when transient movement, paresthesias, and/or speech arrest with counting occurs. For lesions involving the dominant hemisphere, language mapping is typically done first with picture-naming tasks. However, it should be stressed that motor and language functions are being tested simultaneously and continuously.

Once the mapping thresholds are identified in the cortex, resection takes place simultaneously with mapping where stimulation followed by resection occurs repetitively in the cortical and subcortical space. As long as stimulation is negative for eliciting deficits, resection continues. Visual field mapping is done similarly as previously described.[1,2,3,4,17] The patient is shown serial pictures in the quadrant to be preserved and the diagonal quadrant with their primary focus on the center of the screen depicted by a red cross (▶ Fig. 16.2). For example, when surgical resection is occurring in the left posterior temporal lobe, the location of the image of interest is in the right superior quadrant and the diagonal image is in the left inferior quadrant. The patient is instructed to maintain focus on a cross in the center of the screen. The examiner makes sure the patient's gaze is fixed on the cross in the center and there are no eye movements in order to accurately assess their visual fields. A positive mapping occurs when the patient experiences a subjective transient visual disturbance within the contralateral hemifield

(i.e., right superior quadrant) that prevents naming, but not in the ipsilateral diagonal quadrant (i.e., left inferior quadrant). These visual disturbances can be any combination of blurriness, ring or spot of light (also called phosphenes), and/or darkness. In general, phosphenes are referred to as positive effects, while blurred vision and darkness are referred to as negative effects. Both of these effects can happen with stimulation. An inability to name both objects typically implies a language or cognitive deficit rather than a visual field deficit. Resection is stopped for visual field preservation when these deficits in visual fields are elicited with direct electrical stimulation. Once the lesion is disconnected from known eloquent areas (vision, motor, sensory, and/or language), the patient is put back to sleep and the remaining portion of the tumor is resected. The dura, bone, and skin are closed in standard fashion. The patient undergoes a postoperative MRI within 48 hours of surgery and a formal visual field test approximately 3 months after surgery.

16.5.3 Hierarchical Visual Function Mapping

The mapping of hierarchical visual function is still in its infancy.[1,2,3,4,9,17] The majority of these components are mapped indirectly by assessing language functions.[1,2,3,4,9,17] For example, object naming requires visualization and object recognition which involves the optic pathway and the ventral visual stream in addition to memory, semantics, and phonology, among others.[1,2,3,4,9,17] As a result, we advocate for continuous mapping of several different simultaneous functions including object

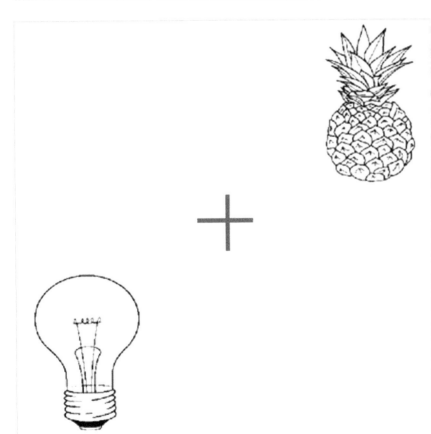

Fig. 16.2 Intraoperative visual field testing. The patients are shown several different images and are told to focus on the red cross in the center to assess their visual fields and minimize eye movement. For a left temporal/occipital lesion, the primary object of concern is in the top right corner. The patients are asked to name the two objects they see, and if they see lights or phosphenes (positive effect) or shadowing or blurriness (negative effects) with the object that prevents naming, it constitutes positive mapping and resection of this area should be avoided. Inability to name both objects constitutes an elicited language deficit and not necessarily a visual field deficit.

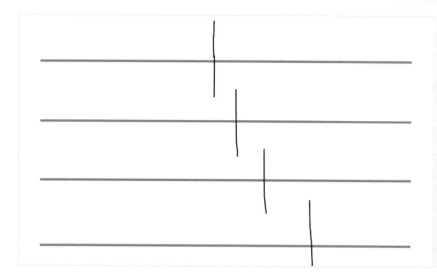

Fig. 16.3 Line bisection test. This test is done mainly to assess awareness and sensory neglect primarily in the right parieto–temporal junction and dorsal stream of visual hierarchical function. The patient is asked to draw a line through the center, and with increasing stimulation they become more neglectful of the left side with parieto–temporal junctional stimulation of part II of the superior longitudinal fasciculus. This results in a rightward deviation of the line as seen here.

naming, motor strength, and visual fields all concurrently. However, a knowledge of the common cortical and subcortical white matter tracts that can potentially be involved will allow the surgeon a heightened awareness of potential deficits elicited during direct electrical stimulation. These functions are absolutely critical for certain occupations and are significant components of one's quality of life.

Intraoperative mapping can help identify involvement of the dual streams by mapping white matter tracts that subserve these functions.[9] As stated previously, in this dual-stream model, the ventral stream is involved with object identification and recognition, while the dorsal stream is involved with spatial location.[9] The ventral stream and the ILF can be evaluated intraoperatively by showing images of facial expressions and reading, where stimulation can impair facial expression recognition and/or dyslexia.[9] These functions are absolutely critical for normal quality of life, especially for certain occupations such as police officers.[9] The dorsal stream and SLF II can be evaluated intraoperatively by a line bisection test.[9] With stimulation especially at the right parietotemporal junction, there will be a rightward deviation with line bisection (▶ Fig. 16.3).[9] In addition, stimulation can induce vertigo especially at different regions of the right SLF II at the insular–parietal cortex, sensorimotor cortex, and visual cortex.[9] Damage to this dorsal stream area can lead to significant incoordination, and these functions are critical for musicians and athletes.[9]

16.6 Case Example

This is a 57-year-old right-handed male pilot with a history of hypertension and coronary artery disease who presented with seizures. He was in his usual state of health but developed acute-onset progressive headaches. Head computed tomography was done and a lesion in the right posterior temporal-occipital region was detected. This was followed by an MRI with contrast that confirmed this subcortical lesion within the posterior temporal and occipital lobe with mild vasogenic edema

(▶ Fig. 16.4). DTI was not done. Formal visual field testing showed intact visual fields bilaterally without deficits. The patient underwent an awake right craniotomy with direct electrical stimulation. The motor cortex was identified with positive mapping by eliciting facial twitching at 3 mA. This amplitude was used for the remainder of the case. The patient was presented visual field images with intermittent facial expression images (▶ Fig. 16.4). Direct electrical stimulation resulted in phosphenes at the medial aspect of the tumor and resection was stopped. Intermittent prosopagnosia was also elicited at this area. Postoperative MRI showed gross total resection of the lesion. Pathology was an isocitrate dehydrogenase (IDH) wild-type, methylguanine DNA methyltransferase methylated glioblastoma. Visual field testing done at 3 months postoperatively confirmed bedside full visual field exams. He underwent radiation and temozolomide chemotherapy and is 18 months out from surgery without signs of recurrence. He has resumed flying planes and has maintained his normal quality of life. Another example of a case involving the visual cortex, visual tract, and right parieto-occipital junction involved in spatial awareness is seen in ▶ Fig. 16.5.

16.7 Conclusion

Vision is an important function for our daily quality of life. It is a complex process that is more than just visualizing an object. It involves object recognition, naming, detection of motion, and memory, among others. These functions involve several different brain areas including the retina, optic nerve, thalamus, primary visual cortex of the occipital lobe, and hierarchical visual processing areas of the dorsal and ventral streams involving the parietal, temporal, and frontal lobes. Lesions within the brain can endanger these functions and removing these lesions can further put these areas at risk. An ability to identify and avoid these areas during neurosurgical procedures can be accomplished with awake brain mapping and direct electrical stimulation, as long as one understands and tests these functions intraoperatively.

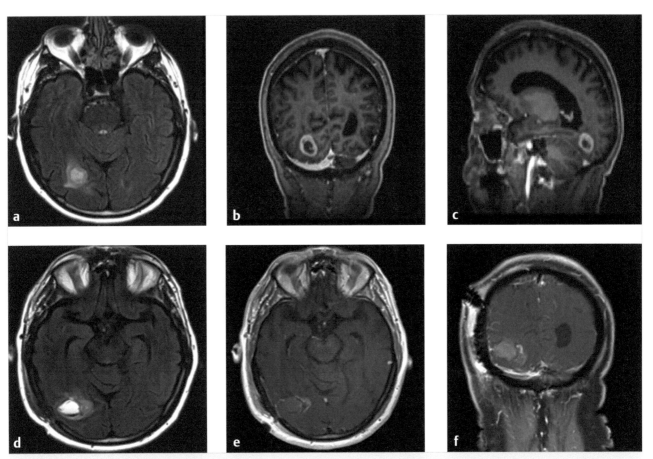

Fig. 16.4 Example of a case involving the visual tracts. This is a 57-year-old right-handed male pilot who presented with headaches. Magnetic resonance imaging showed a contrast-enhancing right posterior temporal-occipital glioblastoma (T2-weighted axial fluid-attenuated inversion recovery [FLAIR] (**a**), T1-weighted axial (**b**), and sagittal (**c**) with contrast). The patient underwent an awake surgery with direct electrical stimulation involving assessment of the sensorimotor cortex to identify positive mapping parameters. The patient was then assessed for visual fields as well as facial expression identification. Positive sites were found for both at the deepest, most medial portion of the tumor. Patient underwent gross total resection of the lesion without neurological deficits (T2-weighted axial FLAIR (**d**), T1-weighted axial (**e**), and sagittal (**f**) with contrast).

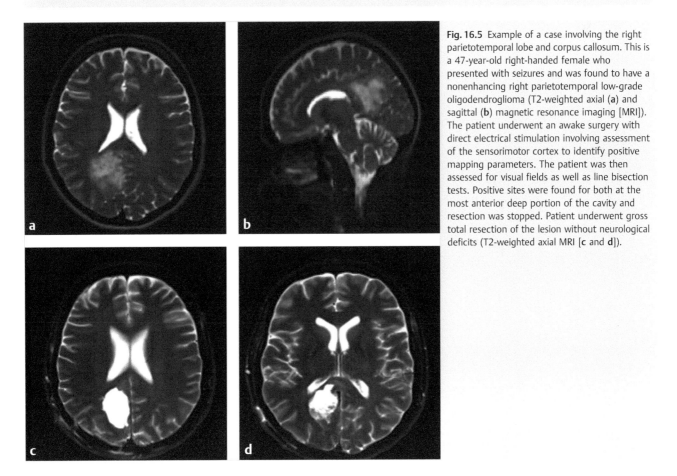

Fig. 16.5 Example of a case involving the right parietotemporal lobe and corpus callosum. This is a 47-year-old right-handed female who presented with seizures and was found to have a nonenhancing right parietotemporal low-grade oligodendroglioma (T2-weighted axial (**a**) and sagittal (**b**) magnetic resonance imaging [MRI]). The patient underwent an awake surgery with direct electrical stimulation involving assessment of the sensorimotor cortex to identify positive mapping parameters. The patient was then assessed for visual fields as well as line bisection tests. Positive sites were found for both at the most anterior deep portion of the cavity and resection was stopped. Patient underwent gross total resection of the lesion without neurological deficits (T2-weighted axial MRI [**c** and **d**]).

References

[1] Bartolomeo P, Thiebaut de Schotten M, Duffau H. Mapping of visuospatial functions during brain surgery: a new tool to prevent unilateral spatial neglect. Neurosurgery. 2007; 61(6):E1340

[2] Duffau H, Velut S, Mitchell MC, Gatignol P, Capelle L. Intra-operative mapping of the subcortical visual pathways using direct electrical stimulations. Acta Neurochir (Wien). 2004; 146(3):265–269, discussion 269–270

[3] Gras-Combe G, Moritz-Gasser S, Herbet G, Duffau H. Intraoperative subcortical electrical mapping of optic radiations in awake surgery for glioma involving visual pathways. J Neurosurg. 2012; 117(3):466–473

[4] Duffau H. Intraoperative monitoring of visual function. Acta Neurochir (Wien). 2011; 153(10):1929–1930

[5] Chaichana KL, Jackson C, Patel A, et al. Predictors of visual outcome following surgical resection of medial sphenoid wing meningiomas. J Neurol Surg B Skull Base. 2012; 73(5):321–326

[6] De Moraes CG. Anatomy of the visual pathways. J Glaucoma. 2013; 22 Suppl 5:S2–S7

[7] Ribas EC, Yagmurlu K, Wen HT, Rhoton AL, Jr. Microsurgical anatomy of the inferior limiting insular sulcus and the temporal stem. J Neurosurg. 2015; 122(6):1263–1273

[8] Rubino PA, Rhoton AL, Jr, Tong X, Oliveira Ed. Three-dimensional relationships of the optic radiation. Neurosurgery. 2005; 57(4) Suppl:219–227, discussion 219–227

[9] Rauschecker JP. Where, when, and how: are they all sensorimotor? Towards a unified view of the dorsal pathway in vision and audition. Cortex. 2018; 98: 262–268

[10] Hana A, Husch A, Hana A, Boecher-Schwarz H, Hertel F. DTI of the visual pathway in cerebral lesions. Bull Soc Sci Med Grand Duche Luxemb. 2012; (2):15–24

[11] Shi Y, Toga AW. Connectome imaging for mapping human brain pathways. Mol Psychiatry. 2017; 22(9):1230–1240

[12] Saeki N, Murai H, Kubota M, et al. Heavily T2 weighted MR images of anterior optic pathways in patients with sellar and parasellar tumours—prediction of surgical anatomy. Acta Neurochir (Wien). 2002; 144(1):25–35

[13] Speckter H, Bido J, Hernandez G, et al. Inversion recovery sequences improve delineation of optic pathways in the proximity of suprasellar lesions. J Radiosurg SBRT. 2018; 5(2):115–122

[14] Watanabe K, Kakeda S, Yamamoto J, et al. Delineation of optic nerves and chiasm in close proximity to large suprasellar tumors with contrast-enhanced FIESTA MR imaging. Radiology. 2012; 264(3):852–858

[15] Dotto PF, Berezovsky A, Cappellano AM, et al. Visual function assessed by visually evoked potentials in optic pathway low-grade gliomas with and without neurofibromatosis type 1. Doc Ophthalmol. 2018; 136(3):177–189

[16] Kurozumi K, Kameda M, Ishida J, Date I. Simultaneous combination of electromagnetic navigation with visual evoked potential in endoscopic transsphenoidal surgery: clinical experience and technical considerations. Acta Neurochir (Wien). 2017; 159(6):1043–1048

[17] Shahar T, Korn A, Barkay G, et al. Elaborate mapping of the posterior visual pathway in awake craniotomy. J Neurosurg. 2018; 128(5):1503–1511

[18] Duffau H. Long-term outcomes after supratotal resection of diffuse low-grade gliomas: a consecutive series with 11-year follow-up. Acta Neurochir (Wien). 2016; 158(1):51–58

[19] McGirt MJ, Chaichana KL, Attenello FJ, et al. Extent of surgical resection is independently associated with survival in patients with hemispheric infiltrating low-grade gliomas. Neurosurgery. 2008; 63(4):700–707, author reply 707–708

[20] Chaichana KL, Cabrera-Aldana EE, Jusue-Torres I, et al. When gross total resection of a glioblastoma is possible, how much resection should be achieved? World Neurosurg. 2014; 82(1–2):e257–e265

[21] Chaichana KL, Chaichana KK, Olivi A, et al. Surgical outcomes for older patients with glioblastoma multiforme: preoperative factors associated with decreased survival. Clinical article. J Neurosurg. 2011; 114(3):587–594

[22] Chaichana KL, Garzon-Muvdi T, Parker S, et al. Supratentorial glioblastoma multiforme: the role of surgical resection versus biopsy among older patients. Ann Surg Oncol. 2011; 18(1):239–245

[23] Chaichana KL, Halthore AN, Parker SL, et al. Factors involved in maintaining prolonged functional independence following supratentorial glioblastoma resection. Clinical article. J Neurosurg. 2011; 114(3):604–612

[24] Chaichana KL, Jusue-Torres I, Navarro-Ramirez R, et al. Establishing percent resection and residual volume thresholds affecting survival and recurrence for patients with newly diagnosed intracranial glioblastoma. Neuro-oncol. 2014; 16(1):113–122

[25] McGirt MJ, Chaichana KL, Gathinji M, et al. Independent association of extent of resection with survival in patients with malignant brain astrocytoma. J Neurosurg. 2009; 110(1):156–162

[26] McGirt MJ, Mukherjee D, Chaichana KL, Than KD, Weingart JD, Quinones-Hinojosa A. Association of surgically acquired motor and language deficits on overall survival after resection of glioblastoma multiforme. Neurosurgery. 2009; 65(3):463–469, discussion 469–470

[27] Eseonu CI, Rincon-Torroella J, ReFaey K, et al. Awake craniotomy vs craniotomy under general anesthesia for peri-Rolandic gliomas: evaluating perioperative complications and extent of resection. Neurosurgery. 2017; 81(3):481–489

[28] Eseonu CI, Rincon-Torroella J, ReFaey K, Quiñones-Hinojosa A. The cost of brain surgery: awake vs asleep craniotomy for peri-Rolandic region tumors. Neurosurgery. 2017; 81(2):307–314

[29] De Witt Hamer PC, Robles SG, Zwinderman AH, Duffau H, Berger MS. Impact of intraoperative stimulation brain mapping on glioma surgery outcome: a meta-analysis. J Clin Oncol. 2012; 30(20):2559–2565

[30] Eseonu CI, ReFaey K, Garcia O, John A, Quiñones-Hinojosa A, Tripathi P. Awake craniotomy anesthesia: a comparison of the monitored anesthesia care and asleep-awake-asleep techniques. World Neurosurg. 2017; 104:679–686

[31] Rolland A, Herbet G, Duffau H. Awake surgery for gliomas within the right inferior parietal lobule: new insights into the functional connectivity gained from stimulation mapping and surgical implications. World Neurosurg. 2018; 112:e393–e406

17 Seizure Mapping Surgery

John P. Andrews and Edward F. Chang

Abstract

Controlling seizures is a critical aspect of many surgeries for epilepsy or brain tumors. In this chapter, we review techniques for intraoperative seizure mapping to improve seizure outcomes for patients with uncontrolled seizures. Specifically, we discuss the use of intraoperative electrocorticography to localize interictal epileptiform discharges, and the use of tailored resections to address them.

Keywords: Seizures, epilepsy, electrocorticography, mapping

17.1 Introduction

The use of electrodes to directly record from the cortex is intricately intertwined with the genesis of epilepsy surgery. The utility of electrocorticography (ECoG) for demarcating seizure-onset zones during chronic, extraoperative intracranial studies is the gold standard for localizing seizure onset, but the use of intraoperative ECoG—limited mostly to interictal epileptiform activity—to intuit epileptogenicity or make judgements about sufficiency of resection is nuanced. As with many aspects of neurosurgical technique, these can vary by institution and surgeon preference.

Whether the desired curative effects from surgery are mediated solely through removal of the offending substrate or rather through a more nuanced disruption of epileptogenic networks, is a subject of ongoing research. Regardless, seizures are an electrophysiologic phenomenon, and while macroscopic lesions are often their cause, electrographic study still offers the most accurate lens through which to delineate epileptiform activity. Intraoperative ECoG can be a useful tool for implicating areas of the brain as parts of the seizure network. It has been a critical part of the epilepsy surgeon's armamentarium since Wilder Penfield's pioneering work. The techniques have evolved to certain degree with technology, but they retain many of the same key aspects and tools that they had in the beginning. This chapter will detail some of the limitations, advantages, and considerations regarding intraoperative ECoG for epilepsy surgery.

17.2 Considerations and Limitations

A knowledge of the limitations of intraoperative ECoG is critical for deciding how best to use such techniques. One restriction to note is the limited window of recording offered during surgery. In contrast to chronic recordings made extraoperatively through implanted subdural electrodes, the time constraints inherent to surgery do not allow one to wait for a patient's habitual seizures intraoperatively. Thus, inferences made in ECoG are drawn from interictal data. Interictal spikes and sharp waves do not necessarily correlate with ictal onset zone. Although likely representing an irritative zone broader and encompassing the ictal onset zone to some degree, they should

not be conceptualized as directly representative of a focus of ictal epileptogenesis.[1,2,3,4] This is a critical distinction to make, because it contextualizes intraoperative ECoG as a supplement to other extraoperative seizure-mapping studies, rather than a stand-alone diagnostic tool that can be the sole guide for resectional epilepsy surgery.

Another unique feature of intraoperative ECoG is the interplay of anesthesia with background activity and epileptiform discharges.[5] For example, opioid medications may enhance epileptiform activity in the cortex, increasing spike frequency such that areas with spike activity might be more easily recognized.[6] On the other hand, propofol, benzodiazepines, barbiturates, and etomidate are all reported to suppress epileptiform activity, which could interfere with the goals of ECoG.[7] Questions remain as to how well pharmacoactivated spikes correlate with native spike activity.[8] An example anesthesia protocol leading up to intraoperative ECoG might involve local anesthesia, nitrous oxide, narcotics, and dexmedetomidine. Anesthesiologists working on these cases should be familiar with the goals and phases of surgery so as to plan appropriately.

The importance of multidisciplinary interplay in planning for intraoperative ECoG cannot be overemphasized (▶ Fig. 17.1). The usefulness of intraoperative ECoG depends critically on being able to interpret the electrographic output of the studies in real time. As with other aspects of epilepsy surgery and decision-making at a large tertiary referral center for epilepsy, the input of specialized neurology colleagues is invaluable. A team of epileptologists trained in interpretation of electroencephalography (EEG) and ECoG should be available in the operating room to assist the surgeon in incorporating the data from ECoG into the surgical plan in real time (▶ Fig. 17.1).

17.3 Generalities of Technique

As discussed in the next section, the specifics of technique for ECoG depend on the question that the study is being used to ask. There are, however, some generalities that may be applied. Recording from the cortical surface can be carried out using either flexible strips or grids of electrodes that are composed of flat discs (the electrode contacts) of platinum, silver, or stainless steel imbedded in Teflon or silastic sheaths[9] (▶ Fig. 17.2). These are advantageous because of their flexibility and low profile. They can be slid into the subdural spaces beyond the margins of the craniotomy to record from areas more difficult to openly expose[10] (▶ Fig. 17.3). Moreover, these electrodes are usually designed to be used for chronic monitoring, so the decision to leave electrodes in for a long-term intracranial study can be made seamlessly during surgery. Alternatively, a fixed array of electrodes can be secured to the skull intraoperatively in a circular frame. Individual, rigid, wire electrodes can be positioned and repositioned strategically on the cortical surface, each of which are covered at the tip by a conductive material like carbon.[11] This form of ECoG is only possible intraoperatively but is particularly useful for mapping of eloquent regions of cortex. The fixed array also has the advantage of being reusable.

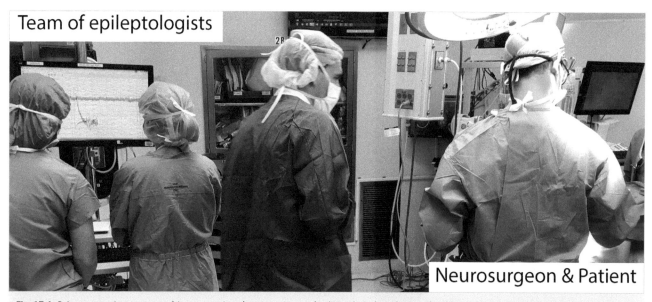

Team of epileptologists

Neurosurgeon & Patient

Fig. 17.1 Seizure-mapping teams and intraoperative electrocorticography (ECoG). Epileptologists should accompany an electroencephalography technologist in the operating room during intraoperative ECoG. Thought should be given to the position of this team so that they can have a reasonable view of the operative field to see where electrodes are placed. A close working relationship between epilepsy surgeons and epilepsy neurology colleagues is critical for safe and effective ECoG.

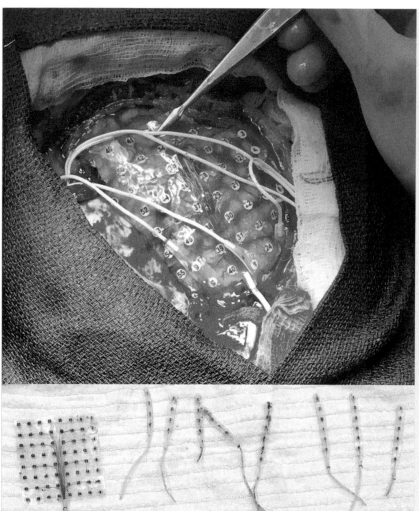

Fig. 17.2 *Top*: 64-contact electrode grids can be used intraoperatively for electrocorticography as well as for chronic implantation for staged intracranial studies prior to resection. Ideally, the grid covers all the area of cortex exposed by the craniotomy. Four or six-contact electrode strips are also supplementing coverage in this example after being slipped beneath the margins of the craniotomy. *Bottom*: Explanted strips and grids comparing a 64-contact grid with 6 and 4-contact electrode strips.

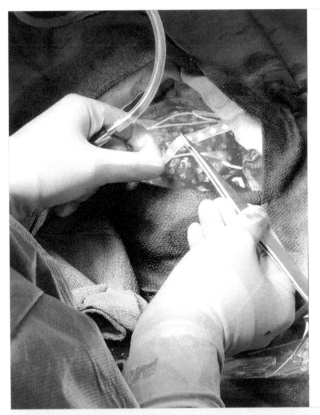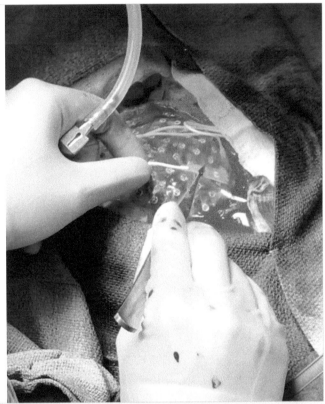

Fig. 17.3 Flexible strip electrodes are effective tools for extending coverage beyond margins of the craniotomy. Due to their narrow profile and flexible material, they will conform to the gross contours of the brain. Longer electrode strips can be used to curve around hard to reach areas such as the anterior temporal pole.

Time is an important factor to take into consideration when performing ECoG, and standard surgical considerations regarding management of extended exposure of the cortex should be considered. There is no set time as to how long one must record from a specific area in order to characterize epileptiform activity. Immediate and early identification of epileptiform activity may immediately answer the question of whether spikes are generated in an area, but when ruling out the involvement of cortex, it may be more difficult to decide how long is sufficient. Studies using ECoG to weigh against the involvement of lateral temporal cortex in temporal lobe epilepsy (TLE) have used 5 minutes as a rough cut-off, and this seems to be a reasonable time-frame.[12]

17.4 Questions

Intraoperative ECoG is most useful when it is employed to answer a specific question. The technique used for ECoG will depend on the question that is being posed. Questions can be asked with ECoG prior to intracranial EEG that guide placement of electrodes for chronic intracranial EEG monitoring. ECoG can be used intraoperatively prior to—or during—resection to implicate cortical areas as possible epileptogenic nodes in a seizure network. Likewise, ECoG can be used as evidence that areas of cortex are not involved in epileptogenicity and can therefore be spared from resection.[13] Pre- and postresection intraoperative ECoG is also sometimes employed as a way to monitor the

effect a resection has had on interictal activity observed in areas of interest, though the prognostic value of pre- and post-resection spikes is a topic of debate.[14,15,16]

17.5 Guiding the Placement of Electrodes

Intraoperative ECoG may be used as an element of the first surgical phase of a staged surgical epilepsy work-up where long-term subdural recordings and extraoperative seizure-mapping is planned prior to a second-stage resection. Extraoperative seizure-mapping is addressed in detail in another chapter, but it should be noted that such extraoperative mapping begins with intraoperative recordings. The question that is asked intraoperatively may be as simple as "Are the electrodes working once they are in place?" The surgery for initial implantation of subdural electrodes or stereotactic depth electrodes should not be completed until it has been verified that the electrodes are recording adequately for interpretation and with an acceptable level of noise. Ideally, this determination can be made by the epilepsy team members who will be interpreting the recordings during the patient's stay. Measuring the electrode impedance while recording can verify electrode contact with the cortex. For example, such measurements can be used to adjust electrode position should large veins lie between electrodes and the cortical surface.[9] Grids or strips may need to be repositioned until recordings are deemed appropriate. In addition, if depth electrodes are being placed, checking the impedance intraoperatively can give clues as to whether any contacts might be within a ventricle if one was traversed.

Responsive neurostimulation (RNS) through implanted intracranial electrodes is becoming a more prominent option for patients with epilepsy who either are not candidates for focal resections or perhaps have already had failed resectional intervention. In such cases, the positioning of electrodes is paramount to the possible effects of stimulation. ECoG input on the precise location for cortical strips, for example, can be very valuable not only to guide diagnostics, but also for the efficacy of this developing therapy.

MRI-negative neocortical epilepsy presents a conundrum because it may represent a diffuse process as opposed to a focal one. If the epileptogenic substrate is distributed widely throughout the cortex, then even ECoG-guided resection will be unlikely to sufficiently localize the epileptogenic zone. Should these patients meet surgical criteria, they should likely undergo chronic intracranial monitoring to localize the lesion. If the focus is not well localized on chronic monitoring, then resection may not be a curative option. However, in this case, intraoperative ECoG may be useful during a second stage of surgery during electrode removal, for searching for sites that might have been missed or sites that could potentially be candidates for RNS strips. ▶ Fig. 17.2 and ▶ Fig. 17.3 show an example from a patient with frontal lobe epilepsy who underwent chronic subdural monitoring. Seizures were found to be multifocal in origin and often originating at the margins of the grid, making it impossible to determine whether the grid was detecting the true first onset or spread from an uncovered onset. At the time of the second stage, the electrodes were moved and distributed more posteriorly to see if there was evidence of epileptiform activity beyond the original grid placement margins, so as to get the information about where to put an RNS stimulator later on (see **Video 17.1**).

17.6 Guiding Extent of Resection

ECoG is generally not necessary for standard resections in patients with TLE and MRI-evident mesial temporal sclerosis (MTS).[17] Anteromesial temporal resections have become a standard procedure that can be performed for patients with TLE and MTS with high rates of seizure freedom without ECoG guidance. A caveat comes with addition of suspected malformations of cortical development (MCDs) in the ipsilateral neocortex that may serve as the epileptogenic focus in what has been termed dual pathology.[18,19] There is some evidence that in cases of MRI-negative TLE, complete resection of baseline interictal discharges may improve seizure freedom.[12,20,21] In the MRI-negative TLE cohort, intraoperative ECoG has been used with some success to support the hypothesis of a mesial TLE syndrome that would respond best to a standard anteromedial resection.[20] In such cases, if there is evidence of mesial onset and other preoperative studies point toward mesial onset, but no MRI lesion is seen, ECoG may be used intraoperatively to screen for epileptiform activity in the lateral cortex. Epileptiform activity in lateral cortex (or lack of epileptiform activity in the mesial structures) can be used as evidence for moving toward a staged

operation with chronic intracranial monitoring, while absence of spikes laterally may be used to support proceeding with anteromedial resection. Determining such facts involves adequate monitoring from both anteromesial and lateral structures, as well as extending to parietal-occipital and subfrontal areas.

Cortical dysplasia is a feature of neocortical epilepsy which may or may not be detected by MRI. Completeness of resection of these lesions has been shown to be the best prognostic factor with regard to seizure freedom.[22] While MRI and intraoperative registration can greatly facilitate resection of these lesions, there may also be generators of interictal spike activity that can be detected using ECoG.[22] Intraoperative ECoG may provide insight on the margins of resection during surgery for refractory epilepsy associated with a lesion such as a malformation of cortical development. Studies suggest that dysplastic tissue is a source of epileptogenicity, and that resection of this irritative zone showing spike activity on ECoG can increase seizure-free outcomes.[23,24,25]

One pitfall to avoid, however, is blindly chasing spikes. While spike activity can suggest epileptogenicity, it is by no means diagnostic. Evidence does not generally support extending resections with the goal of proceeding until all spikes are silenced.[14] On the other hand, framing the question in a more refined way during preoperative planning can restrain one from falling into this trap. As with many of the techniques discussed here, definitive data on ECoG-guided resection for tumor-associated epilepsy is mixed, but there are many reports of its usefulness particularly in regard to low-grade glial tumors.[26,27,28,29] Surgeon preference plays a prominent role in this, as with other aspects of these surgeries, where superiority of one technique may be difficult to prove quantitatively, but good outcomes can be obtained through different techniques.[30,31,32]

17.7 Conclusion

In summary, intraoperative ECoG can be used for a variety of purposes with regard to seizure-mapping. Studies of this type yield the most useful data when specific questions are asked, such that the question is focused with a narrow scope and combined with preoperative and extraoperative findings.

References

[1] de Curtis M, Avanzini G. Interictal spikes in focal epileptogenesis. Prog Neurobiol. 2001; 63(5):541–567

[2] Staley KJ, Dudek FE. Interictal spikes and epileptogenesis. Epilepsy Curr. 2006; 6(6):199–202

[3] Schramm J, Clusmann H. The surgery of epilepsy. Neurosurgery. 2008; 62(2) Suppl 2:463–481, discussion 481. SHC--463-SHC-481

[4] Schramm J. Temporal lobe epilepsy surgery and the quest for optimal extent of resection: a review. Epilepsia. 2008; 49(8):1296–1307

[5] Kuruvilla A, Flink R. Intraoperative electrocorticography in epilepsy surgery: useful or not? Seizure. 2003; 12(8):577–584

[6] Wass CT, Grady RE, Fessler AJ, et al. The effects of remifentanil on epileptiform discharges during intraoperative electrocorticography in patients undergoing epilepsy surgery. Epilepsia. 2001; 42(10):1340–1344

[7] Herrick IA, Gelb AW. Anesthesia for temporal lobe epilepsy surgery. Can J Neurol Sci. 2000; 27 Suppl 1:S64–S67, discussion S92–S96

[8] Chui J, Manninen P, Valiante T, Venkatraghavan L. The anesthetic considerations of intraoperative electrocorticography during epilepsy surgery. Anesth Analg. 2013; 117(2):479–486

[9] Voorhies JM, Cohen-Gadol A. Techniques for placement of grid and strip electrodes for intracranial epilepsy surgery monitoring: pearls and pitfalls. Surg Neurol Int. 2013; 4:98

[10] Cohen-Gadol AA, Spencer DD. Use of an anteromedial subdural strip electrode in the evaluation of medial temporal lobe epilepsy. Technical note. J Neurosurg. 2003; 99(5):921–923

[11] Yang T, Hakimian S, Schwartz TH. Intraoperative electrocorticography (ECog): indications, techniques, and utility in epilepsy surgery. Epileptic Disord. 2014; 16(3):271–279

[12] Burkholder DB, Sulc V, Hoffman EM, et al. Interictal scalp electroencephalography and intraoperative electrocorticography in magnetic resonance imaging-negative temporal lobe epilepsy. JAMA Neurol. 2014; 71(6):702–709

[13] McKhann GM, II, Schoenfeld-McNeill J, Born DE, Haglund MM, Ojemann GA. Intraoperative hippocampal electrocorticography to predict the extent of hippocampal resection in temporal lobe epilepsy surgery. J Neurosurg. 2000; 93(1):44–52

[14] Wray CD, McDaniel SS, Saneto RP, Novotny EJ, Jr, Ojemann JG. Is postresective intraoperative electrocorticography predictive of seizure outcomes in children? J Neurosurg Pediatr. 2012; 9(5):546–551

[15] Cascino GD, Hulihan JF, Sharbrough FW, Kelly PJ. Parietal lobe lesional epilepsy: electroclinical correlation and operative outcome. Epilepsia. 1993; 34 (3):522–527

[16] Leijten FS, Alpherts WC, Van Huffelen AC, Vermeulen J, Van Rijen PC. The effects on cognitive performance of tailored resection in surgery for nonlesional mesiotemporal lobe epilepsy. Epilepsia. 2005; 46(3):431–439

[17] Schwartz TH, Bazil CW, Walczak TS, Chan S, Pedley TA, Goodman RR. The predictive value of intraoperative electrocorticography in resections for limbic epilepsy associated with mesial temporal sclerosis. Neurosurgery. 1997; 40 (2):302–309, discussion 309–311

[18] Lévesque MF, Nakasato N, Vinters HV, Babb TL. Surgical treatment of limbic epilepsy associated with extrahippocampal lesions: the problem of dual pathology. J Neurosurg. 1991; 75(3):364–370

[19] Ho SS, Kuzniecky RI, Gilliam F, Faught E, Morawetz R. Temporal lobe developmental malformations and epilepsy: dual pathology and bilateral hippocampal abnormalities. Neurology. 1998; 50(3):748–754

[20] Luther N, Rubens E, Sethi N, et al. The value of intraoperative electrocorticography in surgical decision making for temporal lobe epilepsy with normal MRI. Epilepsia. 2011; 52(5):941–948

[21] Quigg M. The reliability of intraoperative electrocorticography in magnetic resonance imaging-negative temporal lobe epilepsy: spikes mark the spot. JAMA Neurol. 2014; 71(6):681–682

[22] Krsek P, Maton B, Jayakar P, et al. Incomplete resection of focal cortical dysplasia is the main predictor of poor postsurgical outcome. Neurology. 2009; 72 (3):217–223

[23] Palmini A, Gambardella A, Andermann F, et al. Intrinsic epileptogenicity of human dysplastic cortex as suggested by corticography and surgical results. Ann Neurol. 1995; 37(4):476–487

[24] Wang DD, Deans AE, Barkovich AJ, et al. Transmantle sign in focal cortical dysplasia: a unique radiological entity with excellent prognosis for seizure control. J Neurosurg. 2013; 118(2):337–344

[25] Chang EF, Wang DD, Barkovich AJ, et al. Predictors of seizure freedom after surgery for malformations of cortical development. Ann Neurol. 2011; 70(1): 151–162

[26] Chang EF, Clark A, Smith JS, et al. Functional mapping-guided resection of low-grade gliomas in eloquent areas of the brain: improvement of long-term survival. Clinical article. J Neurosurg. 2011; 114(3):566–573

[27] Tran TA, Spencer SS, Javidan M, Pacia S, Marks D, Spencer DD. Significance of spikes recorded on intraoperative electrocorticography in patients with brain tumor and epilepsy. Epilepsia. 1997; 38(10):1132–1139

[28] Pilcher WH, Silbergeld DL, Berger MS, Ojemann GA. Intraoperative electrocorticography during tumor resection: impact on seizure outcome in patients with gangliogliomas. J Neurosurg. 1993; 78(6):891–902

[29] Berger MS, Ghatan S, Haglund MM, Dobbins J, Ojemann GA. Low-grade gliomas associated with intractable epilepsy: seizure outcome utilizing electrocorticography during tumor resection. J Neurosurg. 1993; 79(1): 62–69

[30] Salanova V, Andermann F, Olivier A, Rasmussen T, Quesney LF. Occipital lobe epilepsy: electroclinical manifestations, electrocorticography, cortical stimulation and outcome in 42 patients treated between 1930 and 1991. Surgery of occipital lobe epilepsy. Brain. 1992; 115(Pt 6):1655–1680

[31] Téllez-Zenteno JF, Hernández Ronquillo L, Moien-Afshari F, Wiebe S. Surgical outcomes in lesional and non-lesional epilepsy: a systematic review and meta-analysis. Epilepsy Res. 2010; 89(2–3):310–318

[32] Wennberg R, Quesney LF, Lozano A, Olivier A, Rasmussen T. Role of electrocorticography at surgery for lesion-related frontal lobe epilepsy. Can J Neurol Sci. 1999; 26(1):33–39

18 Asleep Motor Mapping

Deependra Mahato, Alison U. Ho, and Javed Siddiqi

Abstract

Over the years, neurosurgeons have been developing ways to offer safe maximal resection of lesions, such as cerebral gliomas, adjacent to eloquent cortex via supratentorial craniotomy. In addition to advances in neurosurgical technique, a new age of technology over the past decade has ushered in the innovation of intrasurgical electrostimulation mapping, which has permitted neurosurgeons to operate corresponding to the functional boundary. In this chapter, we will discuss the nuances of intraoperative brain mapping, from preoperative planning to selecting the appropriate method to allow for identification and preservation of the motor cortex for safe, gross-total resection of the identified lesion, during general anesthesia craniotomy.

Keywords: brain mapping, asleep craniotomy, motor cortex

18.1 Introduction

As technology has advanced over recent years, in addition to functional imaging, intraoperative brain mapping techniques have been used widely in patients who undergo craniotomies either awake or under general anesthesia.[1] Unlike functional localization in an awake craniotomy, brain mapping under general anesthesia for tumor resection in eloquent areas requires a more detailed process. Intraoperative somatosensory-evoked potentials (SSEPs) phase reversal and electrical stimulation mapping have been the preferred methods for guiding neurosurgeons to optimize gross total resection, in order to reduce tumor burden and increase survival.[2] At the same time, care must be taken to avoid resultant postoperative neurological deficits, since there is a lack of patient interaction and feedback under general anesthesia as maximal territory is targeted for resection.

18.2 Motor Pathways

The primary motor cortex is an area of the brain located in the frontal lobe in the precentral gyrus and is of principal importance in motor function. This area generates neural impulses that progress along a complex pathway to produce neural excitations, which originate in giant pyramidal cells, known as Betz cells, leading to movement.[3]

Signals travel along this tract and cross the midline, and, as such, signals from the right hemisphere control motor activity on the left side of the body. In addition, the body is represented in a somatotopic arrangement, with a specific amount of brain matter devoted to a body part. Additional areas of the cortex also influence motor functions, such as the posterior parietal is involved in interpreting visual information for motor guidance, and the premotor cortex, just anterior and lateral to MC, is involved in sensory guidance of movement and control of truncal and proximal limb muscles. Associated with the premotor cortex are the cingulate motor area (CMA) and the supplementary motor area (SMA).[4] The SMA is medial and superior to the premotor cortex and is involved in planning complex and dual-handed movements. Neurons from the cortex compose pyramidal tract fibers. These fibers project into well-defined portions of the postcommissural putamen and the subthalamic nucleus (STN).[4] Motor cortex projects to the dorsolateral STN, the SMA, and the premotor cortex, and the CMA projects to the dorsomedial STN.[4] These upper motor neurons (UMNs) send signals from the cerebral cortex to the midbrain and medulla oblongata. The UMNs of motor cortex, via the corticospinal tract, descend to the posterior limb of the internal capsule, through the crus cerebri, to the pons and then to the medullary pyramids where the majority of the axons cross the midline to the contralateral side at the decussation.[3] At this point, they descend as either the lateral corticospinal tract which is responsible for controlling appendicular muscles or the anterior corticospinal tract which is responsible for controlling muscles of the trunk.[3] The anterior corticospinal tracts do not cross in the medulla, instead descending ipsilaterally in the brainstem and entering spinal cord, synapsing at that level with lower motor neurons (LMNs).[3] The lateral corticospinal tract synapses with ventromedial LMNs of the spinal cord. These LMNs innervate the skeletal muscles. The corticobulbar tracts follow a similar path as described above, except when reaching the medulla, the fibers do not cross, remain ipsilateral, and exit at the level of the brainstem to synapse on LMNs of cranial nerves (CNs), specifically the nonocular central nervous system.[3] Fibers of the corticobulbar tract are also involved in sensory information, ending in sensory nuclei of the brainstem, for example, the gracile nucleus.[3]

18.3 Indications

Neurophysiologic brain mapping offers live assessment of cortical and subcortical function to increase specificity in identification of the essential regions of the brain. It is crucial for the neurosurgeon to determine the right corridor to resect tumors that are in eloquent areas and preserve function (▶ Fig. 18.1). In order to determine the eloquent area, such as primary motor cortex, primary somatosensory cortex, language areas such as Broca's and Wernicke's, and visual areas, brain mapping must be done. Of these modalities, only motor mapping may be performed under general anesthesia, as all other forms of mapping inherently require the patient to be awake to participate in providing feedback during testing.

Asleep motor brain mapping is indicated for those who have pathologic lesions (vascular, tumor, epileptogenic focus), and who are not able to engage reliably or productively during an awake craniotomy. This may include patients with comorbidities such as anxiety, developmental delay, or any form of preclusion from communication. Asleep mapping may be contraindicated in persons with medical issues that would make conversion to general anesthesia challenging, such as obesity, obstructive sleep apnea, or any condition creating a difficult airway.[5]

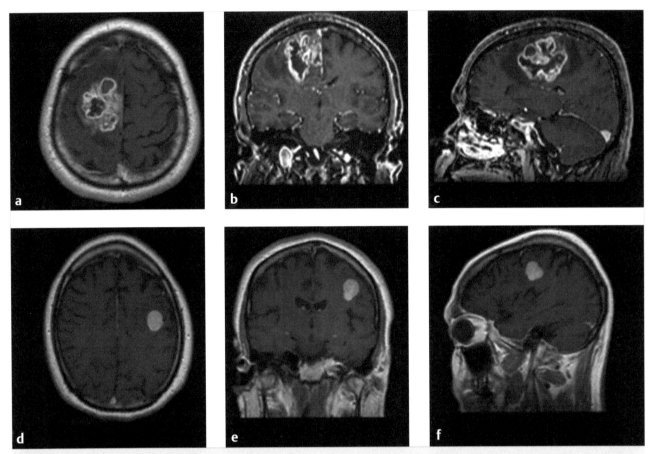

Fig. 18.1 (a) Axial, (b) coronal, and (c) sagittal T1-weighted images with gadolinium showing a contrast-enhancing right frontal lesion involving motor cortex. (d) Axial, (e) coronal, and (f) sagittal T1-weighted images with gadolinium show a contrast-enhancing left frontal lesion involving premotor cortex.

18.4 Preoperative Imaging

It is important for one to be comfortable recognizing the anatomy of regions in question, thereby allowing for conservation of the eloquent areas, including the primary motor cortex. Radiographic review of neuroanatomy on a computed tomography (CT), CT angiogram (CTA), magnetic resonance imaging (MRI), MR angiogram (MRA), and catheter angiography has traditionally been fundamental in aiding preoperative planning in neurosurgery. The above radiographic forms can be utilized in this planning phase, and each offers its own varied aids and advantages compared to the others during this process. Plain CT reveals the overall brain matter, gyral pattern, abnormal attenuation, and mass effect. It also provides especially important views of the cranial vault for any tumor involvement, destructive lesions, or presence of hemorrhagic tumor core.

In 1982, Lee and colleagues first reported the use of an intraoperative CT scanner both in morphologic and in functional stereotactic surgery, and later the use of MRI in selected functional and tumor cases.[6] Localizing the lesion can be approached in a stepwise manner using known anatomical landmarks. On plain CT and T1- and T2-weighted MRI sequences, the superior frontal sulcus posteriorly is seen to end at the precentral gyrus, where on axial imaging, the "omega sign" correlates with the motor hand area on each side, and anterior to

the marginal ramus of the cingulate sulcus, which when taken in view bilaterally forms the "pars bracket sign," is the central sulcus (CS; ► Fig. 18.2).[7]

CTA is a noninvasive way to visualize a tumor's feeding vessels, as well as illustrate the surrounding vasculature, and plays an important role in preoperative planning and surgical approach. However, though CTA has a high degree of specificity in regard to identifying the vasculature, the "gold standard" remains cerebral angiography. MRA offers the same visualization benefit as CT without the risk of radiation exposure or intravenous contrast use, thus making this modality a better alternative for those patients with contraindications to intravenous contrast and radiation, such as, but not limited to, those with a prominent radiographic contrast allergy, or compromised kidney function; though the risk of nephrogenic systemic fibrosis with renal failure may preclude the use of gadolinium that at times may provide additional detail beyond the noncontrast time-of-flight or phase-contrast MRA techniques.

Blood-oxygen-level-dependent functional MRI (BOLD fMRI) is used to localize regions of sensorimotor or language functions when one is actively performing tasks.[8] This is elucidated by detecting the amount of deoxyhemoglobin (paramagnetic compared to oxyhemoglobin) in the capillary and venous structures in brain regions responsible for carrying out movement, sensory perception, or speech generation while said actions are

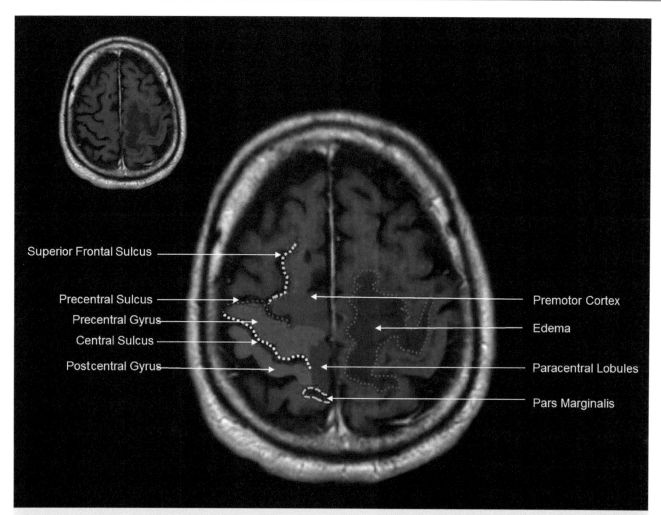

Fig. 18.2 Motor cortex is identified by first finding the superior frontal sulcus (*green dotted line*), which leads to the precentral sulcus (*purple dotted line*). Behind the precentral sulcus is the precentral gyrus, a.k.a. motor cortex (*green shaded area*), which leads more posteriorly to the central sulcus (*yellow dotted line*) followed by the postcentral gyrus, a.k.a. sensory cortex (*blue shaded area*). Finally, the paracentral lobule (*purple shaded area*) is just anterior to the pars marginalis which is a short sulcus that is an extension of the cingulate sulcus posterosuperiorly that reaches the apex but does not extend laterally (*blue dotted line*). Premotor cortex is an area that is directly anterior to the primary motor cortex in the frontal lobe. In this figure, there is also pathology on the left side which shows the edema (*blue dotted line*).

performed.[7] This is feasible, because while oxygen extraction from hemoglobin is increased in activated brain tissue, the amount of increased oxygenated blood flow and volume in response to activity is disproportionately greater, leaving a lesser amount of deoxyhemoglobin in the regions sampled compared to times of inactivity. However, according to Glover, BOLD fMRI faces limitations with low temporal resolution, signal dropout, and/or spatial distortion in frontal, orbital, and lateral parietal regions. This is caused by the approximately 9 ppm difference in magnetic susceptibility at interfaces between air and brain tissue, resulting in lack of BOLD signal in ventral, temporal, and prefrontal cortex regions. Moreover, poor data quality can also result from excessive movement and poor task performance. The scanner's loud noise associated with switched magnetic fields can cause deranged results in studies of audition and resting state networks, though this can be combated with certain techniques.[9,10] The most staggering limitation of fMRI has been in language lateralization, with poor sensitivity noted (only 22% in naming tasks and 36% in verb generation tasks).[7]

Other imaging techniques, including diffusion-weighted imaging (DWI) and diffusion tensor imaging (DTI), are noninvasive MRI sequences that allow preoperative visualization and incorporation of the pyramidal tracts for intraoperative navigation to facilitate localization of lesions in eloquent areas.[7] It is essential to consider that while utilizing neuronavigation during the surgical procedure with the use of mannitol and dexamethasone intraoperatively, changes in tissue volumes and amount of brain shift can alter the correlation between real-time visualization and preoperative images.[7] Therefore, it is essential to keep this phenomenon in mind while utilizing neuronavigation during the surgical procedure. In addition, one must also account for the brain's ability to undergo anatomical and functional reorganization to compensate for pathological damage, that is, brain plasticity.[11,12] Thus, the normal eloquent anatomy identified in preoperative images might not undertake the same function anticipated in case of lesions that have been growing in eloquent areas. DTI and DWI sequences purely provide preoperative prediction of pyramidal tracking, which can be superimposed with real-time, intraoperative mapping, providing real-time detection of the eloquent functional relocation, ensuring a safe and optimal resection.[7]

18.5 Anesthesia Considerations

The ultimate goal for general anesthesia during brain mapping is to minimize the interference with functional mapping, while ensuring the patient's safety during the procedure. The use of volatile agents is not recommended, since these have dual properties of reducing spike activities in epileptic patients and also epileptogenic properties at higher doses.[5] Intravenous general anesthetic agents, along with short-acting paralytics,[13] such as, succinylcholine, atracurium besylate, and rocuronium bromide, are preferred for induction;[14] although, if possible, total avoidance of paralytic agents is recommended.[14,15] Of note, all paralytic agents should be reversed and confirmed with train-of-four monitoring prior to brain mapping procedures.[13] The most common general anesthetic regimens include a combination of propofol or dexmedetomidine with fentanyl, remifentanil, sufentanil, or alfentanil.[13,14,15,16]

18.6 Intraoperative Mapping

Since Food and Drug Administration's approval in 2002, intraoperative mapping has been widely used and has yielded excellent results.[17] This is especially true regarding patients with brain tumors; it provides assistance to safe resection of tumor to the extent of achieving gross total resection, reduced risk of motor deficits, and ultimately improved patient survival.[15,17,18] Unfortunately, it is not suitable for patients who already have significant deficits prior to surgery, since motor-evoked potentials (MEPs) cannot be adequately generated to produce a reliable recording.[19,20]

SSEPs phase reversal and electrical stimulation mapping through direct cortical stimulation (DCS) have been the customary methods to localize central sulcus and peri-Rolandic gyrus.[14] Sensorimotor mapping through SSEPs phase reversal is only applicable for identification of the central sulcus in peri-Rolandic lesions that have distorted the normal central sulcus topography. After reversal of paralytic agents confirmed with train-of-four testing, a strip with 10-mm electrode spacing or a 5 × 4 grid electrode perpendicular to the presumed central sulcus is place on the cortical surface.[14] The neurodiagnostic equipment averages the cortical action potentials generated by contralateral peripheral nerve stimulation. The central sulcus is identified at the point where inversion of a postcentral negative and a precentral positive peak is noted.[15,21] This opposite polarity of recording signals is what is reported as a phase reversal. As shown in ▶ Fig. 18.1, there is a difference of latency between the greatest positivity and negativity. For this reason, some refer to this as a pseudo-phase reversal (▶ Fig. 18.3).

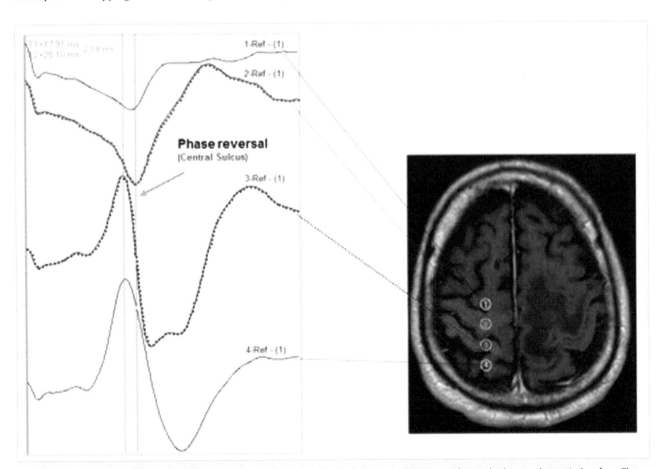

Fig. 18.3 The central sulcus is identified by placing a 10-mm lead perpendicularly across the presumed central sulcus on the cortical surface. The central sulcus (*purple dotted line*) is identified at the point where inversion of a postcentral (*blue shaded region*) negative (*blue dotted line*) and a precentral (*green shaded region*) positive peak, (*red dotted line*) is noted. The central sulcus is noted between 2-Ref and 3-Ref.

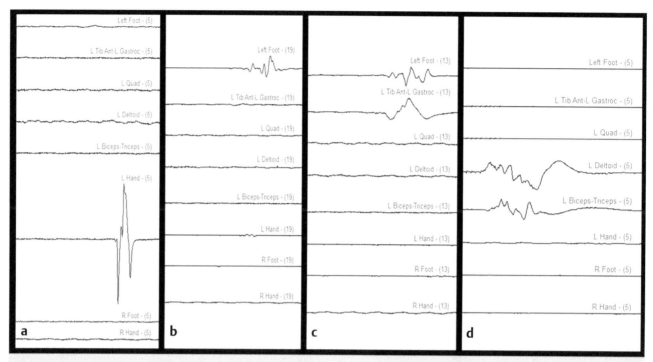

Fig. 18.4 Direct cortical stimulation can elicit a motor response in a single muscle group. **(a)** Left hand, **(b)** left foot, or multiple muscle groups—**(c)** left foot and left gastrocnemius, and **(d)** left deltoid, biceps, and triceps.

To collect well-defined waveforms, one may need to reposition the strip multiple times for interpretation of data and to decrease the chance of a nonobtainable phase reversal record. A cortical SSEP baseline provides valuable information, such as expected latency of the maximum polarity of waves, and needed stimulation intensities and parameters. Phase reversal recording identifies only the central sulcus itself in cases of an infiltrative or pericentral lesion causing anatomical distortion of the central sulcus; however, phase reversal SSEPs offer limited directional information on the particular distribution of motor function on the adjacent exposed cerebral structure. Thus, after the central sulcus is identified by phase reversal SSEPs, direct cortical MEPs (dcMEPs) can be used for identification of motor cortex. The location variation of phase reversals can be up to 10 mm or one sulcus away from central sulcus.[20]

dcMEPs or DCS has been the gold standard for mapping brain function in eloquent areas. In an asleep craniotomy, DCS can only be used for motor mapping. A current is sent either by constant 250 rectangular pulses at a rate of 50.1 Hz for a 0.1 millisecond duration or by repetitive pulses at 3.17 Hz during 0.3 millisecond using a constant-current, biphasic square-wave 60-Hz bipolar stimulator[15] (Ojemann-5 mm distant between electrodes) or a monopolar probe (1.6-mm electrode with monophasic current up to 22 mA).[13] The intensity is increased by increments of 2 mA (maximum of 20[13]–30 mA[14]) until contralateral thumb movement is observed or detected on MEPs, via signal from needle or stick-on electrodes of the median nerve.[14] All expected primary motor cortex areas are stimulated at the lowest intensity before proceeding to higher level of stimulation, noting that diseased cortex may have a higher threshold level. Recorded muscles vary based on the area of exposure. There are two methods of recording muscles activity.

Two needles per muscle provide more specific recording with reduced stimulation artifact; however, this method may limit the number of monitored muscles. In order to enhance the sensitivity of motor mapping with broader muscle-group coverage, a single-needle-per-muscle set-up is preferred. Subcortical motor mapping can be continued during tumor resection. Low-intensity monopolar cathodal stimulation can be transferred to the subcortical white matter. Resultant MEP signals help achieve the goal of maximal safe resection of tumor. ▶ Fig. 18.4a–d show functional motor mapping. Based on the stimulation site and intensity of stimulation, we may see contraction of one muscle or a group of muscles.

One can apply DCS in two ways: negative and positive mapping. In positive mapping, the motor cortex is identified when the current yields muscle action potentials or movement of contralateral target muscles from the face, upper or lower extremities. This allows for surgeon to avoid that area and find a corridor that does not have eloquent area for maximal tumor resection.[21]

In negative mapping, the area of the brain that has no eloquence is confirmed and the resection is carried out until the stimulation yields muscle action potentials. A false negative in this domain of mapping can have serious, adverse consequences in asleep craniotomies, since other eloquent sites, such as language areas (Broca and Wernicke), primary visual areas, the angular gyrus, and mesial temporal regions for memory, are not detected.[2,22] Studies have reported patients with persistent deficits (language, visual, and motor) who had no positive sites detected prior to their resection, and the positive cortex was not exposed during surgery for positive control in these cases.[2,22] Therefore, it is recommended to obtain a wider bone flap to gain access to systematic positive mapping.[21] The

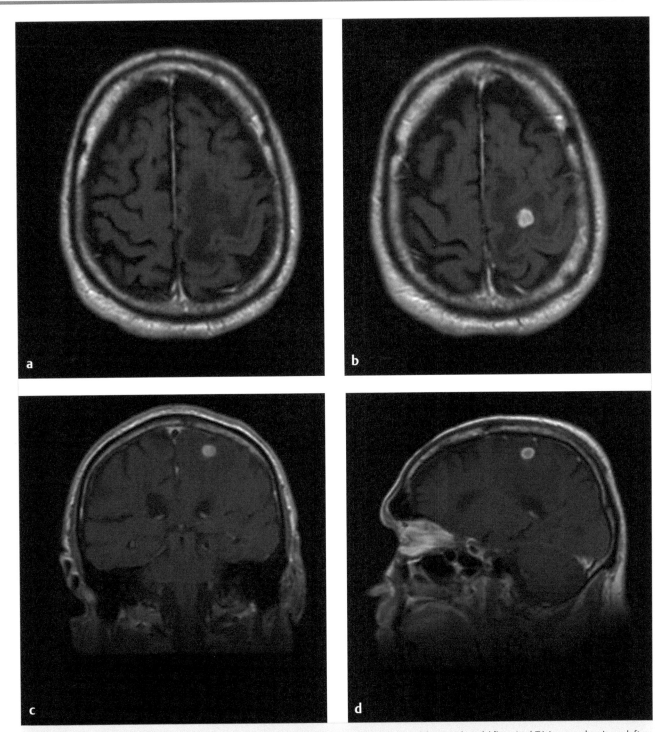

Fig. 18.5 (a) T1-weighted axial image without contrast, (b) T1 axial image with gadolinium, (c) coronal, and (d) sagittal T1 images showing a left frontal contrast-enhancing left frontal lesion at junction of the primary motor cortex and peripheral subcortical tissue.

combination of both positive and negative mapping can better define the cortical limits of tumor resection, especially with low-grade gliomas.

An important common intraoperative brain mapping complication has been intraoperative seizure with DCS. This complication, however, is documented in studies as a low risk (4%).[13] The seizure can be quickly terminated within 5–10 seconds by applying cold Ringer's solution[13,15,23] with the addition of intravenous abortive medications, such as benzodiazepines.[13,15] Another observed complication is a transient postoperative motor deficit, observed in 33% of patients by Raabe and colleagues.[13] The deficit was temporary in most, but 3% of patients had remaining deficit after 3 months due to vascular injury and not from inaccurate mapping of the corticospinal tract.[13]

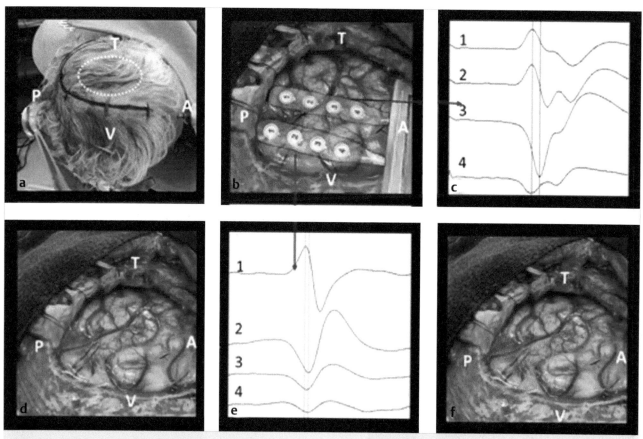

Fig. 18.6 **(a)** Patient positioned with left side up, and his head immobilized in a 3-pin Mayfield holder with a reverse question mark planned incision (*black line*) and planned bone flap removal (*white dotted line*). **(b)** Two cortical lead strips with 10 mm spacing for SSEP phase-reversal testing are placed on the predicted area of the brain where the central sulcus is located. The strip closest to temporal region (T) showed a **(c)** phase reversal between leads 2 and 3, while the strip closest to vertex (V) showed a **(e)** phase reversal between leads 1 and 2. **(d)** The primary cortex is identified as the gyrus **(f)** anterior to central sulcus (*shaded green*). A, anterior; P, posterior; T, temporal region; V, vertex of the head.

18.7 Case Presentation

This is a 65-year-old right-handed male, with a past medical history of sleep apnea, who presented with right arm weakness for 2 weeks (see **Video 18.1**). A noncontrast head CT revealed a small focus of hyperdensity with surrounding hypodensity in the left frontoparietal region. This was followed by an MRI with and without contrast that demonstrated a left subcortical frontal enhancing lesion with surrounding mild vasogenic edema (▶ Fig. 18.5). Given his history of long-term sleep apnea, and short, wide-girth neck, he was not a candidate for an awake craniotomy. Consequently, he underwent an asleep, left craniotomy with motor mapping. The motor cortex was identified by phase reversal SSEPs (▶ Fig. 18.6), and through DCS (▶ Fig. 18.7). In this patient, DCS was initiated using 5 mA, with progression to 7 mA, which elicited a response in the electromyography (EMG). Utilizing DCS, hand, forearm, and facial muscle control on the right was identified based on both the EMG tracings and the visualized motor response of the patient (▶ Fig. 18.7). Negative brain mapping was employed to identify a silent area for surgical approach for resection of the lesion. During resection, there was electrical activity suggestive of seizures; therefore, the field was flooded with cold irrigation lactate ringer,

and he was given benzodiazepine until epileptiform discharges stopped. Resection was continued until gross total resection was achieved. This was confirmed by postoperative MRI.

18.8 Conclusion

Brain mapping for general anesthetic craniotomy is limited to motor mapping at present. During surgical resection, it is recommended to select the shortest surgical corridor through non-eloquent cortex, and avoid sacrificing the important cortical draining veins and arterial structures.[20] A well-formulated plan from presurgical functional imaging, to choice of general anesthetic agents, to intraoperative brain mapping, is necessary to minimize the operative morbidity and postoperative sequelae.[24] Though there have been documented immediate postoperative neurological deficits in patients undergoing intraoperative brain mapping in resection of tumors in eloquent brain areas, the majority of patients recovered to baseline function by 3 to 6 months.[13,25] Studies have shown that intraoperative brain mapping has made total resection of brain masses possible for cases in which this may not otherwise have been possible safely, including patients with well-infiltrated brain tumors, such as

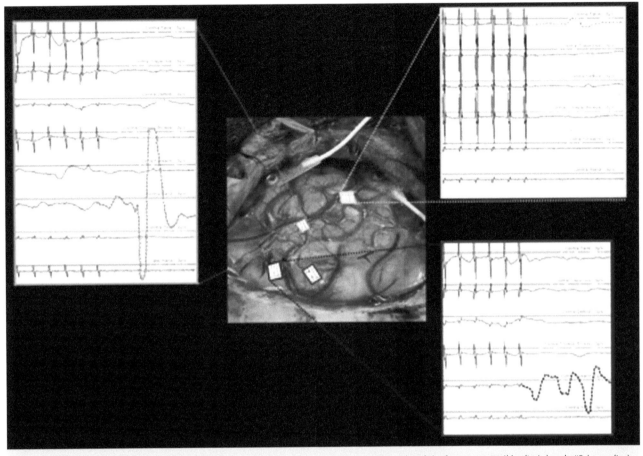

Fig. 18.7 Direct cortical mapping using a 7-mA stimulus elicited a response in electromyography of the forearm at #1 (*blue line*), hands #2 (*green line*), and face #3 (*yellow line*). Based on navigation, the tumor was localized at #4 (*red square*).

low-grade gliomas. Not only has brain mapping made such resections feasible, it has also improved patient survival throughout the years.

References

[1] Zakaria J, Prabhu VC. Cortical mapping in the resection of malignant cerebral gliomas. In: De Vleeschouwer S, ed. Glioblastoma. Codon Publications; 2017

[2] Quinones-Hinojosa, AM. Schmidek & Sweet Operative Neurosurgical Techniques: Indications, Methods, and Results. 1st ed. Elsevier Saunders

[3] Lemaster M. Antomy and Physiology. Oregon State University; 2018

[4] Winn, RH. Youmanns Neurological Surgery. 6th ed. Elsevier Saunders; 2011: 721-729

[5] Piccioni F, Fanzio M. Management of anesthesia in awake craniotomy. Minerva Anestesiol. 2008; 74(7-8):393–408

[6] Lee JY, Lunsford LD, Subach BR, Jho HD, Bissonette DJ, Kondziolka D. Brain surgery with image guidance: current recommendations based on a 20-year assessment. Stereotact Funct Neurosurg. 2000; 75(1):35–48

[7] Waldau B, Haglund MM. Motor, Sensory, and Language Mapping and Monitoring for Cortical Resections | Clinical Gate. Available at: https://clinicalgate.com/motor-sensory-and-language-mapping-and-monitoring-for-cortical-resections/#bib58. Accessed: 21st July 2018

[8] Blumenfeld, H. Introduction to clinical neuroradiology. In: Bluemenfeld H, ed. Neuroanatomy Through Clinical Cases. Sutherland: Sinauer Associates; 2010, 85–123

[9] Glover GH. Overview of functional magnetic resonance imaging. Neurosurg Clin N Am. 2011; 22(2):133–139, vii

[10] Janecek JK, Swanson SJ, Sabsevitz DS, et al. Language lateralization by fMRI and Wada testing in 229 patients with epilepsy: rates and predictors of discordance. Epilepsia. 2013; 54(2):314–322

[11] Duffau H. Brain plasticity and tumors. Adv Tech Stand Neurosurg. 2008; 33: 3–33

[12] Duffau H. Brain plasticity: from pathophysiological mechanisms to therapeutic applications. J Clin Neurosci. 2006; 13(9):885–897

[13] Raabe A, Beck J, Schucht P, Seidel K. Continuous dynamic mapping of the corticospinal tract during surgery of motor eloquent brain tumors: evaluation of a new method. J Neurosurg. 2014; 120(5):1015–1024

[14] Romstöck J, Fahlbusch R, Ganslandt O, Nimsky C, Strauss C. Localisation of the sensorimotor cortex during surgery for brain tumours: feasibility and waveform patterns of somatosensory evoked potentials. J Neurol Neurosurg Psychiatry. 2002; 72(2):221–229

[15] Sarmento SA, de Andrade EM, Tedeschi H. Strategies for resection of lesions in the motor area: preliminary results in 42 surgical patients. Arq Neuropsiquiatr. 2006; 64(4):963–970

[16] Tharin S, Golby A. Functional brain mapping and its applications to neurosurgery. Neurosurgery. 2007; 60(4) Suppl 2:185–201, discussion 201–202

[17] Stecker MM. A review of intraoperative monitoring for spinal surgery. Surg Neurol Int. 2012; 3 Suppl 3:S174–S187

[18] McGirt MJ, Chaichana KL, Gathinji M, et al. Independent association of extent of resection with survival in patients with malignant brain astrocytoma. J Neurosurg. 2009; 110(1):156–162

[19] Winn HR. Youmans Neurological Surgery. 1st ed. Elsevier Saunders; 2011: 743–753

[20] Kim S-M, Kim SH, Seo D-W, Lee K-W. Intraoperative neurophysiologic monitoring: basic principles and recent update. J Korean Med Sci. 2013; 28(9): 1261–1269

[21] Simon MV. Intraoperative neurophysiologic sensorimotor mapping and monitoring in supratentorial surgery. J Clin Neurophysiol. 2013; 30(6):571–590

[22] Sanai N, Mirzadeh Z, Berger MS. Functional outcome after language mapping for glioma resection. N Engl J Med. 2008; 358(1):18–27

[23] Sartorius CJ, Berger MS. Rapid termination of intraoperative stimulation-evoked seizures with application of cold Ringer's lactate to the cortex. Technical note. J Neurosurg. 1998; 88(2):349–351

[24] Berger MS, Ojemann GA. Intraoperative brain mapping techniques in neuro-oncology. Stereotact Funct Neurosurg. 1992; 58(1–4):153–161

[25] Duffau H, Capelle L, Denvil D, et al. Usefulness of intraoperative electrical subcortical mapping during surgery for low-grade gliomas located within eloquent brain regions: functional results in a consecutive series of 103 patients. J Neurosurg. 2003; 98(4):764–778

19 Brainstem and Spinal Cord Mapping

Mohammad Hassan A. Noureldine, Nir Shimony, Rechdi Ahdab, and George I. Jallo

Abstract

During the past few decades, the continuous advancement of intraoperative neuromonitoring and mapping (IONMM) techniques have been pushing forward the limits of surgical resection of brainstem and intramedullary spinal cord (IMSC) lesions. Monitoring modalities such as brainstem auditory evoked potentials, somatosensory-evoked potentials, motor-evoked potentials, D-wave recordings, and free-running electromyography have provided real-time monitoring of the functional integrity of neural tissue, and mapping techniques using hand-held probes and modified surgical instruments allowed for accurate identification of important neuroanatomical structures, paving the way for extensive surgical resection of brainstem and IMSC lesions without compromising neurological function and patient outcomes. The sensitivities and specificities of these modalities in detecting impending neural injury significantly increase when multiple modalities are combined rather than utilized individually. The single most important factor that determines the success of IONMM is employing a multidisciplinary and team-based approach, where open communication between the surgeon, neurophysiologist, and anesthesiologist allows for identifying and controlling possible contributors to changes in the IONMM signal and preventing neural damage before it becomes irreversible.

Keywords: monitoring, mapping, brainstem, spinal cord, somatosensory-evoked potentials, motor-evoked potentials, D-waves

19.1 Introduction

Surgical procedures targeting brainstem and intramedullary spinal cord (IMSC) lesions remain among the most challenging interventions, even after decades of neurosurgical advancements, detailed neuroanatomical descriptions, and optimization of microsurgical techniques. Gross total resection (GTR) is not always possible, and the risk of postoperative complications is relatively high compared to other anatomical locations. Conservative approaches sometimes deter the surgeon from resecting the tumor, thus limiting his or her surgical options to performing an excisional biopsy. Although most cases cannot be cured by surgical resection alone, since other interventions (chemotherapy, radiotherapy, etc.) have failed to show significant benefit on long-term follow-up, achieving maximal safe resection with minimal tumor residual load is still the best initial step for oncological treatment in many cases. This understanding, among others, created motivation for the development of intraoperative neuromonitoring and mapping (IONMM) techniques over the past three decades, encouraging the surgeon to more aggressively, yet safely, resect brainstem and IMSC lesions with better patient outcomes. The goal of this chapter is to provide a brief overview of the IONMM modalities that are utilized during surgeries for resection of brainstem and IMSC lesions as well as to highlight the roles and significance of effective communication between the neurophysiologist, the surgeon, and the anesthesiologist, allowing for safe maximal resection of these challenging lesions.

19.1.1 Pathophysiology of Surgically Induced Nerve Injury

Nerve injury can be broadly categorized into demyelinating and axonal (▶ Fig. 19.1). In the case of demyelinating injury, the axons remain intact and rapid recovery is the rule, usually within a few weeks. On the other hand, axonal injury has a grimmer prognosis since axonal regrowth is slow and often incomplete. At a mechanistic level, early compression initially injures the myelin sheath; if corrective measures are undertaken at this stage, full recovery is the rule. With more severe compression, the axons are eventually damaged, and this may lead to a permanent neurological deficit. Alternatively, ischemic injury is fundamentally different since it affects the axons first, and if corrective measures are not undertaken promptly, it leads to permanent damage. At the earliest stages of ischemia and compression, the axon and myelin sheath are structurally intact but unable to function normally. If the underlying insult is removed immediately, quick recovery is expected within seconds to minutes (▶ Fig. 19.2). The objective of IONMM is to detect the injury at this very early stage.

19.2 Intraoperative Neuroimaging and Mapping Modalities

In general, the neurophysiological techniques utilized to evaluate the functional integrity of the brainstem and spinal cord may fall into one of two main categories: monitoring or mapping. Monitoring modalities provide continuous, real-time data about the functional status of different portions of the brainstem and spinal cord, whereas mapping techniques are based on using a hand-held probe to identify anatomical structures within the surgical field and prevent iatrogenic neural injury. Recently, different surgical tools such as the suction device and bipolar have been modified to allow for continuous, real-time mapping.[1,2]

19.2.1 Monitoring Techniques

Brainstem Auditory Evoked Potentials

Brainstem auditory evoked potentials (BAEPs) test the integrity of the auditory pathways from the auditory nerve to the inferior colliculus through a sequence of stereotyped waveforms generated from multiple axonal pathways in the auditory brainstem. These waves are evoked by auditory stimuli and occur within 10 ms in normal subjects.[3] Interpretation of the BAEPs usually involves measuring the absolute latency of the three most prominent vertex positive peaks I, III and V, along with their relative interpeak latencies. Based on our current understanding of the generators of BAEPs and the pattern of BAEP changes, the site of dysfunction may be roughly inferred.

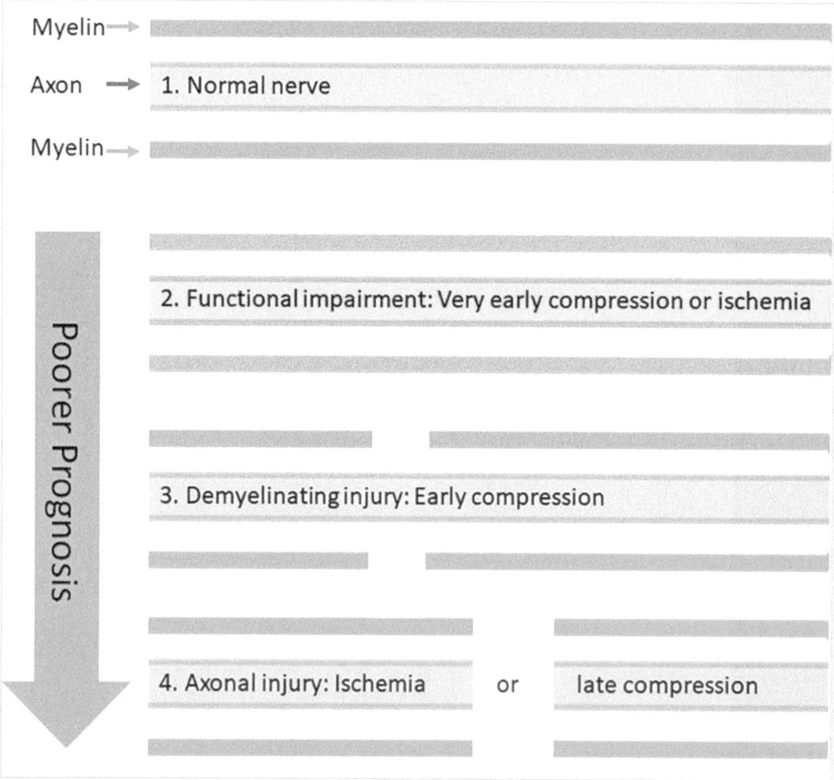

Myelin →

Axon → 1. Normal nerve

Myelin →

↓ Poorer Prognosis

2. Functional impairment: Very early compression or ischemia

3. Demyelinating injury: Early compression

4. Axonal injury: Ischemia   or   late compression

Fig. 19.1 Nerve injury types, mechanisms, and prognosis.

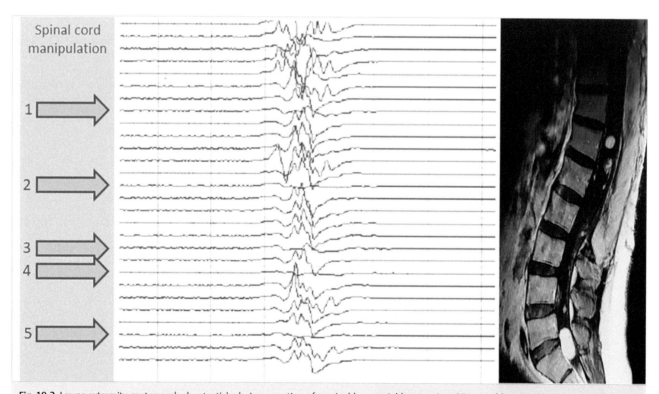

Spinal cord manipulation

1
2
3
4
5

Fig. 19.2 Lower extremity motor-evoked potentials during resection of a spinal hemangioblastoma in a 35-year-old man with Von Hippel–Lindau disease. An abrupt amplitude loss exceeding 90% (*arrow 1*) was first observed when applying traction to the tumor in an attempt to detach it from the surrounding tissue. The waves promptly recovered a few seconds after the pressure was released, indicating transient functional nerve injury. Subsequently, each attempt to manipulate the tumor was associated with a similar amplitude drop (*arrows 2–5*).

The generators of waves I, III, and V are the cochlea/distal auditory nerve, cochlear nucleus/trapezoid body, and the inferior colliculus, respectively. As such, selective loss of wave V is indicative of brainstem injury. On the other hand, abrupt loss of all three waves is seen in ischemia to the cochlea and distal auditory nerve due to injury to the internal auditory artery.

The stimuli are highly recurrent clicks delivered through ear inserts at an intensity of 60 to 70 dB above the patient's hearing threshold.[4] The recording electrode is placed on the ipsilateral earlobe (or mastoid) and referred to an electrode placed on the vertex (Cz according to the International 10–20 System of Electroencephalography [EEG] Electrode Placement).[3] Hundreds of individual trials are averaged to obtain good quality recordings. For more details about the technique and interpretation of the results, please refer to American Clinical Neurophysiology (ACNS) Guidelines: Guideline 9C[3] and Petrova et al.[4]

Indications for intraoperative BAEPs include surgical resection of lesions involving cranial nerve (CN) VIII or the auditory pathways up to the inferior colliculus,[5,6] microvascular decompression for trigeminal/glossopharyngeal neuralgia and hemifacial spasm,[7,8] other cerebellopontine angle surgeries involving the use of cerebellar retractors,[9] which may impose an ischemic risk to the auditory nerve from overstretching, as well as surgical resection of brainstem lesions (tumors, arteriovenous malformations, etc.) located between the pontomedullary junction and inferior colliculus.[10] Some authors have also utilized BAEPs in other procedures that may be associated with risk of brainstem injury (e.g., decompression for Chiari malformation[11]).

BAEPs are sensitive indicators of damage to the auditory pathway, and the absence of wave V at the end of surgery is highly predictive of hearing loss. On the other hand, the predictive value for more subtle changes of wave V is harder to establish and there are no universally recognized warning criteria to date. This is particularly true in acoustic neuroma surgery, where hearing loss tends to occur regardless of the extent of change observed in wave V. It is generally accepted, however, that a 50% amplitude drop and/or a 0.5 to 1 ms increase in wave V latency is predictive of nerve injury.[12,13] Nevertheless, these criteria may be too conservative in some types of surgeries, such as microvascular decompression, where the chance of hearing loss is highest when wave V is completely and permanently lost.[14,15] As such, the definition of warning criteria should take into account the type of surgery, especially whether the case is an acoustic neuroma or a different nearby lesion. It is also important to note that BAEPs are specific to the auditory tracts and do not detect injury to other nearby structures.

Somatosensory-Evoked Potentials

Somatosensory-evoked potentials (SSEPs) evaluate the integrity of the fast-conducting large sensory fiber pathways, whereas injury to the slow-conducting small fiber pathways that convey pain and temperature cannot be detected.[16] SSEPs are classically recorded by stimulating the median nerve at the wrist (upper extremity SSEP) or the posterior tibial nerve behind the medial malleolus (lower extremity SSEP) using a brief current delivered via a self-adhesive surface electrode. This triggers a sensory potential that ascends through the ipsilateral dorsal column up to the nucleus cuneatus, decussates near the cervicomedullary junction, ascends by means of the contralateral medial lemniscus up to the thalamus, and finally projects to the contralateral parietal sensory cortex. Recording electrodes placed at specific locations pick up this electrical activity at three different levels: peripheral nerve, spinal level, and cortical level, where the latter response is most relevant to IONMM. Averaging of 500 to 1,500 responses is usually necessary to obtain good quality recordings. Consequently, it may take several minutes to update the SSEP data, which is one of the major drawbacks of the technique. This may significantly delay the detection of nerve injury and increase the risk of permanent damage.[17] In addition, SSEPs are very sensitive to electrical power interference. The abundance of electrical equipment in the operating theater can significantly affect the quality of the waves and further prolong the recording time (▶ Fig. 19.3). For

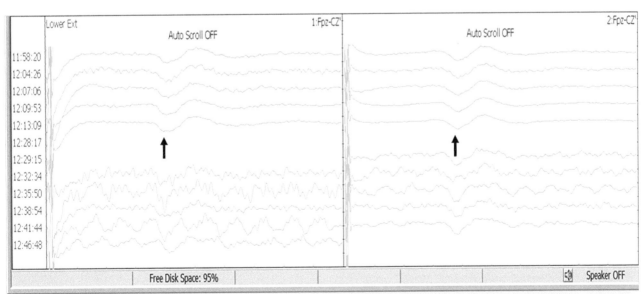

Fig. 19.3 Lower extremity somatosensory-evoked potential (SSEP) monitoring during intramedullary spinal cord (IMSC) tumor resection. Excellent quality waveforms were recorded on both sides (*arrows*) before the microscope was turned on (*upper four waveforms*). The lower five waveforms illustrate the negative impact of electrical equipment on the quality of SSEP recordings.

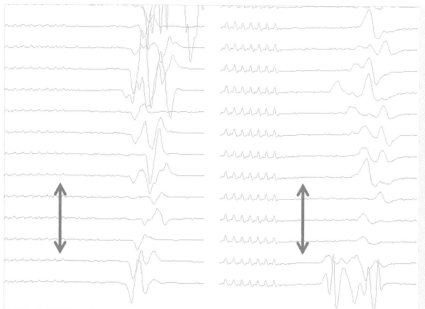

Fig. 19.4 Lower extremity motor-evoked potential monitoring during resection of a brainstem intra-axial tumor. An amplitude drop (*arrows*) was observed before opening the dura mater. Taken out of context, this drop may represent injury to the corticospinal tract. In this particular case, these deteriorating responses were not due to surgical injury but rather due to a confounding factor—the surgeon asked for a short period of muscle relaxation during initial exposure. A similar amplitude drop in the upper extremities was observed (*not shown*), which further confirms the role of a confounding factor rather than surgical injury.

more details about the technique and interpretation of the results, please refer to ACNS Guidelines: Guideline 9D.[18]

Compared to baseline values obtained at the beginning of the surgery, a latency delay of 10% and/or amplitude reduction of 50% of the cortical response are considered critical changes in SSEP signals.[19]

Trigeminal SSEPs

Trigeminal stimulation and effective recording of long-latency SSEPs have been performed in awake patients with different neurological conditions since the 1970s.[20] However, attempts to record trigeminal SSEP responses in patients under general anesthesia were not as successful as those in awake patients.[21] A recent study was able to optimize the neurophysiological and anesthetic conditions and record stable and reliable intraoperative responses of trigeminal SSEPs.[22] In brainstem surgery, the clinical utility of trigeminal SSEPs is yet to be elucidated and more studies are required to evaluate its significance compared to other IONMM modalities.

Transcranial Motor-Evoked Potentials

Transcranial motor-evoked potentials (TcMEPs) are used to monitor the integrity of the corticospinal tracts (CSTs). Transcranial activation of the motor cortex generates a motor potential that follows the descending motor tracts down to the corresponding muscle. Therefore, normal TcMEPs depend on the integrity of the corticospinal fibers, the lower motor neuron, and the neuromuscular junction. When the motor cortex is exposed (e.g., during brain tumor surgery), MEPs can be elicited by stimulating the motor cortex using epidural or subdural electrodes or a hand-held probe.

Trains of electrical pulses are delivered to the motor cortex using scalp electrodes (needle, corkscrew, or regular EEG cup electrodes) placed at C1/C2 or C3/C4 scalp positions of the 10–10 EEG system.[23] The more dorsomedial C1/C2 montage is the preferred montage for eliciting responses in the lower extremities, whereas the C3/C4 montage is used for the upper extremities. In general, the C3/C4 montage causes more current penetration and is therefore more potent; however, it causes more patient movements. It also has the disadvantage of activating the jaw muscles and, therefore, exposes the patient to bite injuries.[24] Recording is done using surface or needle electrodes inserted into the target muscles. It is advisable to choose muscles with heavy corticospinal innervation such as the intrinsic hand muscles, abductor hallucis, tibialis anterior, or extensor hallucis muscles. Although surgical injury to the CSTs will only affect MEPs below the level of surgery, it is recommended to also monitor MEPs above the surgical level. The latter will serve as a control condition to differentiate between surgically induced injury and other confounding factors[25] (▶ Fig. 19.4). MEPs are very sensitive to anesthetics and various other systemic factors such as systemic hypotension, anemia, hypoxemia, and hypothermia.[25] When the upper extremities are included, the recordings provide monitoring and protection for the brachial plexus and peripheral nerves (▶ Fig. 19.5). For more details about the technique and interpretation of results, please refer to Legatt et al.[25]

MEPs are polyphasic waveforms and have a latency of approximately 20 ms for the hands and 45 ms for the feet[26] (▶ Fig. 19.6). MEPs often display significant intertrial variability in morphology and amplitude. Therefore, judging whether any change in MEP amplitudes is related to variability or surgical injury is not always straightforward, and this explains why there are no universally accepted warning criteria. Some programs adopt the "All or Nothing" rule,[26] and others would consider a 50 to 80% drop in amplitude as significant.[27] While a 50% amplitude drop may be significant in cases with perfectly stable MEP throughout the surgery, it could be purely physiological when highly variable MEPs are recorded at baseline (▶ Fig. 19.7). In summary, latency-based criteria for MEPs are not reliable as stand-alone criteria.[28] Compared to SSEPs, TcMEPs have the major advantage of being instantaneous since

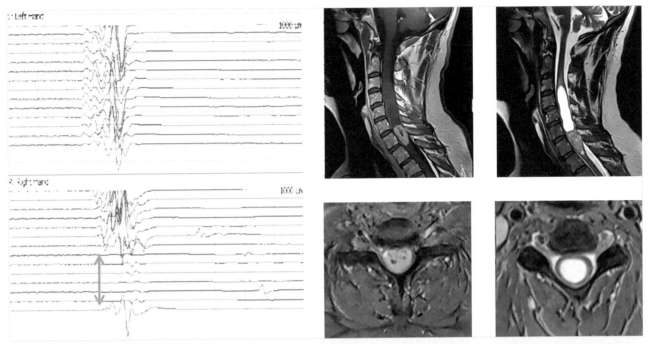

Fig. 19.5 Motor-evoked potential monitoring in the setting of thoracic (T9–T12) spine ependymoma resection. A selective amplitude drop occurred in the right abductor pollicis brevis muscle (*arrow*), whereas responses were unchanged in the other lower and upper extremity muscles (*not shown*). A median nerve injury was suspected. Few minutes after removing the blood pressure cuff and repositioning the right upper extremity, the responses returned to normal.

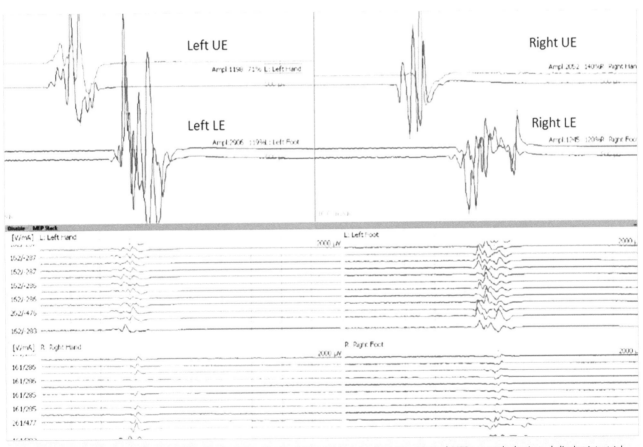

Fig. 19.6 Normal motor-evoked potential (MEP) recordings in the upper and lower extremities. Normal MEPs are polyphasic and display intertrial variability of shape. Once recorded, MEPs are subsequently stacked (*inferior part of the figure*) to allow for comparison with the previous responses. LE, lower extremity; UE, upper extremity.

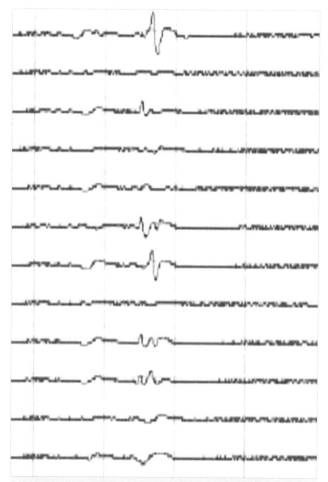

Fig. 19.7 Example of motor-evoked potential (MEP) intertrial variability. MEPs were obtained 10 times in a row using the same stimulation parameters and before any surgical manipulation. Significant changes in the amplitude of MEPs are observed, which at times exceed 95% of the baseline amplitude. Although most cases are less dramatic than this one, intertrial variability often complicates the interpretation of MEPs.

no averaging is needed. Thus, data can be updated very rapidly, and injury can be detected very early. However, one disadvantage of TcMEPs is that these cause patient movements, which could be hazardous in some surgical settings. Other issues include specific anesthetic requirements for MEPs such as the need to avoid muscle relaxing agents, which may cause discomfort for the surgeon.

Corticobulbar MEPs

Following the same concept of TcMEPs, corticobulbar MEP (CoMEP) monitoring provides a real-time functional assessment of corticobulbar pathways from the descending corticobulbar tracts to the CN nuclei and CNs, the significance of which is highest during brainstem surgery. A train of pulses is applied to the dorsolateral aspect of the motor cortex using scalp electrodes (C3/C4[29] or C5/C6[30]). Recordings can be obtained from trigeminal, facial, and bulbar muscles. One drawback of this technique is that given the lateral position of the stimulating electrodes, the CNs can be activated directly by the

spreading of current to the base of the skull. When this occurs, the current shortcuts the corticobulbar tracts leading to false negative results. Switching to monopulse stimulation should abolish CoMEPs and help differentiate between these two scenarios. For detailed description of the technique, please refer to Deletis and Fernández-Conejero[29] and Deletis et al.[31]

D-wave Recording

The D-wave technique involves activating the motor cortex transcranially and recording CST responses from the spinal cord via recording electrodes placed epidurally/subdurally through a laminectomy or using a percutaneous (Touhy) needle. If the lesion is above T10–T11, the electrodes are placed caudal and rostral to the surgical site, the latter serving as a control. D-wave is more reliable when recorded at a cervical and mid-to-upper thoracic spine level because the CST becomes progressively thinner as fibers leave the motor tract at each spinal level.[26] D-waves are perfectly reproducible, less affected by various confounding factors, and can be recorded in patients under neuromuscular blockade; all of these are significant advantages over MEPs. Therefore, D-waves are regarded as the gold standard in terms of CST monitoring when performing intra-axial spinal cord tumor resection. A drop of 50% in peak-to-peak amplitude is a major alarming criterion.[25] The utility of combining D-wave and MEPs includes continuous monitoring of D-wave. As long as the D-wave signal is normal, or the decrease is less than 50%, the deficit in MEPs may be disregarded and in the worst-case scenario, it may lead to transient postoperative deficits. Nevertheless, surgeons should interpret D-wave signal changes cautiously; for example, if D-wave signal amplitudes drop by 30%, surgeons should consider halting the resection, changing the site of resection, and/or releasing retraction, as well as being cognizant that a permanent postoperative deficit may occur if they resume resection in the same site.

Descending Neurogenic Evoked Potentials

Descending neurogenic evoked potentials (dNEPs) are recorded in lower extremity nerves (mostly sciatic nerve at the popliteal fossa), and stimulation is applied at the level of the spinal cord (either epidurally or indirectly by placing needle electrodes between consecutive spinous processes). dNEPs are also referred to as "neurogenic MEPs" since the technique was initially thought to monitor motor responses.[32] Subsequent studies, however, showed that the recorded signals are due to retrograde conduction within the spinal dorsal columns and may not show changes if the CSTs are injured.[33,34] Therefore, dNEPs are of limited use in IMSC surgeries, unless complemented by other monitoring modalities.

Free-running Electromyography

The free-running electromyography (EMG) technique involves recording spontaneous nerve discharges that occur when the nerve is irritated. The abnormal activity is recorded by needle electrodes inserted into the muscle. Not all types of free-running activity are predictive of injury. For example, single potentials or regularly occurring train of triphasic waves are frequently observed with harmless mechanical and thermal insults such as cold fluid irrigation and nerve manipulation.

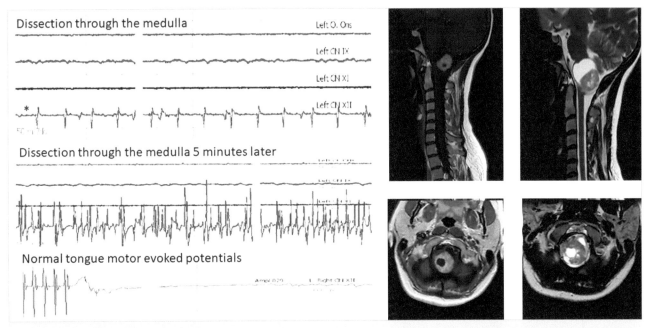

Fig. 19.8 Free-running electromyography (EMG) activity in a case of spinal cord tumor extending into the medulla. While dissecting through the medulla, spontaneous activity in the tongue was recorded (*). This activity is composed of sinusoidal waves discharging at a rate of 20 Hz. Although this type of activity is usually not threatening, the surgeon was informed that he was dissecting in close proximity to the hypoglossal nerve/nucleus. Five minutes later, the firing pattern changed; it was more reminiscent of neurotonic discharges, and the surgeon was asked to stop. Given the significant false positive rates of free-running EMG, tongue motor-evoked potentials (MEPs) were tested and found to be normal. Dissection was carefully resumed under close MEP monitoring.

Their occurrence, however, could be helpful in the sense that they demonstrate that the nerve is functional, muscle relaxation has worn off, and equipment is set up properly. Free-running activity also informs unwary surgeons that they are operating in close proximity to a nerve root. This is particularly important when normal anatomy is distorted by a pathological process. On the other hand, the so-called neuromyotonic discharges are more predictive of injury and should be taken more seriously. But even then, false positive results are frequent (▶ Fig. 19.8); therefore, overreliance on this technique should be avoided.[35,36,37]

Other Monitoring Techniques

Brainstem reflexes may be transiently affected postoperatively despite lack of abnormal signals on different IONMM modalities. Although these reflexes are completely suppressed under general anesthesia, some authors proposed methodologies to elicit the blink reflex[38] as well as record the master H-reflex[29] intraoperatively. Such methodologies, however, require further validation with larger studies, and the value of intraoperative brainstem reflex testing is not established yet.

19.2.2 Mapping Techniques

Dorsal Column Mapping

In IMSC procedures, understanding the exact location of the dorsal columns is crucial to decide on the myelotomy site and point of entry to the cord. Recognizing the surface vascular anatomy is usually helpful, since superficial veins dive into the cord along the midline between the two dorsal columns. In some cases, however, the midline may be difficult to delineate due to IMSC lesions distorting the physiologic anatomy. Dorsal column mapping (DCM) can be utilized in such scenarios to accurately identify the dorsal median raphe prior to performing a midline myelotomy. This is accomplished by using a hand-held probe to stimulate the anatomically distorted area at fine intervals from lateral to medial until phase reversal of the waveform is observed on SSEP recording electrodes applied to the scalp.[39] With practice and experience, DCM may also be helpful in recognizing the resection plane and deciding on the extent of resection.[40,41] Although other techniques of DCM— such as peripheral nerve stimulation and using strip electrodes applied to the spinal cord to record orthodromic sensory conduction;[42] fine-interval stimulation of the spinal cord and recording retrograde sensory conduction at peripheral nerves bilaterally[43]—have been reported, it seems that the first technique is more practical since the same SSEP montage may be used for both monitoring and mapping as well as it is reliable in generating signals within a relatively short duration.

Brainstem Mapping

Brainstem surgery ranks high among the critical neurosurgical procedures due to the neuroanatomical convergence of all the descending and ascending cortical pathways as well as the presence of most of the CN nuclei and CNs in a relatively small area. The presence of a space-occupying lesion in the brainstem distorts the intricate normal anatomy and makes it very difficult even for highly skilled surgeons to visually identify anatomical landmarks. Therefore, the main goal behind intraoperative brainstem mapping is to provide a tool to objectively localize the CN nuclei, CNs and critical brainstem pathways such as CSTs. To our knowledge, Strauss and colleagues were the first to describe the technique of direct electrical stimulation (DES) for mapping of the floor of the fourth ventricle,[44] though electrical stimulation was utilized in earlier studies to adjust the probe position in brainstem biopsies as well as during chronic pain procedures in awake patients.[45,46] Subsequent studies further improved the methodology and fine-tuned the neurophysiological parameters for DES of brainstem structures intraoperatively.[47,48] Finally, the approach for mapping and localization of the CSTs have also been described,[49] and it would be of utmost value during surgical resection of lesions involving the cerebral peduncles and ventral portion of the medulla.

During surgical resection of brainstem lesions, the surgeon has few possible corridors to enter into the brainstem parenchyma. Entry points, such as the midline above the facial colliculus or supra- or infrafacial triangle, demand meticulous brainstem mapping and a very thorough understanding of brainstem anatomy and the structural organization of brainstem nuclei (mainly the motor nuclei). During the mapping step, it is important to localize especially the motor CNs (e.g., VI and VII). After the initial myelotomy is done, ongoing monitoring of the CST and CNs is usually pursued.

19.3 Single- Versus Multi-modality IONMM

Each of the IONMM techniques described in the previous sections monitor and map the functional integrity of distinct anatomical structures and pathways at the levels of brainstem and spinal cord. It is imperative, therefore, to state that no single technique would be sufficient to provide full and accurate prophylaxis against neural tissue injury when utilized alone, especially during IMSC and brainstem surgeries. This has been demonstrated in studies revealing increased sensitivity and specificity when multiple modalities are utilized simultaneously.[50,51] The choice and combination of modalities should be tailored according to individual cases based on the surgeon's clinical judgment and surgical approach as well as the experience of the neurophysiologist with operating a multimodality IONMM.

For example, surgical resection of brainstem and/or cerebellopontine angle lesions may require monitoring using a combination of BAEPs if the lesion involves the auditory nerve/pathways; SSEPs and TcMEPs in almost all cases; and/or CoMEPs, with or without free-running EMG, where recording electrodes are situated in bulbar muscles innervated by CNs that are susceptible to injury (i.e., extraocular muscles for CNs III, IV, and VI, masseter/temporalis for CN V, facial muscles for CN VII, laryngeal muscles for CN X, trapezius for CN XI, and genioglossus for CN XII monitoring).[43] These modalities may also be complemented by intermittently mapping the surgical field using DES before manipulating the distorted anatomical landmarks.[52] The same rule applies to spinal procedures as well.[53] It is noteworthy that sensitivity for detection of injury is more important than the specificity since the surgeon must be warned about signal changes suggesting increased likelihood of occurrence of damage before substantial injury has already occurred. While the sensitivity of single/double modality for detecting impending injury may be relatively low compared to

their specificity,[54] multimodal approaches have yielded sensitivities as high as 99.6%.[55] Not only patients with IMSC lesions[56] will benefit from a multimodality IONMM, but also those undergoing surgery for intradural extramedullary tumors,[57] syringomyelia[58] and tethered cords.[59]

19.4 A Team-based Approach

IONMM requires a team-based approach, where an open and continuous communication between the neurophysiologist, surgeon, and anesthesiologist is essential to maximize the efficacy of IONMM and warrant a successful, noneventful surgery. Nevertheless, it is important to keep in mind that even with multimodal IONMM and experienced teams, there is always a margin of uncertainty in IONMM and injuries may go undetected on real-time monitoring, resulting in postoperative deficits.[60,61]

19.4.1 Role of the Neurophysiologist

The neurophysiologist's role extends beyond discussing the choice of IONMM modalities with the surgeon, ensuring an accurate setup of the electrodes and monitoring machines, and interpreting the obtained signals intraoperatively in real time. Knowledge of the various steps and stages of the surgery is equally important in predicting neural tissue irritation or injury when signal alterations occur, and it helps in differentiating between real damage and shortcomings in the IONMM setup or process, for example, disconnection or change of electrode position, electrocauterization artifacts, physiological variability of responses, etc. When alarming signals arise or a significant change in signal appears on the monitoring screen, the neurophysiologist should promptly warn both the surgeon and the anesthesiologist, and should inquire about any possible surgical maneuver or anesthetic intervention that could have caused this change. Finally, continuous troubleshooting of the monitoring setup and open communication with the surgeon throughout the surgery helps in detecting neural injury early on and before it becomes irreversible.

19.4.2 Role of the Surgeon

The objective nature of IONMM do have a significant impact on the surgeon's decision-making intraoperatively, and signal deterioration may lead to subtotal resection and termination of surgery, which may require a second attempt to surgically resect the rest of the lesion.[62] Therefore, the surgeon's role starts with a thorough discussion with the patient/family about the goals of the surgery, extent of surgical resection of the IMSC or brainstem lesion, and expected postoperative outcomes. These goals will reflect the decision on what threshold in signal change will inform the surgeon about when to terminate the surgery, even if GTR has not been achieved. Indeed, significant changes in intraoperative signals have been shown to predict postoperative outcomes after surgical resection.[63] The anatomical location of the lesion and extent of involvement of the neural structures/pathways will affect the surgeon's choice of the monitoring modalities, and whether mapping techniques should be employed intraoperatively as well. Of important note is the fact that IONMM is never meant to replace the surgeon's knowledge of anatomy, surgical skills, and expertise in resecting IMSC and brainstem lesions, but rather provide a means of objective assessment of the functional integrity of the neural tissue at moments of hesitation and doubt, and when an objective answer to these doubts will facilitate intraoperative decision-making. Surgeons should be familiar with all the monitoring modalities being used in the specific surgery they are performing, as well as the interpretation of the various alarms and results of the IONMM.

When the IONMM signal suddenly disappears or significantly deteriorates below critical values, the first reaction is to understand the meaning of the specific modality that it is down (e.g., drop in MEPs while D-waves remain intact in IMSC surgery). In cases where the change in the IONMM is significant, the surgeon should temporarily stop the resection and remove any traction on the surgical bed; continuous monitoring will provide an estimation of the injury and inform the surgeon whether further resection is acceptable or it may lead to irreversible damage.[28] There is no consensus on how much time should the surgery be stopped for, but some authors propose a 30 minutes waiting time after a significant drop or disappearance in the TcMEP and D-wave signals during resection of IMSC lesions.[64] Irrigation of the surgical field with warm normal saline also helps by washing away blood products, cellular metabolites, and potassium, which may alter the conduction of impulses along a vulnerable neural tissue. It also helps by excluding functional conduction blocks of nerve conduction that occur with cooling of the spinal cord/brainstem below physiological levels. Preoperative administration of steroids could be of benefit in patients with tumors associated with neurological deficits secondary to vasogenic edema,[40] but the effect of intraoperative steroid administration after IONMM signal loss have not been elucidated yet.

19.4.3 Role of the Anesthesiologist

Anesthesia has a paramount role in the team-based approach to an efficient IONMM. The suppressive effects of most anesthetic agents on EEG[65] as well as on signals obtained from different IONMM modalities have been consistently reported.[66] Modern inhalational agents inhibit neuronal excitability by activating the two-pore-domain potassium channels,[67] where the greatest inhibition was reported by using isoflurane and nitric oxide,[68] followed by sevoflurane,[69] and desflurane.[70] Therefore, the best anesthetic approach is to avoid these agents whenever possible. Very low doses (0.3–0.4 MAC) of these agents are recommended if their use in IONMM is unavoidable.[66] On the other hand, total intravenous anesthesia (TIVA) (i.e., use of propofol and opioid drugs) has been shown to be consistently superior to inhalational agents, demonstrating a less suppressive profile on IONMM signals.[68,71,72] Short-acting neuromuscular blocking agents may be used during induction of anesthesia but should be stopped completely afterwards to prevent IONMM signal loss when TcMEPs and mapping techniques are utilized. Not only does the choice of anesthetic agents affect the success of IONMM, but also the anesthesiologist's skills in keeping a stable anesthetic background, especially during critical portions of the surgery, such as tumor resection, where signal changes are more likely to reflect neural injury.

In addition, the anesthesiologist's role is to provide an optimal physiological milieu for IONMM signal recording. The control of mean arterial pressure (MAP) plays a significant role during IONMM. As in most of the neurosurgical procedures, increasing the MAP is avoided in IMSC and brainstem surgeries due to continuous oozing of venous blood, which obscures the surgical field. However, when IONMM signals change due to neural injury, increasing the MAP (above 60 mm Hg[73] or even 80 mm Hg, if injury is documented[74]) may be helpful by improving local perfusion and preventing ischemia, and has been associated with favorable outcomes in multiple studies.[63,75,76] Hypoxemia and hypocapnia ($PaCO_2$ less than 20 mm Hg) could also produce signal changes,[77,78] and baseline IONMM recordings prior to anticipated hypocapnia (i.e., due to induced hyperventilation) are recommended. Keeping a hematocrit value above 32% is considered safe and should not cause signal alterations until hematocrit levels fall below 20% and 15%, leading to decrease in amplitude and increase in latency of SSEPs, respectively.[79] Physiologic blood levels of other metabolites (electrolytes, glucose, etc.) should be optimized to avoid signal alterations as well.[80] Hypothermia will cause SSEPs latency prolongation and MEPs signal delay, and the opposite is seen in hyperthermia; thus, the patient's core temperature is ideally kept within 2 to 3 °C of their baseline to prevent IONMM signal changes.[81] Finally, the anesthesia team should keep an open communication with the neurophysiologist and the surgeon about any change in these physiologic parameters, which may lead to IONMM signal alterations that affect intraoperative decision-making.

19.5 Conclusion

There has been continuous advancement of IONMM techniques that has increased the ability to safely and more effectively resect lesions within the brainstem and spinal cord. These monitoring modalities include BAEPs, SSEPs, MEPs, D-wave recordings, and free-running electromyography that provide real-time information about the functional integrity of neural tissue. In addition, mapping techniques using hand-held probes and modified surgical instruments allow for accurate identification of important neuroanatomical structures. The sensitivities and specificities of these modalities in detecting impending neural injury significantly increase when these modalities are combined. More important than this is the need to employ a multidisciplinary and team-based approach, with open communication between the surgeon, neurophysiologist, and anesthesiologist.

References

[1] Pallud J, Rigaux-Viode O, Corns R, et al. Direct electrical bipolar electrostimulation for functional cortical and subcortical cerebral mapping in awake craniotomy. Practical considerations. Neurochirurgie. 2017; 63(3):164–174

[2] Raabe A, Beck J, Schucht P, Seidel K. Continuous dynamic mapping of the corticospinal tract during surgery of motor eloquent brain tumors: evaluation of a new method. J Neurosurg. 2014; 120(5):1015–1024

[3] American Clinical Neurophysiology Society. Guideline 9C: guidelines on short-latency auditory evoked potentials. J Clin Neurophysiol. 2006; 23(2):157–167

[4] Petrova LD. Brainstem auditory evoked potentials. Am J Electroneurodiagn Technol. 2009; 49(4):317–332

[5] Bischoff B, Romstöck J, Fahlbusch R, Buchfelder M, Strauss C. Intraoperative brainstem auditory evoked potential pattern and perioperative vasoactive treatment for hearing preservation in vestibular schwannoma surgery. J Neurol Neurosurg Psychiatry. 2008; 79(2):170–175

[6] Radtke RA, Erwin CW, Wilkins RH. Intraoperative brainstem auditory evoked potentials: significant decrease in postoperative morbidity. Neurology. 1989; 39(2 Pt 1):187–191

[7] Polo G, Fischer C, Sindou MP, Marneffe V. Brainstem auditory evoked potential monitoring during microvascular decompression for hemifacial spasm: intraoperative brainstem auditory evoked potential changes and warning values to prevent hearing loss–prospective study in a consecutive series of 84 patients. Neurosurgery. 2004; 54(1):97–104, discussion 104–106

[8] Hatayama T, Møller AR. Correlation between latency and amplitude of peak V in the brainstem auditory evoked potentials: intraoperative recordings in microvascular decompression operations. Acta Neurochir (Wien). 1998; 140 (7):681–687

[9] Møller AR, Jannetta PJ. Monitoring auditory functions during cranial nerve microvascular decompression operations by direct recording from the eighth nerve. J Neurosurg. 1983; 59(3):493–499

[10] Legatt AD. Mechanisms of intraoperative brainstem auditory evoked potential changes. J Clin Neurophysiol. 2002; 19(5):396–408

[11] Zamel K, Galloway G, Kosnik EJ, Raslan M, Adeli A. Intraoperative neurophysiologic monitoring in 80 patients with Chiari I malformation: role of duraplasty. J Clin Neurophysiol. 2009; 26(2):70–75

[12] American Electroencephalographic Society. Guideline eleven: guidelines for intraoperative monitoring of sensory evoked potentials. J Clin Neurophysiol. 1994; 11(1):77–87

[13] Legatt AD. Brainstem auditory evoked potentials. In: Husain A, ed. A Practical Approach to Neurophysiologic Intraoperative Monitoring. 2nd ed. New York, NY: Demos Medical Publishing, LLC; 2015:46–54

[14] Thirumala PD, Carnovale G, Loke Y, et al. Brainstem auditory evoked potentials' diagnostic accuracy for hearing loss: systematic review and meta-analysis. J Neurol Surg B Skull Base. 2017; 78(1):43–51

[15] Park S-K, Joo B-E, Lee S, et al. The critical warning sign of real-time brainstem auditory evoked potentials during microvascular decompression for hemifacial spasm. Clin Neurophysiol. 2018; 129(5):1097–1102

[16] Halonen J-P, Jones SJ, Edgar MA, Ransford AO. Conduction properties of epidurally recorded spinal cord potentials following lower limb stimulation in man. Electroencephalogr Clin Neurophysiol. 1989; 74(3):161–174

[17] Schwartz DM, Auerbach JD, Dormans JP, et al. Neurophysiological detection of impending spinal cord injury during scoliosis surgery. J Bone Joint Surg Am. 2007; 89(11):2440–2449

[18] American Clinical Neurophysiology Society. Guideline 9D: guidelines on short-latency somatosensory evoked potentials. J Clin Neurophysiol. 2006; 23 (2):168–179

[19] Nuwer MR, Dawson EG, Carlson LG, Kanim LE, Sherman JE. Somatosensory evoked potential spinal cord monitoring reduces neurologic deficits after scoliosis surgery: results of a large multicenter survey. Electroencephalogr Clin Neurophysiol. 1995; 96(1):6–11

[20] Stöhr M, Petruch F. Somatosensory evoked potentials following stimulation of the trigeminal nerve in man. J Neurol. 1979; 220(2):95–98

[21] Stechison MT. The trigeminal evoked potential: part II. Intraoperative recording of short-latency responses. Neurosurgery. 1993; 33(4):639–643, discussion 643–644

[22] Malcharek MJ, Landgraf J, Hennig G, Sorge O, Aschermann J, Sablotzki A. Recordings of long-latency trigeminal somatosensory-evoked potentials in patients under general anaesthesia. Clin Neurophysiol. 2011; 122(5):1048–1054

[23] American Electroencephalographic Society. Guideline thirteen: guidelines for standard electrode position nomenclature. J Clin Neurophysiol. 1994; 11(1): 111–113

[24] Szelényi A, Kothbauer KF, Deletis V. Transcranial electric stimulation for intraoperative motor evoked potential monitoring: stimulation parameters and electrode montages. Clin Neurophysiol. 2007; 118(7):1586–1595

[25] Legatt AD, Emerson RG, Epstein CM, et al. ACNS guideline: transcranial electrical stimulation motor evoked potential monitoring. J Clin Neurophysiol. 2016; 33(1):42–50

[26] Macdonald DB, Skinner S, Shils J, Yingling C, American Society of Neurophysiological Monitoring. Intraoperative motor evoked potential monitoring - a position statement by the American Society of Neurophysiological Monitoring. Clin Neurophysiol. 2013; 124(12):2291–2316

[27] Langeloo DD, Lelivelt A, Louis Journée H, Slappendel R, de Kleuver M. Transcranial electrical motor-evoked potential monitoring during surgery for spinal deformity: a study of 145 patients. Spine. 2003; 28(10):1043–1050

[28] Deletis V, Sala F. Intraoperative neurophysiological monitoring of the spinal cord during spinal cord and spine surgery: a review focus on the corticospinal tracts. Clin Neurophysiol. 2008; 119(2):248–264

[29] Deletis V, Fernández-Conejero I. Intraoperative monitoring and mapping of the functional integrity of the brainstem. J Clin Neurol. 2016; 12(3):262–273

[30] Verst SM, Sucena AC, Maldaun MV, Aguiar PH. Effectiveness of C5 or C6-Cz assembly in predicting immediate postoperative facial nerve deficit. Acta Neurochir (Wien). 2013; 155(10):1863–1869

[31] Deletis V, Fernández-Conejero I, Ulkatan S, Rogić M, Carbó EL, Hiltzik D. Methodology for intra-operative recording of the corticobulbar motor evoked potentials from cricothyroid muscles. Clin Neurophysiol. 2011; 122(9):1883–1889

[32] Owen JH, Laschinger J, Bridwell K, et al. Sensitivity and specificity of somatosensory and neurogenic-motor evoked potentials in animals and humans. Spine. 1988; 13(10):1111–1118

[33] Minahan RE, Sepkuty JP, Lesser RP, Sponseller PD, Kostuik JP. Anterior spinal cord injury with preserved neurogenic 'motor' evoked potentials. Clin Neurophysiol. 2001; 112(8):1442–1450

[34] Toleikis JR, Skelly JP, Carlvin AO, Burkus JK. Spinally elicited peripheral nerve responses are sensory rather than motor. Clin Neurophysiol. 2000; 111(4): 736–742

[35] Romstöck J, Strauss C, Fahlbusch R. Identification of cranial nerve nuclei. Muscle Nerve. 2000; 23(9):1445–1446

[36] Romstöck J, Strauss C, Fahlbusch R. Continuous electromyography monitoring of motor cranial nerves during cerebellopontine angle surgery. J Neurosurg. 2000; 93(4):586–593

[37] Prell J, Strauss C, Rachinger J, et al. The intermedius nerve as a confounding variable for monitoring of the free-running electromyogram. Clin Neurophysiol. 2015; 126(9):1833–1839

[38] Deletis V, Urriza J, Ulkatan S, Fernandez-Conejero I, Lesser J, Misita D. The feasibility of recording blink reflexes under general anesthesia. Muscle Nerve. 2009; 39(5):642–646

[39] Simon MV, Chiappa KH, Borges LF. Phase reversal of somatosensory evoked potentials triggered by gracilis tract stimulation: case report of a new technique for neurophysiologic dorsal column mapping. Neurosurgery. 2012; 70 (3):E783–E788

[40] Mehta AI, Mohrhaus CA, Husain AM, et al. Dorsal column mapping for intramedullary spinal cord tumor resection decreases dorsal column dysfunction. J Spinal Disord Tech. 2012; 25(4):205–209

[41] Cheng JS, Ivan ME, Stapleton CJ, Quinones-Hinojosa A, Gupta N, Auguste KI. Intraoperative changes in transcranial motor evoked potentials and somatosensory evoked potentials predicting outcome in children with intramedullary spinal cord tumors. J Neurosurg Pediatr. 2014; 13(6):591–599

[42] Yanni DS, Ulkatan S, Deletis V, Barrenechea IJ, Sen C, Perin NI. Utility of neurophysiological monitoring using dorsal column mapping in intramedullary spinal cord surgery. J Neurosurg Spine. 2010; 12(6):623–628

[43] Kim K, Cho C, Bang MS, Shin HI, Phi JH, Kim SK. Intraoperative neurophysiological monitoring: a review of techniques used for brain tumor surgery in children. J Korean Neurosurg Soc. 2018; 61(3):363–375

[44] Strauss C, Romstöck J, Nimsky C, Fahlbusch R. Intraoperative identification of motor areas of the rhomboid fossa using direct stimulation. J Neurosurg. 1993; 79(3):393–399

[45] Bullard DE, Makachinas TT, Nashold BS, Jr. The role of monopolar stimulation during computed-tomography-guided stereotaxic biopsies. Appl Neurophysiol. 1988; 51(1):45–54

[46] Young RF, Tronnier V, Rinaldi PC. Chronic stimulation of the Kölliker-Fuse nucleus region for relief of intractable pain in humans. J Neurosurg. 1992; 76 (6):979–985

[47] Morota N, Deletis V, Epstein FJ, et al. Brain stem mapping: neurophysiological localization of motor nuclei on the floor of the fourth ventricle. Neurosurgery. 1995; 37(5):922–929, discussion 929–930

[48] Morota N, Deletis V. The importance of brainstem mapping in brainstem surgical anatomy before the fourth ventricle and implication for intraoperative neurophysiological mapping. Acta Neurochir (Wien). 2006; 148(5):499–509, discussion 509

[49] Deletis V, Sala F, Morota N. Intraoperative neurophysiological monitoring and mapping during brain stem surgery: a modern approach. Operat Tech Neurosurg.. 2000; 3(2):109–113

[50] Gunnarsson T, Krassioukov AV, Sarjeant R, Fehlings MG. Real-time continuous intraoperative electromyographic and somatosensory evoked potential recordings in spinal surgery: correlation of clinical and electrophysiologic findings in a prospective, consecutive series of 213 cases. Spine. 2004; 29(6): 677–684

[51] Manninen PH, Patterson S, Lam AM, Gelb AW, Nantau WE. Evoked potential monitoring during posterior fossa aneurysm surgery: a comparison of two modalities. Can J Anaesth. 1994; 41(2):92–97

[52] Slotty PJ, Abdulazim A, Kodama K, et al. Intraoperative neurophysiological monitoring during resection of infratentorial lesions: the surgeon's view. J Neurosurg. 2017; 126(1):281–288

[53] Verla T, Fridley JS, Khan AB, Mayer RR, Omeis I. Neuromonitoring for intramedullary spinal cord tumor surgery. World Neurosurg. 2016; 95:108–116

[54] Hamilton DK, Smith JS, Sansur CA, et al. Scoliosis Research Society Morbidity and Mortality Committee. Rates of new neurological deficit associated with spine surgery based on 108,419 procedures: a report of the scoliosis research society morbidity and mortality committee. Spine. 2011; 36(15):1218–1228

[55] Thuet ED, Winscher JC, Padberg AM, et al. Validity and reliability of intraoperative monitoring in pediatric spinal deformity surgery: a 23-year experience of 3436 surgical cases. Spine. 2010; 35(20):1880–1886

[56] Nadkarni TD, Rekate HL. Pediatric intramedullary spinal cord tumors. Critical review of the literature. Childs Nerv Syst. 1999; 15(1):17–28

[57] Ghadirpour R, Nasi D, Iaccarino C, et al. Intraoperative neurophysiological monitoring for intradural extramedullary tumors: why not? Clin Neurol Neurosurg. 2015; 130:140–149

[58] Pencovich N, Korn A, Constantini S. Intraoperative neurophysiologic monitoring during syringomyelia surgery: lessons from a series of 13 patients. Acta Neurochir (Wien). 2013; 155(5):785–791, discussion 791

[59] Kothbauer KF, Novak K. Intraoperative monitoring for tethered cord surgery: an update. Neurosurg Focus. 2004; 16(2):E8

[60] Lesser RP, Raudzens P, Lüders H, et al. Postoperative neurological deficits may occur despite unchanged intraoperative somatosensory evoked potentials. Ann Neurol. 1986; 19(1):22–25

[61] Molaie M. False negative intraoperative somatosensory evoked potentials with simultaneous bilateral stimulation. Clin Electroencephalogr. 1986; 17(1):6–9

[62] Kothbauer KF, Deletis V, Epstein FJ. Motor-evoked potential monitoring for intramedullary spinal cord tumor surgery: correlation of clinical and neurophysiological data in a series of 100 consecutive procedures. Neurosurg Focus. 1998; 4(5):e1

[63] Skinner SA, Nagib M, Bergman TA, Maxwell RE, Msangi G. The initial use of free-running electromyography to detect early motor tract injury during resection of intramedullary spinal cord lesions. Neurosurgery. 2005; 56(2) Suppl:299–314, discussion 299–314

[64] Sala F, Bricolo A, Faccioli F, Lanteri P, Gerosa M. Surgery for intramedullary spinal cord tumors: the role of intraoperative (neurophysiological) monitoring. Eur Spine J. 2007; 16(2) Suppl 2:S130–S139

[65] Purdon PL, Sampson A, Pavone KJ, Brown EN. Clinical electroencephalography for anesthesiologistspart I: background and basic signatures. Anesthesiology. 2015; 123(4):937–960

[66] Glover CD, Carling NP. Neuromonitoring for scoliosis surgery. Anesthesiol Clin. 2014; 32(1):101–114

[67] Patel AJ, Honoré E, Lesage F, Fink M, Romey G, Lazdunski M. Inhalational anesthetics activate two-pore-domain background K+ channels. Nat Neurosci. 1999; 2(5):422–426

[68] Pechstein U, Nadstawek J, Zentner J, Schramm J. Isoflurane plus nitrous oxide versus propofol for recording of motor evoked potentials after high frequency repetitive electrical stimulation. Electroencephalogr Clin Neurophysiol. 1998; 108(2):175–181

[69] Chong CT, Manninen P, Sivanaser V, Subramanyam R, Lu N, Venkatraghavan L. Direct comparison of the effect of desflurane and sevoflurane on intraoperative motor-evoked potentials monitoring. J Neurosurg Anesthesiol. 2014; 26 (4):306–312

[70] Martin DP, Bhalla T, Thung A, et al. A preliminary study of volatile agents or total intravenous anesthesia for neurophysiological monitoring during posterior spinal fusion in adolescents with idiopathic scoliosis. Spine. 2014; 39 (22):E1318–E1324

[71] Lo Y-L, Dan Y-F, Tan YE, et al. Intraoperative motor-evoked potential monitoring in scoliosis surgery: comparison of desflurane/nitrous oxide with propofol total intravenous anesthetic regimens. J Neurosurg Anesthesiol. 2006; 18 (3):211–214

[72] Taniguchi M, Nadstawek J, Pechstein U, Schramm J. Total intravenous anesthesia for improvement of intraoperative monitoring of somatosensory evoked potentials during aneurysm surgery. Neurosurgery. 1992; 31(5):891–897, discussion 897

[73] Choi I, Hyun S-J, Kang J-K, Rhim S-C. Combined muscle motor and somatosensory evoked potentials for intramedullary spinal cord tumour surgery. Yonsei Med J. 2014; 55(4):1063–1071

[74] Ahn H, Fehlings MG. Prevention, identification, and treatment of perioperative spinal cord injury. Neurosurg Focus. 2008; 25(5):E15

[75] Hyun S-J, Rhim S-C. Combined motor and somatosensory evoked potential monitoring for intramedullary spinal cord tumor surgery: correlation of clinical and neurophysiological data in 17 consecutive procedures. Br J Neurosurg. 2009; 23(4):393–400

[76] Polo A, Tercedor A, Paniagua-Soto J, Acosta F, Cañadas A. Monitorización neurofisiológica en la cirugía de escoliosis con hipotensión controlada. Rev Esp Anestesiol Reanim. 2000; 47(8):367–370

[77] Grundy BL, Heros RC, Tung AS, Doyle E. Intraoperative hypoxia detected by evoked potential monitoring. Anesth Analg. 1981; 60(6): 437–439

[78] Gravenstein MA, Sasse F, Hogan K. Effects of hypocapnia on canine spinal, subcortical, and cortical somatosensory-evoked potentials during isoflurane anesthesia. J Clin Monit. 1992; 8(2):126–130

[79] Nagao S, Roccaforte P, Moody RA. The effects of isovolemic hemodilution and reinfusion of packed erythrocytes on somatosensory and visual evoked potentials. J Surg Res. 1978; 25(6):530–537

[80] Sloan TB, Heyer EJ. Anesthesia for intraoperative neurophysiologic monitoring of the spinal cord. J Clin Neurophysiol. 2002; 19(5):430–443

[81] Oro J, Haghighi SS. Effects of altering core body temperature on somatosensory and motor evoked potentials in rats. Spine. 1992; 17(5):498–503

Section III

Postoperative Brain Mapping for Recovery of Function

20 Importance of Rehabilitation after Eloquent Brain Surgery

Kenneth Ngo, Andrea J. Davis, Russell Addeo, Jodi Morgan, Jennifer Walworth, and Sarah Chamberlin

Abstract

Rehabilitation has a very important role in caring for patients after eloquent brain surgery. In a rehabilitation hospital, the patient has the unique experience of a team of rehabilitation professionals working closely together to help optimize a patient's complex medical conditions and improve their cognitive and functional abilities. These impairments are often more evident after eloquent brain surgery, where patients often have impairments in cognitive, communicative, mobility, and self-care skills. In addition to functional impairments, medical complications can occur and risk of increasing medical comorbidities increases after surgery. Therefore, having a team of healthcare professionals to address their medical and functional needs helps optimize medical conditions and maximize functional potentials.

Keywords: rehabilitation, brain injury, occupational therapy, physical therapy, speech therapy

20.1 Introduction

After eloquent brain surgery, patients often need to be transferred to an acute inpatient rehabilitation hospital for close medical monitoring and intensive therapy. Patients often require a hospital level of care, where nursing and physicians are readily available to address their complex medical needs. A rehabilitation team is often led by a physiatrist, a medical physician specializing in physical medicine and rehabilitation (a medical subspecialty within the American Boards of Medical Specialties).[1] In the context of neurological rehabilitation, a physiatrist has specialized training in evaluating and treating cognitive and functional impairments due to complex neurological conditions. At major rehabilitation centers, availability of board-certified brain injury specialists (CBIS) is often present to care for patients with complex brain conditions. The physiatrist works together with the rehabilitation team as well as a medical team, which may include medical internists and other medical subspecialists, to optimize patient care. In addition to understanding the cognitive and functional sequelae of neurological conditions and their recovery patterns, a physiatrist also has expertise in understanding the therapy approaches to rehabilitation and direct the rehabilitation team to optimize functional recovery.

20.2 Rehabilitation Team

A comprehensive rehabilitation team in an acute inpatient rehabilitation hospital includes the patient and families, a physiatrist, neuropsychologist/psychologist, rehabilitation nurse, speech–language pathologist, physical therapist, occupational therapist (OT), respiratory therapist, registered dietician, case manager/social worker/care coordinator, recreational therapist,

and chaplain.[2] The team works closely together with an interdisciplinary approach that is patient-centric, and often communicates with one another on a daily basis about patient's progress and any barriers to progress in functional improvement. The goals are defined early in the rehabilitation process, reviewed periodically, and each team member has high accountability for the progress toward defined goals. This highly organized model of care is most successful in the inpatient rehabilitation setting (**see** ▶ Table 20.1).

The patient's goal of rehabilitation post–eloquent brain surgery is often restoration of cognition, speech–language skills,

Table 20.1 Members of a rehabilitation team

Physiatrist	• A medical physician specializing in physical medicine and rehabilitation, who leads the rehabilitation team in diagnosing of medical conditions and functional impairments, establishing and executing rehabilitation plans of care, and addressing any barriers to help maximize patients' functional potentials
Rehabilitation nurse	• Has additional qualified training in rehabilitation nursing, who provides nursing care to patients/families with emphasis on their rehabilitation needs
Neuropsychologist, psychologist	• Determines psychological factors that influence recovery, and designs and implements psychological interventions to help patients and families
Speech–language pathologist	• Diagnose and treats swallowing disorders, speech–language and cognitive/communication disorders
Physical therapist	• Assesses motor and mobility impairments, establishes and executes treatment plans designed to maximize functional mobility
Occupational therapist	• Utilizes therapeutic activities to maximize independence in the areas of activities of daily living, work, and leisure activities
Social worker, case manager	• Assesses and addresses social barriers to recovery and ensures optimal care transitions between acute care hospital, rehabilitation facilities, home, and other settings
Respiratory therapist	• Optimizes acute and chronic cardiopulmonary function of a patient, including teaching patients/families on how to optimize their cardiopulmonary function and quality of life
Dietician	• Assesses nutritional needs of patients with various medical conditions and disease states to provide individualized dietary education plans to patients and families
Chaplain	• Assesses and addresses emotional and spiritual well-beings of patients and families
Music therapist	• Uses music interventions to establish a therapeutic relationship with patients to address speech/language, cognitive, physical, and social needs
Recreational therapist	• Utilizes recreational and leisure activities as therapeutic interventions to help improve function and quality of life

mobility, and self-care skills. From a medical standpoint, the goal is to optimize medical comorbidities and address primary, secondary, and tertiary prevention issues to minimize medical complications that may affect recovery. A speech–language pathologist typically addresses patient's impairments in swallowing, language, cognitive, and communication skills. A physical therapist and OT typically address impairments in mobility, transfers, and self-care skills. A rehabilitation nurse often has additional training to address rehabilitation needs, including expertise in wound care, bowel and bladder management, medication teaching especially those that affect cognition and function, and patient and family education. A care manager, often a social worker or a nurse case manager, helps coordinate the patient's care with the rehabilitation team and identify resources to help the patient receive the appropriate rehabilitation services in their recovery. This well-coordinated interdisciplinary approach to patient care maximizes the chance of recovery for a patient undergoing eloquent brain surgery.

This highly effective inpatient interdisciplinary rehabilitation approach to care can be modeled in the outpatient and home care settings. Sometimes, a patient post–eloquent brain surgery may be able to be discharged directly to their home. Rehabilitation can be instituted in the patient's home if a patient has difficulty getting to an outpatient rehabilitation center. Nursing and all therapy disciplines can provide rehabilitative services in the patient's home. For those who are able to go to the outpatient setting, major rehabilitation outpatient centers are able to provide dedicated programs for patients with neurological conditions. Whether at home or in the outpatient settings, the rehabilitation approaches to care should follow the model as described earlier, and, preferably, should be in collaboration with a physiatrist.

20.3 Rehabilitation Nursing

Rehabilitation nursing embraces the values of compassion, knowledge, poise, sanguinity, and skillfulness. Through these values, nurses care for patients holistically while providing patient-centered care. At the time of admission to inpatient rehabilitation, nurses are often the first person a patient meets and rapport is established very early. This connection between nurse and patient, with the patient's goals for rehabilitation well understood, helps facilitate care throughout their recovery. Positive expression and an optimistic attitude help build trust and respect. A rehabilitation nurse is skilled at giving patients appropriate autonomy, all the while encouraging them to be a strong advocate of their care.

Patients post–eloquent brain surgeries who come to an inpatient rehabilitation hospital often have high medical acuity. Rehabilitation nurses are challenged with the management of health conditions and comorbidities as well as providing education about specific aspects of self-care. They work very closely with physiatrists, therapists, and the rest of the rehabilitation team in a goal-oriented manner. A high level of team collaboration and patient/family education is what distinguishes a rehabilitation nurse from nurses in the acute care setting. Furthermore, the use of evidence-based practices assures that nurses provide age- and development-appropriate education to patients and caregivers to maximize recovery potentials.

Many rehabilitation nurses in major rehabilitation hospitals have additional certification, officially designated as Certified Rehabilitation Registered Nurse credentials (CRRN). Obtaining this certification is evidence of high commitment to excellence in caring for patients with a neurological condition that affect cognition and function. Rehabilitation nurses with CRRN credentials engage in lifelong learning to obtain new knowledge and a skillset that allows them to coach and provide education to promote self-efficacy. In addition, many rehabilitation nurses who take care of patients post–eloquent brain surgeries have additional certification as certified CBIS. This high level of training and skillset makes rehabilitation nurse a highly valued member of the rehabilitation team.

20.4 Neuropsychology/Psychology

A neuropsychologist plays an important role in the rehabilitation process for individuals undergoing eloquent brain surgery, prior to and following surgery.[3] Prior to surgery, a neuropsychological evaluation provides a detailed evaluation of cognitive and emotional functioning. Presurgical evaluations can provide an important baseline to determine the presence, severity, and causes of cognitive impairments (e.g., some cognitive weaknesses could be due to brain lesions, but others may be due to medication effects, prior learning disorders, or prior brain insults) and to determine if there are emotional/psychological factors that need to be addressed.[3] The evaluations are usually conducted within a few weeks and days prior to surgery. The baseline neuropsychological evaluation serves to map the domains of cognitive functioning which may be impaired (e.g., attention, executive functioning, language skills, spatial processing, and memory) and where these weaknesses localize in the brain, similar to what is commonly done in epilepsy patients prior to undergoing surgery.[4] This serves to identify areas of cognition which are weak, how it affects their daily functioning, and which areas may require compensation. The presurgical evaluation of emotional status determines whether there is a significant mood, anxiety, or behavioral disorder which would require intervention. This may also suggest the need of psychopharmacological intervention, psychotherapy/cognitive, and/or behavioral interventions. The assessment can also help with assessing realistic emotional expectations prior to undergoing the surgical procedure.[5]

Following the surgical procedure, in the post–acute phase, a post-neuropsychological evaluation is conducted to determine if there has been any objective and reliable change in cognitive functioning. The evaluation forms the blueprint to guide treatment, to determine whether cognitive/speech therapy services are necessary, and, if so, what specific areas require focus. In addition, the post-neuropsychological evaluation is invaluable to make determinations about whether an individual can return to either school or work. The post-assessment of emotional status also includes additional screening for significant mood, anxiety, or behavioral disorders.[5]

The neuropsychologist also plays a crucial role in determining the psychological factors that influence recovery, and with designing and implementing psychological interventions. This can include cognitive behavioral therapy for the development of coping strategies for adjustment disorders, mindfulness, and relaxation training to address postsurgical anxiety symptoms; more intensive psychotherapy for more entrenched mood disorders; or behavioral interventions to address maladaptive patterns of behavior. There is a role for consideration of medications to help with mood and affective symptoms.

The neuropsychological evaluation can also assist with developing realistic vocational and/or academic pursuits and how this would be best achieved. The role of a neuropsychologist is invaluable for patient's pre– and post–eloquent brain surgery, as well as the inpatient and outpatient settings.

20.5 Speech Language and Cognitive Therapy

Speech–language pathology (SLP) rehabilitation encompasses services necessary for the diagnosis and treatments of swallowing (dysphagia), speech–language, and cognitive–communication disorders that result in communication disabilities. Following eloquent brain surgery, the most common areas a speech–language pathologist treats is in the areas of production (e.g., articulation, apraxia, and dysarthria), resonance (e.g., hypernasality and hyponasality), voice (e.g., phonation quality, pitch, and respiration), fluency (e.g., stuttering), language (e.g., comprehension, expression, reading, writing, pragmatics, semantics, and syntax), cognition (e.g., attention, memory, problem solving, and executive functioning), and swallowing (dysphagia).[6]

Difficulty swallowing is called dysphagia. Swallowing is the process of moving food or liquid from one's mouth to the stomach. It is something we do almost automatically, but is in fact a "multidimensional and complex" process and involves contributions from several neuroanatomical structures including muscles and nerves. Following brain surgery, patients can often experience difficulty swallowing which may affect health, safety, or quality of life. Difficulty swallowing could lead to chest infection, dehydration, or malnutrition, which can be potentially fatal conditions.

A speech–language pathologist would assess anatomy and physiology of swallowing function, determine appropriate and safest nutrition and diet, and develop a comprehensive swallowing therapy program. Various therapeutic techniques can improve swallow function and safety including swallowing exercises to increase resistance, muscle load, strength, coordination of muscles, and increasing swallowing safety. Dysphagia

therapy focuses on task specificity, training in compensatory strategies, and modified diets for safest nutritional means.

About 30 to 50% of patients with primary brain tumors experience aphasia.[7] Aphasia can be defined as a language disorder that affects the ability to read, write, speak, or understand language. Aphasia does not affect intellect. One of the most dramatic impacts of aphasia is on conversational speech and interactions. Treatment of aphasia (expressive or receptive) can address word retrieval, grammatical expression, reading comprehension, writing, language comprehension, and life consequences of aphasia. Therapeutic interventions can vary depending on the person with aphasia, the rehabilitation setting and the stage of recovery. In general, there are two main types of therapies: impairment-based therapies (direct) and nonimpairment-based (communication based) therapies. Impairment-based approaches to treatment focus on directly addressing the language and communication impairment of aphasia such as naming, grammatical expression, or reading impairment (alexia).

When clinicians focus on the life consequences of aphasia in their treatment plan by focusing on helping the individual return to his or her former life activities, such as participating in a book club or community aphasia program, they are focusing on a nonimpairment-based approach to treatment. In recent years, nonimpairment-based therapies have gained in popularity and are embodied in what is known as life participation approach to aphasia or LPAA. The LPAA is a consumer-driven service-delivery approach that supports individuals with aphasia and others affected by it in achieving their immediate and longer-term life goals.[8] Currently in clinical practice, many clinicians focus on a combination of the two approaches to maximize recovery throughout the continuum of care. There is evidence in recent literature supporting language recovery long after the onset of aphasia.

Similar to someone using a wheelchair for mobility difficulties, compensatory communication implies a realistic acceptance of chronic impairment and ability to convey a message or idea. AAC or alternative and augmentative communication can supplement or aid someone who has severe communication deficits following surgery. AAC consists of low-tech and high-tech options. Low-tech options include using a simple yes/no board (▸ Fig. 20.1), pointing to pictures or icons, drawing, and gestures or simplified sign language. High-tech options generally rely on computers with digitized speech options (▸ Fig. 20.2).[9] New technology and

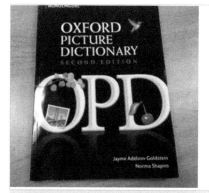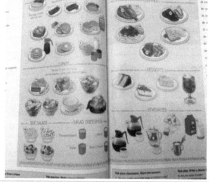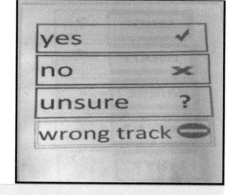

Fig. 20.1 Low-tech options for augmentative and alternative communication.

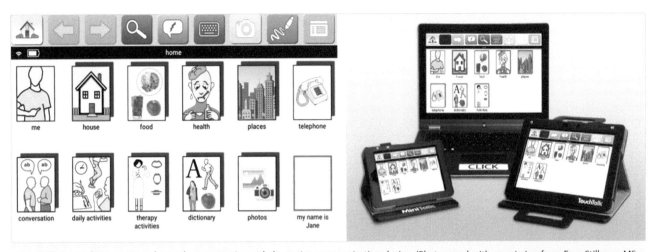

Fig. 20.2 Lingraphica, a more advanced augmentative and alternative communication device. (Photos used with permission from Faye Stillman, MS, CCC-SLP/ATP from Lingraphica.)

applications are now available at low or no cost and are aphasia dedicated. A speech–language pathologist can assess and determine the best option for someone. For many people, the recovery process can include using these devices or applications to supplement speech at some stage in recovery and increase the stimulation of language and skills that are already there.

Language assessment, prognosis, treatment, and recovery patterns of aphasia relating to cancer or surgery may be different from those associated with stroke. It is imperative that SLPs working in medical settings understand the clinical intervention and counselling needs of patients following surgery. Communication rehabilitation as well as aphasia therapy is aimed at helping individuals with aphasia maximize functional communication, life participation, and conveying messages. There are currently growing number of specialized therapies, technologies, resources, aphasia centers, and training that are beneficial in helping a person with loss of communication and their families.

20.6 Physical Therapy

Physical therapy's role following eloquent brain surgery is aimed at restoration of function and reduction of motor impairments. Physical therapists (PTs) assess balance, strength, flexibility, coordination, and muscle tone, as well as analyze movement patterns. Taking into consideration a patient's prior level of function, comorbidities, and goals, a comprehensive treatment plan is developed to maximize function and reduce disability.

The presence of motor deficits can limit a patient's independence, safety, and quality of life. Various therapeutic techniques are used to address primary and secondary motor deficits including the use of neuromuscular electrical stimulation (NMES), forced use of a paretic limb, general strengthening exercises, and stretching.[10] Gait training is initiated in the earliest stages of recovery and can include the use of body weight support to allow for facilitation of noncompensatory movement patterns. Balance is addressed both in the context of gait and transfer training and the use of a tailored balance program based on results from standardized outcome measures. Task practice of other mobility skills including bed mobility; transfers to bed,

toilet, and car; and stair training are also paramount in ensuring successful function at home and in the community.[10]

While the ultimate goal of rehabilitation is the complete recovery of neurological function, PTs have expertise in utilizing appropriate durable medical equipment to facilitate compensation, such as assistive devices or orthotics, to ensure safety, reduce fall risk, and enhance function. The presence of a PT is vital in every rehabilitation setting, whether inpatient, home, or outpatient.

20.7 Occupational Therapy

Similar to SLP and PT, OTs are vital members of the rehabilitation team for all care settings. OTs utilize therapeutic activities to maximize independence in all areas of a patient's life, from activities of daily living (ADLs), work and other productive activities, and play and leisure pursuits. OTs utilize a holistic approach to the rehabilitation of a patient which requires an understanding of how cognitive, physical, sensory, and behavioral impairments may impact various ADLs, consider the patient's prior level of functioning, insight and awareness of current deficit areas, and tailor interventions toward patient-specific goals.

During the intervention process, an OT works toward increasing a patient's independence through a variety of rehabilitative techniques, including constraint-induced movement therapy, NMES, functional neurostimulation of muscles to "retrain" muscle functioning during meaningful activities, and task-analysis to facilitate the relearning of motor, sensory, and cognitive skills in natural environments.[11]

Additionally, compensatory strategies are used as an adjunct to rehabilitative techniques to maximize return to a patient's desired life roles and activities. Compensatory strategies may include the introduction of adaptive equipment during ADLs; recommendations for environment adaptations to compensate for changes in perception, safety awareness, and other cognitive or physical impairments; and caregiver training in cueing and reducing activity demands to support a patient's return to more challenging activities. OTs may also introduce visual compensatory techniques and utilization of physician-prescribed optical devices to compensate for changes in visual acuity, attention, visual field loss, and other oculomotor dysfunctions to promote occupational function and quality of life.[11]

In addition to rehabilitation nursing, neuropsychology/psychology, SLP, PT, OT, other rehabilitation team members include case manager, social worker, vocational and educational rehabilitation counselor, respiratory therapist, recreational therapist, registered dietician, and chaplain.

20.8 Technology in Rehabilitation

Technologies can be used to address communication barriers, promote functional recovery, and allow accessibility at home and in the community. As discussed earlier, a Lingraphica augmentative and alternative communication device can significantly improve a patient's quality of life. Technological devices have become the standard of care in early rehabilitation of limb function and are used to improve motor control and coordination. Devices such as the ArmeoSpring, a robotic arm exoskeleton, provide assist-as-needed to the impaired limb to allow patients to participate in therapeutic exercises disguised as motivating games (► Fig. 20.3). The exercises are designed for patients to practice the movement patterns needed to complete ADLs while providing real-time feedback on the patients' performance.

Devices for lower extremity include functional electrical stimulation devices, such as FES-Bike, Zero G, and Hybrid-Assistive Limb exoskeleton (► Fig. 20.4). These devices are used to harness neuroplasticity for motor and cognitive recovery. Neuroplasticity is defined as the central nervous system's ability to respond to intrinsic and extrinsic stimuli to reorganize its structure, function, and connections.[12] Other advances in rehabilitation technology include virtual reality and robotic devices. These advanced technological devices address the key factors for recovery, including higher intensity of therapy, the manner in which the task is carried out, increased therapy adherence and motivation, and improved progressive feedback of performance. The future of rehabilitation likely will include stem cell therapy, in conjunction with the use of robotic and virtual reality technologies, to minimize impairments and maximize function and quality of life.

20.9 Conclusion

A rehabilitation team involves many professionals from different disciplines, with various areas of expertise, working closely together in an interdisciplinary approach to help patients maximize their functional potential. The ultimate goal of rehabilitation is to return the patient back to daily life with highest functional independence possible, whether it is back to work, school, or leisure activities.

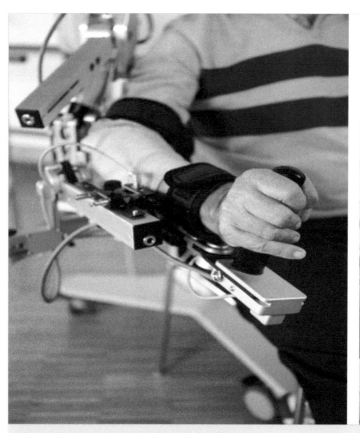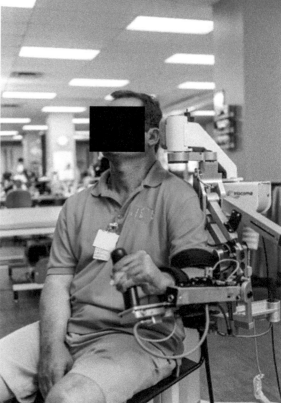

Fig. 20.3 ArmeoSpring robotic device for upper extremity.

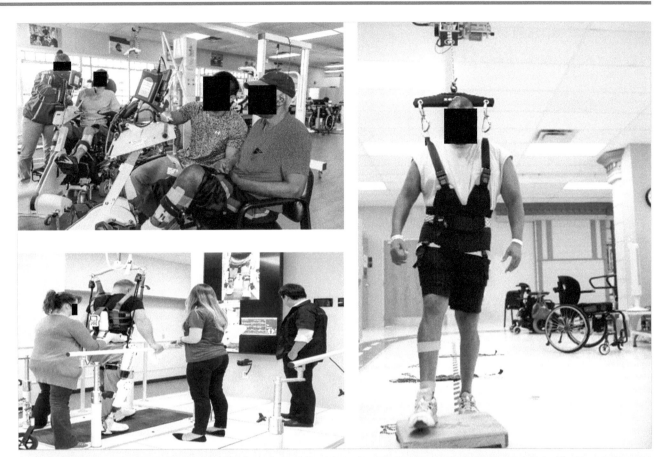

Fig. 20.4 FES-Bike, Zero G, and Hybrid-Assistive Limb exoskeleton.

References

[1] What is a Physiatrist? Available at: https://www.aapmr.org/about-physiatry/about-physical-medicine-rehabilitation/what-is-physiatry. Accessed August 5, 2018

[2] Ivanhoe CB, Durand-Sanchez A, Spier ET. Acute rehabilitation. In: Zasler ND, Katz DI, Zafonte RD, eds. Brain Injury Medicine: Principles and Practice. 2nd ed. New York, NY: Demos Medical Publishing; 2013:385–400

[3] Mishkim M. The practice of neuropsychological assessment. In: Lezak MD, Howieson DB, Loring DW, Hannay HJ, Fischer JS. Neuropsychological Assessment. 4th ed. Oxford: Oxford University Press; 2004:3–13

[4] Lee GP. Neuropsychological assessment of epilepsy. In: Neuropsychology of Epilepsy and Epilepsy Surgery. Oxford: Oxford University Press; 2010:95–131

[5] Sawrie SM. The Neuropsychology of Adult Neuro-Oncology. In: Synder PJ, Nussbaum PD, Robins DL, eds. Clinical Neuropsychology: A Pocket Handbook for Assessment. 2nd ed. Washington, DC: American Psychological Association; 2006

[6] American Speech-Language Hearing Association. Available at: www.asha.org. Accessed July 22, 2019

[7] Davie GL, Hutcheson KA, Barringer DA, Weinberg JS, Lewin, JS. Aphasia in patients after brain tumor resection. Aphasiology. 2009; 23(9):1196–1206

[8] Kagan A, Simmons, Mackie, N, Rowland, A, et al. Counting what counts: A framework for capturing real-life outcomes of aphasia intervention. Aphasiology. 2008; 22(3):258–280

[9] Beukelman DR, Garrett KL, Yorkston KM. Augmentative Communication Strategies for Adults with Acute or Chronic Medical Conditions. Baltimore, MD: Paul H Brookes Publishing; 2007

[10] Kushner, DS, Amidei C, .. Rehabilitation of motor dysfunction in primary brain tumor patients. Neurooncol Pract. 2015; 2(4):185–191

[11] American Occupational Therapy Association. Occupational therapy practice framework: domain and process (3rd ed.). Am J Occup Ther. 2014;; 68(Suppl 1):S1:S48

[12] Cramer SC, Sur M, Dobkin BH, et al. Harnessing neuroplasticity for clinical applications. Brain. 2011; 134(Pt 6):1591–1609

21 Emergence of Deep Learning Methods for Deep Brain Stimulation–Evoked Functional Connectomics

Christine Edwards, Abbas Z. Kouzani, Kendall H. Lee, and Erika Ross

Abstract

Deep brain stimulation (DBS) devices are becoming an increasingly common treatment for refractory Parkinson disease and other movement disorders. With advances in neurotechnologies and neuroimaging, along with an increased understanding of neurocircuitry, there is a rapid rise in the use of DBS therapy as an effective treatment for an increasingly wide range of neurologic and psychiatric disorders. DBS technologies are evolving toward an implantable closed-loop therapeutic neurocontrol system to provide continuous customized neuromodulation for optimal clinical results. Even so, there is much to be learned regarding the pathologies of these neurodegenerative and psychiatric disorders and the latent mechanisms of DBS that provide therapeutic relief. This chapter converges two breakthrough research areas—powerhouse deep learning methods and DBS-evoked functional connectomics—that are expected to advance DBS therapies toward precise neuromodulation for optimal therapeutic relief. This chapter describes the resurgence of artificial intelligence and provides an introduction to its subfield of deep learning, followed by an overview of in vivo neuroimaging modalities and brain mappings. A deeper dive into functional neuroimaging processing and an overview of classical multivariate pattern analysis methods is provided to set the stage for a review of functional neuroimaging studies that leverage deep learning methods. Such methods applied to DBS-evoked functional neuroimaging data are expected to enable the characterization and prediction of patterns of activation, in relationship to electrode placement, stimulation parameters, and behavioral assessment data.

Keywords: deep brain stimulation, deep learning, neuroimaging, connectomics

21.1 Introduction

Modern day deep brain stimulation (DBS) devices are considered pacemakers for the brain, as the devices were developed based on predicate cardiac pacemakers. Similarly, with cardiac pacemakers, DBS devices deliver electrical stimulation to a targeted area via an implanted electrode lead. The electrode lead in the DBS device is subcutaneously connected to a pulse generator controller that is implanted in the chest beneath the clavicle. As with cardiac pacemakers that restore normal cardiac rhythm, brain pacemakers seek to modulate disordered circuitry to restore functionality. Although they share similarities with cardiac pacemakers, the underlying mechanisms are more complex and far less understood. In general, a DBS open-loop system stimulates a targeted subcortical region with a high-frequency pulse (100–250 Hz) to disrupt the disordered neurocircuitry and modulate underlying electrical and chemical changes.[1,2] The target location is dependent on the patient's diagnosis, history, and corresponding symptoms. Modern day

DBS was founded in 1987 and gained traction in the 1990s with Food and Drug Administration (FDA) approval to treat refractory neurological movement disorders, including Parkinson disease (PD), essential tremor (ET), and dystonia.[3,4,5] Building upon advances in technologies and lessons learned over decades of neurosurgery to treat neurological and psychiatric disorders, over 100,000 people worldwide have been implanted with open-loop DBS devices (see ▶ Fig. 21.1).[6]

Today, there is a rapid rise in the use of DBS to treat an increasingly wide range of neurologic and psychiatric disorders.[7] Following a 30-year gap of little to no innovation in DBS technologies, there is now a drive to create an implantable closed-loop therapeutic neurocontrol system to provide continuous customized neuromodulation for optimal clinical results.[8,9,10,11] Even so, there is much to be learned regarding the immediate and long-term mechanisms of DBS therapy and the neurological and neuropsychiatric disorders that it aims to treat. Linking multimodal in vivo neuroimaging with DBS is a powerful combination that reveals new insights into structural, functional, and effective connectivity of brain circuitry under all of these conditions.

In this era of "big data," data science has emerged as a highly valued interdisciplinary field that brings together advances in computational methods and technologies to analyze and

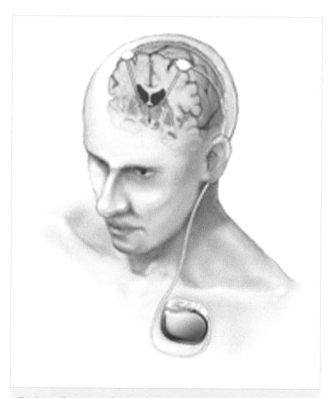

Fig. 21.1 Illustration of an implanted open-loop deep brain stimulation system. (Reproduced with permission from Edwards et al.[12])

discover latent patterns in large-scale heterogeneous datasets. This combination of mathematics, statistics, computer science, and domain expertise is creating opportunities to utilize data-driven techniques to unveil insights that lead to new or refined hypotheses and enable more informed decision-making processes. DBS investigative studies and clinical uses are creating a multimodal data-rich environment that is ripe for discovery of the biological underpinnings of functional and dysfunctional brain circuitry. Powerful breakthrough data science methods, such as deep learning applied to DBS data, are expected to lead to advanced pattern analysis analytics. This multidiscipline approach has potential to transform our understanding of brain circuitry and ultimately usher in breakthroughs in bioelectronics medical technologies to optimize treatments.

This chapter provides a historical perspective and an introduction to deep learning methods, followed by an overview of the growing discipline of connectomics. Furthermore, this chapter includes an overview of in vivo neuroimaging modalities that are utilized to visualize and assess the macroscale connectivity of brain regions where each node of the map represents hundreds of thousands of neurons. A deeper dive into the functional neuroimaging processing is provided to set the stage for a review of multivariate pattern analysis (MVPA) methods for global assessment of DBS-evoked functional connectome data.

21.2 Rise of Deep Learning Methods

Deep learning methods are a subset of machine learning approaches that apply a hierarchy of nonlinear transformations to learn invariant discriminant feature representations of data, for pattern analysis and classification tasks. Such methods are not new, but have experienced a significant revival and are now dominating in application areas such as computer vision, audio processing, and natural language processing.

Deep learning origins date back to, at least, the 1940s when artificial neural networks (ANNs) were first introduced as a connectionist model.[13] Connectionism involves the concept of artificial intelligence (AI) emerging from simple interconnected computational units into a hierarchy. Computational units and their weighted connections are analogous to neurons and the strengths of their synaptic connections, respectively. Meanwhile, Hebbian learning theorized that synchronized firing of neurons strengthens their synaptic connections, whereas neurons firing out of sync experience weakened or nonexistent synaptic connections. Hebbian theory describes a mechanism for brain plasticity, where neurons dynamically adapt their connections during the learning process.[14]

In the 1950s and 1960s, simple ANNs such as perceptrons were created to learn mappings between input data and output values for pattern recognition tasks such as binary classification of images.[15] A perceptron is considered a single layer neural network, as it has one layer of weighted connections between input nodes and an output node. The weights of the perceptron represent the learned linear decision boundary that optimally separates two classes of data for binary classification. If the data are not linearly separable, then the perceptron will not converge on a decision boundary to appropriately classify the data. During that time, it was shown that perceptrons were incapable

of modeling a simple XOR Boolean function, leading to much debate regarding the usefulness of connectionist models.[15,16] At the same time, Hubel and Wiesel conducted a series of significant physiological experiments where they discovered simple and complex cells within the primary visual cortex of a cat and monkey via microelectrode recordings.[17,18,19] Their discoveries of the hierarchical organization of the brain to achieve visual perception earned them the Nobel Prize in Physiology or Medicine in 1981, and inspired decades of vision models and machine learning approaches to teach computers how to recognize visual patterns.[20,21,22,23,24,25,26,27,28,29,30]

In 1986, interests in connectionist models were renewed with the introduction of the backpropagation algorithm which made it possible to train ANNs, such as feed-forward multilayer perceptrons, recurrent neural networks (RNNs), and convolutional neural networks (ConvNets).[21,31,32,33,34] These networks include hidden layers between the input and output layers to model more complex functions (see ▶ Fig. 21.2). During the training process, the input data are first propagated forward through the nodes of the network. The input data may be in the form of raw data such as pixels or voxels, or in the form of feature vectors representing the original data. The computed value of each node in the hidden and output layers is a weighted sum of its inputs passed through a nonlinear activation function (e.g., rectified linear unit). At each output node, an error signal is calculated to measure the difference between the actual output and the expected output. This error signal is then propagated back through the network to compute the delta error at each node. Optimization methods such as stochastic gradient descent are used to determine the optimal weights to minimize the error signal across the network.

According to the universal approximation theorem, an ANN can estimate any sufficiently smooth function.[35] Inspired by the organization of our brain into cortical layers, adding depth (i.e., more hidden layers), rather than simply increasing the width (i.e., more nodes per layer), allows for more complex transformations of input data into patterns for higher-level pattern recognition tasks. Despite the power of the backpropagation algorithm, training neural networks beyond a couple of hidden layers remained difficult, requiring much computational power and training data to learn many parameters that defined the network architecture. Converging on an optimal solution of tuned parameters, without overfitting to training data, was especially challenging. As a result, many steered away from using ANNs for decades, in favor of simpler shallow architectures such as support vector machines (SVMs), which converge to an optimal solution with less training data and computational power requirements.[36]

Despite the so-called AI winter in the 1990s to mid-2000s, a subset of researchers remained committed to pursuing biologically inspired connectionist models for automated pattern analysis tasks and ultimately AI. Pioneers of deep neural networks include Yoshua Bengio (from the University of Montreal), Geoffrey Hinton (from the University of Toronto and Google, Inc.), Yann LeCun (from New York University and Facebook, Inc.), Tomaso Poggio (from the McGovern Institute for Brain Research at MIT), and Terrence Sejnowski (from the Salk Institute for Biological Studies). The Neural Information Processing Systems (NIPS) Conference, established in 1987, with Terrence Sejnowski as its president since 1993, remains the primary conference

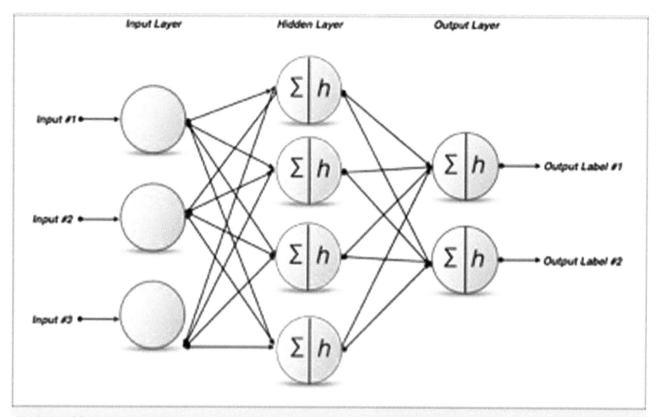

Fig. 21.2 Multilayer perceptrons (MLPs) are the most common type of shallow feed-forward neural networks. MLPs include at least one hidden layer between the input and output layers. At each layer, the nodes compute a weighted sum of their inputs that is then passed onto a nonlinear activation transformation function, such as a hyperbolic tangent or a sigmoid function. Most recently, rectified linear unit (RefigLU; instead of Hodgkin–Huxley) functions are preferred due to computational savings required by deeper networks with many hidden layers. During the training process, optimal weights of the connected nodes are learned using the backpropagation algorithm.

where leaders in connectionism research convene annually. Incremental improvements toward deep neural networks occurred over a decade, while understanding of the hierarchical organization of the primate cerebral cortex significantly increased. For instance, Long Short-Term Memory (LSTM) models were introduced in 1997 to overcome the vanishing gradient problem (i.e., decaying backpropagation error) encountered by previous RNN architectures.[37] Early applications of LSTM models were primarily in the natural language processing domain.[38,39,40] Meanwhile, Van Essen's wiring diagram of the hierarchical distributive organization of cortical areas for perception, which included feed-forward and feedback connections, continued to motivate advances in deep neural network models.[23] This wiring diagram includes at least 30 cortical areas for visual perception. An over simplification of the visual system separates processing into the "where or how" (dorsal stream) and "what" (ventral stream) pathways of the visual cortex, while ignoring feedback mechanisms. The feed-forward ventral visual stream progresses from the retina to the lateral geniculate nucleus of the thalamus, which then relays this information to the primary visual cortex (V1), followed by the visual areas V2, V4, the inferotemporal (IT) cortex, and the prefrontal cortex. This primate visual processing model, coupled with early findings of Hubel and Wiesel, inspired computer vision models such as "Hierarchical Model and X" (HMAX) for feed-forward object recognition.[25,27] Likewise,

ConvNets were largely inspired by biological vision, as their convolutional and max-pooling layers extracted increasingly invariant features that resembled simple and complex cells of the primary visual cortex. Lower levels of the hierarchy are tuned to respond to low-level features (e.g., edges). Ascending the hierarchy, the network nodes combine patterns from lower levels, to respond to increasingly complex patterns, and at the highest level perform tasks such as face and object recognition. Biologically inspired neural networks were increasingly applied to a variety of specific visual recognition tasks, such as LeNet-5 which was a ConvNet fine-tuned to recognize handwritten digits within specific document images.[22] Although these networks were comparable or outperformed other pattern analysis techniques, acquiring sufficiently large annotated datasets and computational power to tune their parameters for visual recognition tasks remained a challenge until the early 2010s.

In 2006, the connectionism research community experienced a turning point—the AI winter was beginning to thaw—with the introduction of a method that enabled faster training of deep neural networks.[41] Rather than starting with random weights, this approach uses generative models, called "restricted Boltzmann machines (RBMs), at each layer to initialize the weights of the network; thus, this unsupervised pretraining of parameters allowed for faster convergence of the network to an optimal solution. Hinton et al demonstrated this method by introducing deep belief networks (DBNs) with an architecture

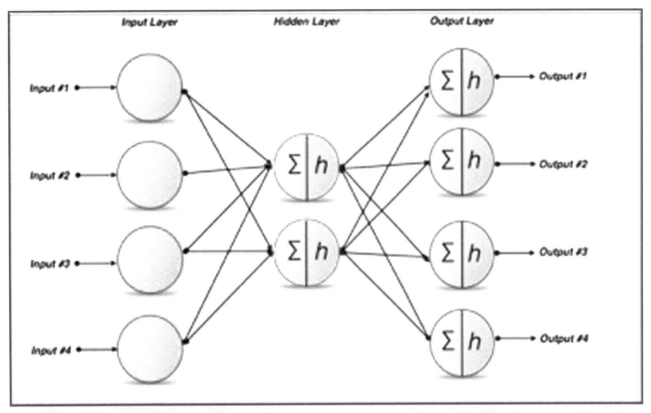

Fig. 21.3 This is an illustration of an autoencoder, where the hidden layer is a compressed version of the input data, and the output layer is a reconstruction of the input data from the compressed version. During training of the network, the error between the input and reconstructed output is minimized. Autoencoders, along with restricted Boltzmann machines, may be used to initialize deep neural networks or stacked as a building block for various deep neural network architectures.

composed of stacked RBMs.[41] Shortly thereafter Bengio et al extended this initialization method to train a deep network of stacked autoencoders[42] (see ▶ Fig. 21.3). Unsupervised training of these generative models at each layer allowed the deep neural networks to learn sparse distributed high-level representations of data to use for dimensionality reduction and more generalized models for pattern analysis tasks.

From the late 2000s, deep neural networks started to advance, and applications were gaining momentum as large-scale labeled datasets and large-scale commodity computing platforms, such as cloud and graphics processing units, were making it possible to train deep generalized models for tasks such as pattern analysis for image understanding. Deep feedforward and RNNs provide significantly surpassing performance on benchmark datasets and rank first place in many pattern recognition and machine learning competitions. Beginning in 2009, Microsoft Research applied deep neural networks to automatically learn high-level abstract features that represent salient representations of data for natural language processing applications. They demonstrated that deep features learned from acoustic spectrograms were superior to long-standing audio features, such as Mel Frequency Cepstral Coefficients for applications such as speech recognition.[43] Deep learning methods (e.g., LSTMs) have dominated multilingual handwriting recognition competitions. In 2011, deep neural networks won a traffic sign recognition competition. While interests in deep

learning were steadily increasing through the late 2000s and early 2010s, the larger machine learning community did not fully embrace this movement until 2012.

Deep learning research catapulted to the limelight in 2012, with renewed interests (and fears) regarding the potential capabilities of AI. During this time the Google Brain project released a paper describing their unsupervised deep autoencoder architecture that learned high-level representations of object categories from an unlabeled dataset of 10 million, 200 × 200 image frames extracted from YouTube videos. This architecture demonstrated the power of learning hierarchical feature representations for applications such as face recognition and compared it to biological neural networks that are believed to have a hierarchy that leads to specific face neurons. Meanwhile, a ConvNet-based method won the ImageNet Large Scale Visual Recognition Competition (ILSVRC) in 2012, which was a catalyst for deep learning efforts that now dominate computer vision and other pattern recognition domains (see ▶ Fig. 21.4).[44] ILSVRC is the benchmark competition (2010–2015) for image classification and object recognition tasks. Its annotated image dataset includes 1.2 million images with 1,000 category labels that semantically map to the WordNet benchmark dataset. To this day, ImageNet is the largest, most diverse, labeled dataset that is publicly available; thus, it has been a game changer for the computer vision community and has fueled the exponential rise in deep computer vision architectures.

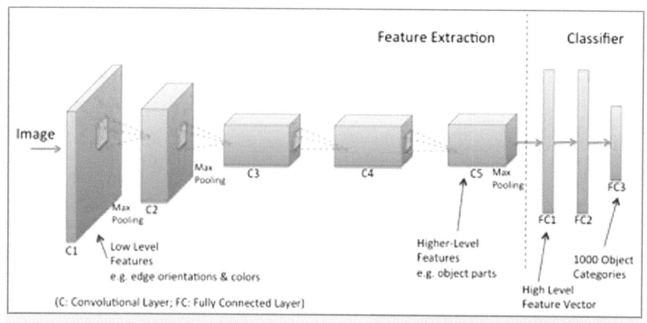

Fig. 21.4 An illustration of a convolutional neural network.[44] A hierarchy of convolutional and subsampling layers transforms the input image into an abstract conceptual feature vector that represents the content of the image. This is followed by a fully connected neural network, which maps the feature vector into a lower dimensional semantic space, where each component of the resulting vector is a probability score corresponding to an ImageNet object category.

Today, deep learning techniques and applications continue to evolve at a rapid pace. The deep learning community is investigating methods that reduce the amount of training data required to learn feature representations and regularization methods to create generalizable models. Transfer learning methods enable the retraining of deep ANNs by reusing the lower level feature representations and fine-tuning the higher-level concept representations. As such, transfer learning is an option to fine-tune deep ANNs for other domains where there may be an insufficient amount of labeled training data. Also, variations of Generative Adversarial Networks (GANs), introduced by Ian Goodfellow in 2014, are changing the landscape of unsupervised learning methods and extending their use to novel applications, such as photo-realistic single-image super-resolution. In addition, deep reinforcement learning methods are advancing toward systems that are capable of processing high-dimensional sensory inputs from their environment and learn the appropriate actions.[45]

21.3 In Vivo Neuroimaging Modalities and Maps

Decades of advances in neuroimaging technologies have resulted in powerful investigative and clinical tools that are providing remarkable noninvasive, in vivo, multimodal views of the brain. Such tools are the basis for the construction of macroscale connectomes that capture the mapping of brain region-to-region wiring diagrams, to reveal the structural, functional, and effective connectivity.[46] Structure and function are interwoven.[47] Structural connectomes characterize and map anatomically connected brain regions, whereas functional connectomes map functionally correlated local and distal brain

regions. Effective connectomes provide a directional mapping to characterize causality of functionally related brain regions.[48] Dynamic brain connectivity is encountered with disease progression and treatment, and this neural plasticity may be characterized by analysis of multimodal connectome data across time scales.[49]

21.4 Structural Neuroimaging

Neuroimaging technologies that capture anatomical structures include computed tomography (CT) and magnetic resonance imaging (MRI). Since the first human CT scan in the 1970s, this technology is commonly used in clinical situations for anatomical assessments, by creating cross-sectional images and three-dimensional (3D) reconstructions from the acquired attenuation X-ray signals passed through the targeted anatomy. In the 1980s, MRI was introduced as a clinical alternative that leverages magnetic susceptibility to differentiate brain tissue, without exposing the patient to ionizing radiation. Rather, a patient positioned within the bore of an MRI scanner is exposed to a strong magnetic field (e.g., 1.5 T), with gradient coils that spatially vary the field strength across the brain. Radiofrequency (RF) transceiver coils transmit pulsed signals tuned to the resonant spin frequency of targeted atomic nuclei, such as hydrogen protons, which are prevalent in living organisms in the form of water molecules. The targeted atomic nuclei absorb energy from the RF signals, exciting them into a higher energy state that is out of alignment with the magnetic field of the scanner. As the protons relax back into their lower energy state, RF energy is released and captured by the RF antenna coil. These MR signals are acquired and transformed into 2D cross-sectional slices and a 3D reconstructed brain volume. Compared to CT images, MRI scans provide a more detailed view of soft tissue. As such, MRI is often used to assess individualized mapping of a patient's brain anatomy prior to DBS implantation, thus enabling more precise identification of DBS anatomical target(s) and trajectory path for the DBS electrode(s). Although MRI does not expose the patient to ionizing radiation, safety guidelines must be closely followed to prevent injuries caused by the interaction of the scanner's strong magnetic field with metallic components of neurostimulation systems. As such, there are only a few institutions that incorporate MRI technologies once the DBS device is implanted. Postoperative CT scans are often used to assess and confirm the placement of the DBS electrode(s). Multimodal approaches may fuse CT and MRI scans to provide a richer anatomical view. In addition to safety measures, intraoperative and postoperative MR imaging must also include imaging protocols to mitigate potential image artifacts surrounding the DBS lead(s).

In general, MRI protocols configure pulse sequence parameters, such as the "time to repetition" (TR) and "time to echo" (TE), in concert with intrinsic tissue properties (e.g., T1 and T2) to adjust the contrast of resulting images based on the targeted applications. TR is the time interval between the RF pulses, and TE is the time interval between the transmission of an RF signal and when the (echo) MR signal is measured. After an RF pulse is applied, T1 is the time required for the atomic nuclei to return to equilibrium, with spins aligned to the scanner's magnetic field. This realignment to recover longitudinal magnetization is an exponential process with time constant T1. At the same time, T2 is the intrinsic property that describes the time it takes for the atomic nuclei to dephase from their excited state, leading to an exponential decay of the transverse magnetization that is typically slower than the T1 rate. The effect of neighboring proton spin interactions is characterized by this T2 property. $T2^*$ is an additional property that encompasses both the intrinsic T2 property and the effect of distortions in the external magnetic field. Spin-echo pulse sequences use an additional 180-degree RF refocusing pulse to reduce the effects of inhomogeneity of the external magnetic field (i.e., reduces $T2^*$ sensitivity), such as at air–tissue interfaces. Fast spin-echo imaging is a variation of spin-echo pulse sequences that allow for faster, more practical acquisition times, primarily to acquire T2-weighted images. Gradient-echo (GRE) imaging uses gradients, rather than an additional refocusing pulse, to generate the echo signal. Variations of GRE pulse sequences are often used for generation of high-resolution anatomical T1- and T2-weighted brain images, as well as for generation of functional $T2^*$-weighted images which will be discussed further. In general, for T1-weighted images, white matter appears brighter than gray matter, and fluids, such as cerebrospinal fluid, appear dark, whereas, in T2-weighted images, white matter appears darker than gray matter, and fluid-filled regions are highlighted. In general, MRI scanners with stronger magnetic fields (e.g., ultrahigh 7.0 T) produce images with a greater dynamic range to acquire finer details that visually discriminate neighboring anatomical brain regions.[50,51] Furthermore, techniques such as echo-planar imaging have made it possible to more rapidly acquire images, which has in turn paved the way for other modalities of MRI that are more time dependent.[52]

MRI technologies continue to evolve and expand to include techniques such as diffusion tensor imaging (DTI) which is sensitive to the diffusion properties of water through specific types of tissues.[53] In particular, DTI is used to visualize and analyze the white matter tracts that connect brain regions.[54,55] Macroscale structural connectomes typically leverage conventional MRI and DTI methods, to define the nodes (e.g., parcellated gray matter regions) and weighted edges (e.g., white matter tracts) of the brain graph, respectively.[56] As previously stated, structure and function are interwoven. This applies to the organization of the brain, and to the evolving neuroimaging technologies used to provide insight into the structure and function of the brain. Structural neuroimaging provides the anatomical context for functional brain data.

21.5 Functional Neuroimaging

Functional neuroimaging includes noninvasive in vivo technologies such as single photon emission computed tomography (SPECT), positron emission tomography (PET), and functional MRI (fMRI). Both SPECT and PET scanners detect energy released from intravenously injected radiopharmaceuticals, as they accumulate and decay within the brain, forming 2D and 3D images that capture cerebral blood flow (CBF) and molecular level metabolic changes, indirectly measuring neural activity. Compared to PET, SPECT is more widely available for clinical uses, as it is less expensive, and its radiotracers are more accessible with a longer half-life; however, PET scans are less prone to image artifacts and have better spatial resolution. A common radiotracer used for PET-based neuroimaging is fludeoxyglucose (FDG), which is processed by the brain as glucose. As such, activated brain regions experience increased blood flow and accumulation of FDG to replenish metabolic energy corresponding to neural activity. Both SPECT and PET technologies continue to evolve as powerful neuroimaging modalities that provide insight into global patterns of targeted neurotransmitter (e.g., dopamine) release corresponding to activated brain circuitry. However, as with anatomical CT scans, these neuroimaging modalities expose the patient to ionizing radiation; thus, DBS clinical and investigated studies to optimize DBS lead location and stimulation parameters settings are limited. Meanwhile, MRI technologies were expanded to include functional neuroimaging modalities, namely, blood oxygen level dependent (BOLD) fMRI in 1990.[57] Compared to SPECT and PET, BOLD fMRI produces 2D and 3D imaging with higher spatial resolution, without exposing the patient to radioactive material. Rather than using an exogenous contrasting agent, BOLD fMRI leverages the paramagnetic properties of deoxyhemoglobin as an endogenous contrasting agent to indirectly capture neural activity by mapping of blood oxygenation. As with conventional MRI techniques, DBS studies that leverage fMRI must follow careful safety precautions and imaging protocols to mitigate risks associated with the interactions between the metallic components of the DBS system and the scanner's strong magnetic field.[58,59,60,61,62]

Additional macroscale in vivo functional neuroimaging technologies include electroencephalography (EEG) and magnetoencephalography (MEG), which use noninvasive sensors on or near the scalp to measure cortical electrical and magnetic changes induced by neuronal activity, respectively. EEG and MEG are advantageous as they have higher temporal resolution (i.e., milliseconds) compared to fMRI, which indirectly measures neural activity and is limited by the hemodynamic response timing that is on the order of seconds. However, fMRI and PET modalities have higher spatial resolution, on the order of millimeters rather than centimeters. Although more invasive, electrocorticography (ECoG) technologies enable direct electrophysiological monitoring by recording global field potentials on the cortical surface, rather than measuring attenuation signals outside the skull. As such, ECoG techniques have higher spatial resolution than EEG, while also having higher temporal resolution. Recently, functional neuroimaging studies combined intraoperative ECoG sensorimotor cortex recordings with subthalamic nucleus (STN) LFP recordings acquired during the implantation of the DBS leads; in doing so, this enabled the discovery of a potential biomarker for PD dysfunctional motor circuitry and a potential feedback mechanism for future closed-loop DBS systems.[63,64,65,66]

Functional connectomics includes the study of intrinsic resting state, as well as stimulus-evoked functional brain networks. Such studies are providing insights into the pathophysiological mechanisms of neurodegenerative and psychiatric disorders and possible clinical biomarkers to aid in diagnosis and treatment.[67,68] Given that fMRI provides a noninvasive in vivo view of the brain in action, with high spatial resolution, it is especially powerful when combined with DBS technologies.[48,69,70,71,72] DBS-evoked functional connectomics based primarily on multivariate analysis of BOLD fMRI data is enabling characterization of spatially distributed patterns of brain activity to optimize DBS therapy.

21.6 Role of Macroscale Connectomics

21.6.1 Connectomics and Deep Learning

Connectomics is the creation and analysis of connectional brain maps, also known as connectomes.[73] The connectome describes the brain's neural connections that give rise to behavior and cognition.[74] Connectomes characterize the structural, functional, and effective connectivity of neural elements within the brain. Furthermore, connectomes are categorized by scale, depending on the number of neurons represented by each of the neural elements in the corresponding brain maps. These wiring diagrams range in resolution from (microscale) synaptic-level over cubic micrometer volumes to (macroscale) parcellated regions distributed over the whole brain.

Microscale connectomes provide neuron-to-neuron wiring diagrams, with a few nanometers of spatial resolution, leveraging in vitro neuroimaging technologies such as serial block-face electron microscopy (EM) and fluorescence microscopy techniques to visualize synaptic circuits.[75,76,77] A single neuron may communicate with thousands of neurons, requiring high-throughput acquisition and processing, resulting in a very densely connected brain map. Currently, only a complete microscale connectome exists for C. elegans, consisting of 302 neurons reconstructed postmortem via EM.[78,79] One of the largest microscale endeavors was the reconstruction of a 100-µm cube of a mouse retina, representing approximately 1,000 neurons and 250,000 synapses.[80] The Open Connectome Project

(OCP) created an open-sourced platform to facilitate connectome data sharing, and incorporated a processing pipeline for EM connectome to automatically annotate and apply graph theoretic techniques for analysis.[81,82,83,84,85,86]

Mesoscale connectomes provide neuronal population-to-population wiring diagrams, with micrometer or submicrometer spatial resolution, mapping local circuitry (e.g., cortical columns), with hundreds to thousands of neurons represented per population node.[87] Microscale and mesoscale data are acquired using advanced technology such as high-throughput EM and volumetric calcium light-field microscopy.[88]

Macroscale connectomes provide a brain region-to-region wiring diagram, with millimeter spatial resolution, leveraging noninvasive in vivo neuroimaging technologies such as MRI and PET. The Human Connectome Project (HCP) is seeking to acquire and map the brain of 1,500 healthy human subjects, using noninvasive in vivo neuroimaging modalities, such as resting-state functional MRI (rs-fMRI), structural MRI, and DTI.[53,89,90,91] Macroscale brain maps approximate global wiring connections across parcellated cortical and subcortical brain regions, whereas mesoscale brain maps provide a zoomed-in view with a more detailed description of localized brain circuitry. Advances in neuroimaging, data science methods, and large-scale computing technologies will enable mapping of dynamic connectomes across scales and modalities, providing insight into the human brain's functional and dysfunctional circuitry over time.[74,92,93,94] The U.S. Intelligence Advanced Research Projects Activity (IARPA) launched a program called "Machine Intelligence from Cortical Networks" (MICrONS) in 2016, funding research that will facilitate the reconstruction and investigation of mesoscale connectomes to inspire next-generation machine learning algorithms.

The human brain is the ultimate computing machine, inspiring a long history of machine learning approaches that attempt to mimic sensory processing, cognition, and intelligence. In turn, such methods are applied to automate pattern analysis tasks of large-scale brain datasets. In particular, deep learning methods (e.g., ConvNets and stacked autoencoders), which are ANNs inspired by our brain's hierarchical organization into cortical areas for sensory processing, are dominating applications such as computer vision, audio processing, and natural language processing.[95] It is not surprising that deep learning methods are increasingly used to automate processing of micro- to macroscale multimodal connectome data. For example, ConvNets are used for segmentation of neural elements to enable the creation of structural EM connectomes[96] and to segment brain tissue in MRI data.[97,98,99] Furthermore, ConvNets, as well as deep neural networks composed of stacked autoencoders or RBMs, have been applied across macroscale structural (e.g., MRI) and functional neuroimaging datasets (e.g., PET, rs-fMRI, and fMRI) to learn multimodal feature representations and discover and classify connectivity patterns.[100,101,102,103,104,105,106]

21.6.2 Connectomics and Deep Brain Stimulation

Linking multimodal macroscale connectomics with DBS is a powerful combination that is expected to significantly advance

DBS technologies and provide more precise effective treatment for refractory movement and psychiatric disorders.[70,107,108] Structural and functional macroscale connectomics are providing insights into the normal functioning brain and the dysfunction that occurs with pathologies of neurodegenerative and psychiatric disorders, leading to potential individualized biomarkers to aid in the diagnosis, and predict optimal treatment.[49,109,110,111,112,113,114,115] Subject-specific structural and functional macroscale connectomes will enable more precise navigation during DBS electrode placement and optimized stimulation parameters, to maximize therapeutic effects and minimize adverse effects.[72,107,116,117] Furthermore, brain mapping techniques enable investigation of the underlying mechanisms of DBS and the modulated brain circuitry that may lead to more effective stimulation targets and parameters.[7,118,119,120,121] In particular, DBS-evoked functional brain maps, such as those acquired using fMRI, allow for the global assessment of the distributed patterns of activation corresponding to electrode placement, stimulation parameters, and behavioral results.[60,71,122,123,124,125,126] An automated large-scale computing pipeline is needed to create and analyze DBS-evoked functional connectomes for clinical and research uses. As deep learning methods continue to dominate machine learning applications, such methods are expected to play a key role in facilitating this pipeline, especially with regard to automatically recognizing patterns of activation and extracting signals of interest.

21.7 Investigation of Multivariate Pattern Analysis Methods for DBS-Evoked Functional Macroscale Connectome Data

Multivariate pattern analysis methods enable investigation of globally distributed patterns of neural activation evoked by DBS of specific components of dysfunctional brain circuitry. Such methods leverage machine learning techniques to discover and classify patterns of activity across functional neuroimaging data as related to experimental conditions. Traditionally, MVPA methods are applied in cognitive neuroscience as a tool to map stimulus-evoked brain responses to cognitive states such as for visual perception understanding experiments. Application of MVPA methods to DBS-evoked functional macroscale connectome data allows for global assessment of functional connectivity associated with electrode placement, stimulation parameters, and behavioral outcomes. Novel MVPA approaches that leverage deep learning techniques are expected to improve recognition of DBS-evoked functional connectivity patterns. As such, linking DBS-evoked functional connectomics with deep learning methods is expected to lead to further insights into the mechanisms of effective neuromodulation, and potentially enable DBS therapy that is optimized to a patient's precise needs.

The following section provides a more detailed description of the acquisition and analysis of BOLD fMRI data. Classical MVPA methods, along with novel deep learning approaches, are presented as applied to fMRI data. This chapter concludes with a discussion on the implications of the expected rise in the use of fMRI with DBS, coupled with the rise in deep learning methods to construct and characterize connectomes.

21.7.1 DBS-Evoked BOLD fMRI Data

BOLD fMRI data acquisition in conjunction with DBS requires careful adherence to safety and imaging protocols, such as using specific fMRI pulse sequences to minimize risk of the DBS leads producing excessive heat and reducing susceptibility artifacts.[62] The BOLD signal is a proxy for neural activity across hundreds of thousands of neurons, where each voxel is on the scale of a cubic millimeter. The temporal dynamics of the hemodynamic response to increase metabolic needs of active neurons, which is on the order of seconds, is a limiting factor for the overall temporal resolution of BOLD fMRI data.[127]

Neurovascular coupling describes how blood flow and neuronal activity are intertwined. This complex relationship is dependent on CBF, cerebral blood volume (CBV), and cerebral metabolic rate of oxygen consumption (CMRO$_2$), along with other factors.[128] In general, there is increased flow of oxygenated blood to compensate for the increased metabolic needs of active neurons. This corresponds to a decrease in deoxyhemoglobin concentration levels that manifest as an increase in the BOLD fMRI signal which peaks between 4 and 6 seconds after the initial onset of neural activity. As the neural activity subsides, the flow of oxyhemoglobin subsides, resulting in increased concentrations of deoxyhemoglobin, and subsequently decreases the BOLD fMRI signal to a level below the baseline. This time to the undershoot peak is typically within 5 to 10 seconds after the peak BOLD signal.

Although the hemodynamic responses may differ across brain regions, experimental conditions, and subjects, a canonical hemodynamic response function (HRF) is often used to predict each voxel's BOLD response.[129] This can be thought of as a linear time-invariant system where the neural activity stimulus signal is convolved with the HRF to produce a predicted hemodynamic response. In addition, upon DBS stimulation, an initial negative dip in the BOLD response has been observed in DBS-fMRI data just prior to an increase in blood flow corresponding to the neural activity. This initial negative dip is not included in the canonical HRF used in most fMRI analysis studies (see ▶ Fig. 21.5).[44] An HRF that includes this initial dip in BOLD signal has potential to increase spatial and temporal specificity, as it is more closely tuned to the neural activity.[130,131,132,133,134,135]

21.7.2 Classical Multivariate Pattern Analysis

MVPA was first introduced as multivoxel pattern analysis, but the acronym has evolved to multivariate pattern analysis.[136,137] In contrast to voxel-wise univariate approaches, which independently evaluate each voxel without considering covariances across voxels, MVPA methods enable the evaluation of global spatiotemporal patterns of activations across the brain simultaneously. Most applications of MVPA are found in cognitive neuroscience studies and are at times referred to as "brain decoding" or "Mind Reading."[138,139,140,141,142] Such studies seek to understand how our brain encodes and decodes information. In general, the goal of MVPA is to learn the relationship

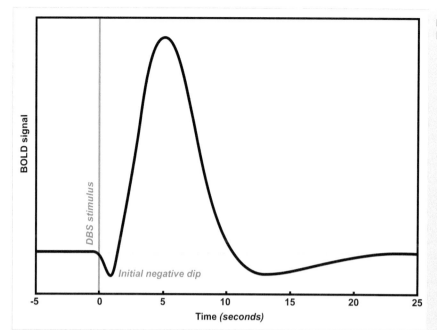

Fig. 21.5 Blood oxygen level dependent (BOLD) hemodynamic response. (Source: William Curry.)

between the patterns of activation and the experimental conditions. MVPA typically leverages conventional supervised machine learning approaches, which include primarily the following steps: (1) feature extraction/selection to represent high-dimensional BOLD data in a lower dimensional feature vector space, (2) classifier training to learn the transformation from feature vector space to experimental conditions, and (3) generalization testing to evaluate the classifier's performance given new datasets.

Feature Representation and Dimensionality Reduction

BOLD fMRI studies require the detection of weak signals within high-dimensional noisy data. The "curse of dimensionality" manifests in supervised machine learning when the dimensions of the feature space are much higher than the number of training samples. As such, resulting models may be overfit to the training data and exhibit poor performance when new data are encountered. Regularization techniques are used to mitigate overfitting models to training data. Reducing the dimensionality of the feature vector space is a typical approach for improving a classifier's performance. Feature representation methods perform feature extraction, selection, or a combination of both to represent the high-dimensional BOLD fMRI data space into a lower dimensional feature space.

Feature extraction approaches include data-driven single-matrix factorization methods such as principal component analysis (PCA) and independent component analysis (ICA).[143,144] PCA transforms the data into a smaller dimensional space defined by orthogonal (uncorrelated) principal components that account for most of the variability within the data. Singular value decomposition of a data matrix is often used to determine the principal components. The first component has the highest eigenvalue, and captures the greatest amount of variability in the data. Depending on the processing steps performed, the largest components may be variations caused by noise rather than the BOLD signal. ICA identifies subsets of voxels that vary together over time, and creates a generative model to characterize separate components of the data. In other words, ICA decomposes the BOLD data into independent components, such as separating activated BOLD responses from physiological noise artifacts. Factor analysis methods such as ICA are powerful data-driven techniques used to discover latent structures within data, such as in rs-fMRI studies to identify intrinsic neural networks.[69]

Feature selection methods select a subset of features from either the high-dimensional data space or the lower dimensional feature vector space. Excluding uninformative nonsignal voxels occurring outside the boundaries of the brain is a good starting point for removing noise. This includes selecting voxels within known anatomical regions of interest.[145,146,147] Univariate voxel-wise statistics may be used to determine which voxels to include in the MVPA, although this may risk discarding voxels with weak responses that contribute information collectively with their neighboring voxels.[148] A searchlight technique may be used to identify neighboring voxels that encode information across a spotlight area of specific radius.[149] Recursive feature elimination is a data-driven approach that selects discriminating voxels by recursively applying a SVM classifier.[150]

Classification of Multivariate Patterns

There are numerous machine learning strategies for recognizing spatiotemporal patterns of activation in BOLD fMRI data.[151] Conventional MVPA approaches use supervised learning techniques to classify spatial patterns of activation across voxels, which require an annotated dataset as the ground truth during the training phase. When there is a limited amount of training data available, techniques such as *k*-fold cross-validation and leave-one-out cross-validation may be used to train and test classifiers. Cross-validation approaches split the data into independent training and test datasets, to learn the parameters of the classifier and to evaluate its performance, respectively. In the context of fMRI analysis, "leave-one-run-out" cross-validation, where k equals the number of runs, is an option. Another strategy is to use "leave-one-stimulus-pair-out" cross-validation, where k equals the number of stimuli. If the classifier performs poorly, then this potentially indicates that the classifier is overfit to the training data and does not generalize to other data. Classifiers with complex nonlinear decision boundaries are vulnerable to overfitting when an insufficient amount of training data is available. Additional algorithm-specific regularization methods are often employed to help mitigate this risk.

SVMs are a common supervised machine learning approach for classification applications.[152,153] During the learning phase, a decision boundary is estimated as a hyperplane with support vectors that maximize the distance between the decision boundary and feature vectors that are near the boundary. Nonlinear SVMs may use a kernel trick (e.g., polynomial kernels and radial basis function [RBF]) to map feature vectors to a feature space where the classes of vectors are more separable. There are several MVPA review papers that compare SVM classifiers, along with other types of classifiers such as Fisher's linear discriminant analysis, Gaussian Naïve Bayes, and k-nearest neighbors (KNN).[154,155,156] Classifier performance metrics can be formulated from a confusion matrix that defines the number of true positives and true negatives on the diagonal, false positives in the upper quadrant, and false negatives in the lower quadrant. From this matrix, the following performance metrics may be derived: accuracy, false discovery rate, precision, recall, sensitivity, and specificity. The receiver operating characteristic (ROC) is also a good alternative for evaluating a classifier's performance, with the area under the curve (AUC) as a typical metric.[156] In general, linear SVM approaches are the classifier of choice for MVPA methods, as they outperformed or were comparable to other classification methods. However, classifier performance is dependent on the quality and quantity of feature vectors used to train and evaluate the classifiers. In contrast to conventional MVPA methods, deep learning methods do not require a feature engineering process that usually requires domain expertise to select features.

21.7.3 Deep Learning Applications

Since its revival in 2012, deep learning methods continue to evolve and remain the dominant machine learning approach in application domains such as computer vision, audio processing, and natural language processing. In general, deep learning methods apply a hierarchy of nonlinear transformations to learn invariant discriminant feature representations of data, for pattern analysis and classification tasks. Deep learning methods are able to discover complex latent feature representations from raw data.[157] A deep learning framework may be used to generate feature vectors from raw data (e.g., voxels) as input to a fully connected feed-forward network or other classifiers (e.g., SVM).

Neuroimaging studies demonstrated that generative RBMs are at least comparable to the state-of-the-art ICA methods, validating that it was able to effectively learn features from raw fMRI data and identify intrinsic networks.[101,158] These studies further validated that adding depth—that is, stacking RBMs to form a DBN—improves classification accuracy as applied to structural MRI data. Each layer of the DBN was pretrained using unsupervised generative RBM, and then fine-tuned using a feed-forward network for classification. The DBN generated features that were then fed into several different classifiers (i.e., RBF-kernel SVM, logistic regression, and KNN) for comparison. All of the classifiers performed significantly better using features generated by the DBN with three hidden layers, compared to more shallow networks.

Neuroimaging task-based and rs-fMRI studies have leveraged deep neural networks that are composed of stacked autoencoders to recognize functional connectivity patterns.[102,105,106] These studies demonstrated that the deep learning methods effectively performed unsupervised feature learning to discover latent structures to represent the data in a lower dimensional feature space. For instance, an rs-fMRI study was able to automatically learn features and identify functional connectivity patterns to differentiate healthy subjects from patients suffering from schizophrenia.[105] Another rs-fMRI study combined the power of a deep autoencoder with a Hidden Markov Model (HMM) to evaluate the dynamic functional connectivity of healthy subjects versus those with a mild cognitive impairment (MCI).[106] In addition, a study demonstrated that a deep neural network was able to learn features from a large fMRI database and classify the brain activity into seven task categories. This network was then used to decode the brain activity of a new subject, achieving a higher accuracy than baseline methods (e.g., SVMs).[159]

Several studies have demonstrated the power of using deep learning techniques for multimodal neuroimaging applications, namely, structural MRI and functional PET data. Using a deep learning approach that used randomized denoising autoencoders, a potential multimodal imaging biomarker was established to predict the progression from MCI to Alzheimer disease (AD).[104] Another study used a deep Boltzmann machine to learn latent features from MRI and PET images and then discover joint features across the modalities. These deep multimodal features were then coupled with an SVM to differentiate between normal controls, AD, and varying degrees of MCI.[103] Furthermore, another study leveraged a 3D CNN deep learning model to predict PET patterns from MRI data, as an effective method to complete and integrate multimodal data.[100]

21.8 Discussion and Concluding Remarks

Although MVPA is a standard tool for fMRI studies, DBS-fMRI studies primarily utilize univariate approaches. There are a small number of groups using modeling approaches such as dynamic causal modeling to investigate effective connectivity, as well as groups that are using tractography to investigate structural connectivity.[46,48] With the recent FDA approval to use a full-body 1.5 T MRI scan with a DBS system, the number of DBS-fMRI studies to investigate functional connectivity is increasing.[62] In general, MVPA approaches are beginning to evolve to leverage deep learning methods, especially to learn feature representations from the raw data, rather than conventional methods that often require domain expertise to select features to represent the input data. Furthermore, as deep learning methods are applicable across modalities, they are enabling the integration and analysis of multimodal functional connectome data.

To this day, the underlying therapeutic mechanisms of DBS are not well understood; even so, DBS therapy is a standard treatment for refractory neurological movement disorders and is emerging as a treatment option for refractory psychiatric disorders. Linking multimodal DBS-evoked connectomics with advanced data science methods is expected to provide invaluable insights into the pathologies of neurodegenerative and psychiatric disorders. Furthermore, studies have demonstrated that therapeutic and adverse effects are driven by stimulation of specific components of the basal ganglia thalamocortical circuitry, which is composed primarily of three segregated circuits. For instance, DBS therapy for PD requires precise electrode contact placement within the STN to stimulate the motor circuitry; deviations from the exact placement within the STN may stimulate the limbic circuitry and cause adverse effects. As such, subject-specific multimodal connectomes will enable more precise navigation during DBS electrode placement and optimize stimulation parameters, to maximize therapeutic effects while minimizing adverse effects.

References

[1] Tye SJ, Frye MA, Lee KH. Disrupting disordered neurocircuitry: treating refractory psychiatric illness with neuromodulation. Mayo Clin Proc. 2009; 84(6):522–532

[2] Lee KH, Blaha CD, Garris PA, et al. Evolution of deep brain stimulation: human electrometer and smart devices supporting the next generation of therapy. Neuromodulation. 2009; 12(2):85–103

[3] Benabid AL, Pollak P, Louveau A, Henry S, de Rougemont J. Combined (thalamotomy and stimulation) stereotactic surgery of the VIM thalamic nucleus for bilateral Parkinson disease. Appl Neurophysiol. 1987; 50(1–6):344–346

[4] Miocinovic S, Somayajula S, Chitnis S, Vitek JL. History, applications, and mechanisms of deep brain stimulation. JAMA Neurol. 2013; 70(2):163–171

[5] Smith KA, Pahwa R, Lyons KE, Nazzaro JM. Deep brain stimulation for Parkinson's disease: current status and future outlook. Neurodegener Dis Manag. 2016; 6(4):299–317

[6] Shen H. Neuroscience: tuning the brain. Nature. 2014; 507(7492):290–292

[7] Lozano AM, Lipsman N. Probing and regulating dysfunctional circuits using deep brain stimulation. Neuron. 2013; 77(3):406–424

[8] Santos FJ, Costa RM, Tecuapetla F. Stimulation on demand: closing the loop on deep brain stimulation. Neuron. 2011; 72(2):197–198

[9] Little S, Pogosyan A, Neal S, et al. Adaptive deep brain stimulation in advanced Parkinson disease. Ann Neurol. 2013; 74(3):449–457

[10] Grahn PJ, Mallory GW, Khurram OU, et al. A neurochemical closed-loop controller for deep brain stimulation: toward individualized smart neuromodulation therapies. Front Neurosci. 2014; 8:169

[11] Hebb AO, Zhang JJ, Mahoor MH, et al. Creating the feedback loop: closed-loop neurostimulation. Neurosurg Clin N Am. 2014; 25(1):187–204

[12] Edwards CA, Kouzani A, Lee KH, Ross EK. Neurostimulation devices for the treatment of neurologic disorders. Mayo Clin Proc. 2017; 92(9):1427–1444

[13] McCulloch WS, Pitts W. A logical calculus of the ideas immanent in nervous activity. 1943. Bull Math Biophys. 1990(1–2):99–115

[14] Hebb DO. The Organization of Behavior. New York, NY: Wiley & Sons; 1949

[15] Rosenblatt F. The Perceptron—A Perceiving and Recognizing Automaton. Cornell Aeronautical Laboratory; 1957

[16] Minsky M, Papert SA. Perceptrons: An Introduction to Computational Geometry. MIT Press; 1969

[17] Hubel DH, Wiesel TN. Receptive fields of single neurones in the cat's striate cortex. J Physiol. 1959; 148:574–591

[18] Hubel DH, Wiesel TN. Receptive fields, binocular interaction and functional architecture in the cat's visual cortex. J Physiol. 1962; 160:106–154

[19] Hubel DH, Wiesel TN. Receptive fields and functional architecture of monkey striate cortex. J Physiol. 1968; 195(1):215–243

[20] Fukushima K. Neocognitron: a self-organizing neural network model for a mechanism of pattern recognition unaffected by shift in position. Biol Cybern. 1980; 36(4):193–202

[21] Lecun Y, Jackel LD, Boser B, et al. Handwritten digit recognition - applications of neural network chips and automatic learning. IEEE Commun Mag. 1989; 27(11):41–46

[22] Lecun Y, Bottou L, Bengio Y, Haffner P. Gradient-based learning applied to document recognition. P IEEE. 1998; 86(11):2278–2324

[23] Felleman DJ, Van Essen DC. Distributed hierarchical processing in the primate cerebral cortex. Cereb Cortex. 1991; 1(1):1–47

[24] Lowe DG. Object Recognition from Local Scale-Invariant Features. International Conference on Computer Vision (ICCV); 1999

[25] Riesenhuber M, Poggio T. Hierarchical models of object recognition in cortex. Nat Neurosci. 1999; 2(11):1019–1025

[26] Arathorn D. Map-Seeking Circuits in Visual Cognition: A Computational Mechanism for Biological and Machine Vision. Stanford: Stanford University Press; 2002

[27] Serre T, Wolf L, Bileschi S, Riesenhuber M, Poggio T. Robust object recognition with cortex-like mechanisms. IEEE Trans Pattern Anal Mach Intell. 2007; 29(3):411–426

[28] George D, Hawkins J. Towards a mathematical theory of cortical micro-circuits. PLOS Comput Biol. 2009; 5(10):e1000532

[29] Rolls ET. Invariant visual object and face recognition: neural and computational bases, and a model, VisNet. Front Comput Neurosci. 2012; 6:35

[30] LeCun Y, Bengio Y, Hinton G. Deep learning. Nature. 2015; 521(7553):436–444

[31] Rumelhart DE, Hinton GE, Williams RJ. Learning representations by back-propagating errors. Nature. 1986; 323(6088):533–536

[32] Werbos PJ. Beyond Regression: New Tools for Prediction and Analysis in the Behavioral Sciences. Harvard University; 1974

[33] Werbos PJ. Generalization of backpropagation with application to a recurrent gas market model. Neural Netw. 1988; 1(4):339–356

[34] McClelland JL. The organization of memory. A parallel distributed processing perspective. Rev Neurol (Paris). 1994; 150(8–9):570–579

[35] Cybenko G. Approximation by superpositions of a Sigmoid function. Math Contr Signals Syst. 1989; 2:303–314

[36] Cortes C, Vapnik V. Support-vector networks. Mach Learn. 1995; 20(3):273–297

[37] Hochreiter S, Schmidhuber J. Long short-term memory. Neural Comput. 1997; 9(8):1735–1780

[38] Graves A, Eck D, Beringer N, Schmidhuber J. Biologically plausible speech recognition with LSTM neural nets. BioADIT. 2004; 3141:127–136

[39] Graves A, Schmidhuber J. Framewise phoneme classification with bidirectional LSTM and other neural network architectures. Neural Netw. 2005; 18(5–6):602–610

[40] Beringer N, Graves A, Schiel F, Schmidhuber J. Classifying unprompted speech by retraining LSTM nets. ICANN. 2005; 3696:575–581

[41] Hinton GE, Osindero S, Teh YW. A fast learning algorithm for deep belief nets. Neural Comput. 2006; 18(7):1527–1554

[42] Bengio Y, Lamblin P, Popovici D, Larochelle H. Greedy Layer-Wise Training of Deep Networks Neural Information Processing Systems. Montreal, Quebec; 2007

[43] Deng L, Li J, Huang J-T, et al. Recent Advances in Deep Learning for Speech Research at Microsoft. ICASSP; 2013

[44] Krizhevsky A, Sutskever I, Hinton G. ImageNet Classification with Deep Convolutional Neural Networks. Paper presented at the Neural Information Processing Systems; 2012; Lake Tahoe

[45] Mnih V, Kavukcuoglu K, Silver D, et al. Human-level control through deep reinforcement learning. Nature. 2015; 518(7540):529–533

[46] Gibson WS, Cho S, Abulseoud OA, et al. The impact of mirth-inducing ventral striatal deep brain stimulation on functional and effective connectivity. Cereb Cortex. 2017; 27(3):2183–2194

[47] Stafford JM, Jarrett BR, Miranda-Dominguez O, et al. Large-scale topology and the default mode network in the mouse connectome. Proc Natl Acad Sci U S A. 2014; 111(52):18745–18750

[48] Kahan J, Urner M, Moran R, et al. Resting state functional MRI in Parkinson's disease: the impact of deep brain stimulation on 'effective' connectivity. Brain. 2014; 137(Pt 4):1130–1144

[49] van Hartevelt TJ, Cabral J, Deco G, et al. Neural plasticity in human brain connectivity: the effects of long term deep brain stimulation of the subthalamic nucleus in Parkinson's disease. PLoS One. 2014; 9(1):e86496

[50] Olman CA, Yacoub E. High-field FMRI for human applications: an overview of spatial resolution and signal specificity. Open Neuroimaging J. 2011; 5: 74–89

[51] Duchin Y, Abosch A, Yacoub E, Sapiro G, Harel N. Feasibility of using ultra-high field (7 T) MRI for clinical surgical targeting. PLoS One. 2012; 7(5): e37328

[52] Hashemi R, Bradley W, Lisanti C. MRI The Basics. 2nd ed. Lippincott Williams & Wilkins; 2004

[53] Uğurbil K, Xu J, Auerbach EJ, et al. WU-Minn HCP Consortium. Pushing spatial and temporal resolution for functional and diffusion MRI in the Human Connectome Project. Neuroimage. 2013; 80:80–104

[54] Lambert C, Zrinzo L, Nagy Z, et al. Confirmation of functional zones within the human subthalamic nucleus: patterns of connectivity and sub-parcellation using diffusion weighted imaging. Neuroimage. 2012; 60(1):83–94

[55] Rozanski VE, Vollmar C, Cunha JP, et al. Connectivity patterns of pallidal DBS electrodes in focal dystonia: a diffusion tensor tractography study. Neuro-image. 2014; 84:435–442

[56] Hagmann P, Kurant M, Gigandet X, et al. Mapping human whole-brain structural networks with diffusion MRI. PLoS One. 2007; 2(7):e597

[57] Ogawa S, Lee TM, Kay AR, Tank DW. Brain magnetic resonance imaging with contrast dependent on blood oxygenation. Proc Natl Acad Sci U S A. 1990; 87(24):9868–9872

[58] Spiegel J, Fuss G, Backens M, et al. Transient dystonia following magnetic resonance imaging in a patient with deep brain stimulation electrodes for the treatment of Parkinson disease. Case report. J Neurosurg. 2003; 99(4):772–774

[59] Henderson JM, Tkach J, Phillips M, Baker K, Shellock FG, Rezai AR. Permanent neurological deficit related to magnetic resonance imaging in a patient with implanted deep brain stimulation electrodes for Parkinson's disease: case report. Neurosurgery. 2005; 57(5):E1063–, discussion E1063

[60] Phillips MD, Baker KB, Lowe MJ, et al. Parkinson disease: pattern of functional MR imaging activation during deep brain stimulation of subthalamic nucleus–initial experience. Radiology. 2006; 239(1):209–216

[61] Arantes PR, Cardoso EF, Barreiros MA, et al. Performing functional magnetic resonance imaging in patients with Parkinson's disease treated with deep brain stimulation. Mov Disord. 2006; 21(8):1154–1162

[62] Kahan J, Papadaki A, White M, et al. The safety of using body-transmit MRI in patients with implanted deep brain stimulation devices. PLoS One. 2015; 10(6):e0129077

[63] Qasim SE, de Hemptinne C, Swann NC, Miocinovic S, Ostrem JL, Starr PA. Electrocorticography reveals beta desynchronization in the basal ganglia-cortical loop during rest tremor in Parkinson's disease. Neuro-biol Dis. 2016

[64] Rowland NC, De Hemptinne C, Swann NC, et al. Task-related activity in sensorimotor cortex in Parkinson's disease and essential tremor: changes in beta and gamma bands. Front Hum Neurosci. 2015; 9:512

[65] de Hemptinne C, Swann NC, Ostrem JL, et al. Therapeutic deep brain stimulation reduces cortical phase-amplitude coupling in Parkinson's disease. Nat Neurosci. 2015; 18(5):779–786

[66] McCracken CB, Kiss ZHT. Time and frequency-dependent modulation of local field potential synchronization by deep brain stimulation. PLoS One. 2014; 9(7):e102576

[67] Castellanos FX, Di Martino A, Craddock RC, Mehta AD, Milham MP. Clinical applications of the functional connectome. Neuroimage. 2013; 80:527–540

[68] Zhan X, Yu R. A window into the brain: advances in psychiatric fMRI. BioMed Res Int. 2015; 2015:542467

[69] Kringelbach ML, Green AL, Aziz TZ. Balancing the brain: resting state networks and deep brain stimulation. Front Integr Nuerosci. 2011; 5:8

[70] Fox MD, Buckner RL, Liu H, Chakravarty MM, Lozano AM, Pascual-Leone A. Resting-state networks link invasive and noninvasive brain stimulation across diverse psychiatric and neurological diseases. Proc Natl Acad Sci U S A. 2014; 111(41):E4367–E4375

[71] Min HK, Ross EK, Lee KH, et al. Subthalamic nucleus deep brain stimulation induces motor network BOLD activation: use of a high precision MRI guided stereotactic system for nonhuman primates. Brain Stimul. 2014; 7(4):603–607

[72] Knight EJ, Testini P, Min HK, et al. Motor and nonmotor circuitry activation induced by subthalamic nucleus deep brain stimulation in patients with Parkinson disease: intraoperative functional magnetic resonance imaging for deep brain stimulation. Mayo Clin Proc. 2015; 90(6):773–785

[73] Sporns O, Tononi G, Kötter R. The human connectome: a structural description of the human brain. PLOS Comput Biol. 2005; 1(4):e42

[74] Betzel RF, Avena-Koenigsberger A, Goñi J, et al. Generative models of the human connectome. Neuroimage. 2016; 124 Pt A:1054–1064

[75] Bock DD, Lee WC, Kerlin AM, et al. Network anatomy and in vivo physiology of visual cortical neurons. Nature. 2011; 471(7337):177–182

[76] Livet J, Weissman TA, Kang H, et al. Transgenic strategies for combinatorial expression of fluorescent proteins in the nervous system. Nature. 2007; 450 (7166):56–62

[77] Lichtman JW, Sanes JR. Ome sweet ome: what can the genome tell us about the connectome? Curr Opin Neurobiol. 2008; 18(3):346–353

[78] White JG, Southgate E, Thomson JN, Brenner S. The structure of the nervous system of the nematode Caenorhabditis elegans. Philos Trans R Soc Lond B Biol Sci. 1986; 314(1165):1–340

[79] Varshney LR, Chen BL, Paniagua E, Hall DH, Chklovskii DB. Structural properties of the Caenorhabditis elegans neuronal network. PLOS Comput Biol. 2011; 7(2):e1001066

[80] Helmstaedter M, Briggman KL, Turaga SC, Jain V, Seung HS, Denk W. Connectomic reconstruction of the inner plexiform layer in the mouse retina. Nature. 2013; 500(7461):168–174

[81] Vogelstein JTQ. Q&A: What is the Open Connectome Project? Neural Syst Circuits. 2011; 1(1):16

[82] Burns R, Roncal WG, Kleissas D, et al. The Open Connectome Project Data Cluster: Scalable Analysis and Vision for High-Throughput Neuroscience. Scientific and statistical database management: International Conference, SSDBM: proceedings International Conference on Scientific and Statistical Database Management; 2013

[83] Vogelstein JT, Gray Roncal W, Vogelstein RJ, Priebe CE. Graph classification using signal-subgraphs: applications in statistical connectomics. IEEE Trans Pattern Anal Mach Intell. 2013; 35(7):1539–1551

[84] Burns R, Vogelstein JT, Szalay AS. From cosmos to connectomes: the evolution of data-intensive science. Neuron. 2014; 83(6):1249–1252

[85] Weiler NC, Collman F, Vogelstein JT, Burns R, Smith SJ. Synaptic molecular imaging in spared and deprived columns of mouse barrel cortex with array tomography. Sci Data. 2014; 1:140046

[86] Harris KM, Spacek J, Bell ME, et al. A resource from 3D electron microscopy of hippocampal neuropil for user training and tool development. Sci Data. 2015; 2:150046

[87] van den Heuvel MP, de Reus MA. Chasing the dreams of early connectionists. ACS Chem Neurosci. 2014; 5(7):491–493

[88] Prevedel R, Yoon YG, Hoffmann M, et al. Simultaneous whole-animal 3D imaging of neuronal activity using light-field microscopy. Nat Methods. 2014; 11(7):727–730

[89] Smith SM, Beckmann CF, Andersson J, et al. WU-Minn HCP Consortium. Resting-state fMRI in the Human Connectome Project. Neuroimage. 2013; 80:144–168

[90] Marcus DS, Harms MP, Snyder AZ, et al. WU-Minn HCP Consortium. Human Connectome Project informatics: quality control, database services, and data visualization. Neuroimage. 2013; 80:202–219

[91] Hodge MR, Horton W, Brown T, et al. ConnectomeDB–Sharing human brain connectivity data. Neuroimage. 2016; 124 Pt B:1102–1107

[92] Sporns O. The human connectome: origins and challenges. Neuroimage. 2013; 80:53–61

[93] Hagmann P, Cammoun L, Gigandet X, et al. MR connectomics: principles and challenges. J Neurosci Methods. 2010; 194(1):34–45

[94] Mišić B, Betzel RF, Nematzadeh A, et al. Cooperative and competitive spreading dynamics on the human connectome. Neuron. 2015; 86(6):1518–1529

[95] Ramakrishnan K, Scholte S, Lamme V, Smeulders A, Ghebreab S. Convolutional neural networks in the brain: an fMRI study. J Vis. 2015; 15(12):371

[96] Arganda-Carreras I, Turaga SC, Berger DR, et al. Crowdsourcing the creation of image segmentation algorithms for connectomics. Front Neuroanat. 2015; 9:142

[97] Guo Y, Wu G, Commander LA, et al. Segmenting hippocampus from infant brains by sparse patch matching with deep-learned features. MICCAI. 2014; 17:308–315

[98] Zhang W, Li R, Deng H, et al. Deep convolutional neural networks for multimodality isointense infant brain image segmentation. Neuroimage. 2015; 108:214–224

[99] Kleesiek J, Urban G, Hubert A, et al. Deep MRI brain extraction: A 3D convolutional neural network for skull stripping. Neuroimage. 2016; 129:460–469

[100] Li R, Zhang W, Suk HI, et al. Deep learning based imaging data completion for improved brain disease diagnosis. Med Image Comput Comput Assist Interv. 2014; 17:305–312

[101] Plis SM, Hjelm DR, Salakhutdinov R, et al. Deep learning for neuroimaging: a validation study. Front Neurosci. 2014; 8:229

[102] Firat O. Deep learning for brain decoding. Paper presented at the Proceeding of the 21st International Conference on Image Processing; 2014; Paris, France

[103] Suk HI, Lee SW, Shen D, Alzheimer's Disease Neuroimaging Initiative. Hierarchical feature representation and multimodal fusion with deep learning for AD/MCI diagnosis. Neuroimage. 2014; 101:569–582

[104] Ithapu VK, Singh V, Okonkwo OC, Chappell RJ, Dowling NM, Johnson SC, Alzheimer's Disease Neuroimaging Initiative. Imaging-based enrichment criteria using deep learning algorithms for efficient clinical trials in mild cognitive impairment. Alzheimers Dement. 2015; 11(12):1489–1499

[105] Kim J, Calhoun VD, Shim E, Lee JH. Deep neural network with weight sparsity control and pre-training extracts hierarchical features and enhances classification performance: Evidence from whole-brain resting-state functional connectivity patterns of schizophrenia. Neuroimage. 2016; 124 Pt A: 127–146

[106] Suk HI, Wee CY, Lee SW, Shen D. State-space model with deep learning for functional dynamics estimation in resting-state fMRI. Neuroimage. 2016; 129:292–307

[107] Hart MG, Ypma RJ, Romero-Garcia R, Price SJ, Suckling J. Graph theory analysis of complex brain networks: new concepts in brain mapping applied to neurosurgery. J Neurosurg. 2016; 124(6):1665–1678

[108] Goodman WK, Insel TR. Deep brain stimulation in psychiatry: concentrating on the road ahead. Biol Psychiatry. 2009; 65(4):263–266

[109] Insel TR. Integrating neuroscience into psychiatric residency training. Asian J Psychiatr. 2015; 17:133–134

[110] Gabrieli JDE, Ghosh SS, Whitfield-Gabrieli S. Prediction as a humanitarian and pragmatic contribution from human cognitive neuroscience. Neuron. 2015; 85(1):11–26

[111] Smith SM. The future of FMRI connectivity. Neuroimage. 2012; 62(2):1257–1266

[112] Zuo XN, Ehmke R, Mennes M, et al. Network centrality in the human functional connectome. Cereb Cortex. 2012; 22(8):1862–1875

[113] Greicius M. Resting-state functional connectivity in neuropsychiatric disorders. Curr Opin Neurol. 2008; 21(4):424–430

[114] Uddin LQ, Kelly AMC, Biswal BB, Castellanos FX, Milham MP. Functional connectivity of default mode network components: correlation, anticorrelation, and causality. Hum Brain Mapp. 2009; 30(2):625–637

[115] Cao M, Wang JH, Dai ZJ, et al. Topological organization of the human brain functional connectome across the lifespan. Dev Cogn Neurosci. 2014; 7:76–93

[116] Lujan JL, Chaturvedi A, Malone DA, Rezai AR, Machado AG, McIntyre CC. Axonal pathways linked to therapeutic and nontherapeutic outcomes during psychiatric deep brain stimulation. Hum Brain Mapp. 2012; 33(4):958–968

[117] Choi KS, Riva-Posse P, Gross RE, Mayberg HS. Mapping the "depression switch" during intraoperative testing of subcallosal cingulate deep brain stimulation. JAMA Neurol. 2015; 72(11):1252–1260

[118] Stefurak T, Mikulis D, Mayberg H, et al. Deep brain stimulation for Parkinson's disease dissociates mood and motor circuits: a functional MRI case study. Mov Disord. 2003; 18(12):1508–1516

[119] Mayberg HS, Lozano AM, Voon V, et al. Deep brain stimulation for treatment-resistant depression. Neuron. 2005; 45(5):651–660

[120] Johansen-Berg H, Gutman DA, Behrens TE, et al. Anatomical connectivity of the subgenual cingulate region targeted with deep brain stimulation for treatment-resistant depression. Cereb Cortex. 2008; 18(6):1374–1383

[121] Giacobbe P, Mayberg HS, Lozano AM. Treatment resistant depression as a failure of brain homeostatic mechanisms: implications for deep brain stimulation. Exp Neurol. 2009; 219(1):44–52

[122] Knight EJ, Min HK, Hwang SC, et al. Nucleus accumbens deep brain stimulation results in insula and prefrontal activation: a large animal FMRI study. PLoS One. 2013; 8(2):e56640

[123] Min HK, Hwang SC, Marsh MP, et al. Deep brain stimulation induces BOLD activation in motor and non-motor networks: an fMRI comparison study of STN and EN/GPi DBS in large animals. Neuroimage. 2012; 63(3):1408–1420

[124] Paek SB, Min HK, Kim I, et al. Frequency-dependent functional neuromodulatory effects on the motor network by ventral lateral thalamic deep brain stimulation in swine. Neuroimage. 2015; 105:181–188

[125] Van Den Berge N, Vanhove C, Descamps B, et al. Functional MRI during hippocampal deep brain stimulation in the healthy rat brain. PLoS One. 2015; 10(7):e0133245

[126] Ross EK, Kim JP, Settell ML, et al. Fornix deep brain stimulation circuit effect is dependent on major excitatory transmission via the nucleus accumbens. Neuroimage. 2016; 128:138–148

[127] Logothetis NK. What we can do and what we cannot do with fMRI. Nature. 2008; 453(7197):869–878

[128] Kim SG, Ogawa S. Biophysical and physiological origins of blood oxygenation level-dependent fMRI signals. J Cereb Blood Flow Metab. 2012; 32(7):1188–1206

[129] Aguirre GK, Zarahn E, D'esposito M. The variability of human, BOLD hemodynamic responses. Neuroimage. 1998; 8(4):360–369

[130] Duong TQ, Kim DS, Uğurbil K, Kim SG. Spatiotemporal dynamics of the BOLD fMRI signals: toward mapping submillimeter cortical columns using the early negative response. Magn Reson Med. 2000; 44(2):231–242

[131] Zarahn E. Spatial localization and resolution of BOLD fMRI. Curr Opin Neurobiol. 2001; 11(2):209–212

[132] Yeşilyurt B, Uğurbil K, Uludağ K. Dynamics and nonlinearities of the BOLD response at very short stimulus durations. Magn Reson Imaging. 2008; 26 (7):853–862

[133] Hu X, Yacoub E. The story of the initial dip in fMRI. Neuroimage. 2012; 62 (2):1103–1108

[134] Watanabe M, Bartels A, Macke JH, Murayama Y, Logothetis NK. Temporal jitter of the BOLD signal reveals a reliable initial dip and improved spatial resolution. Curr Biol. 2013; 23(21):2146–2150

[135] Siero JC, Hendrikse J, Hoogduin H, Petridou N, Luijten P, Donahue MJ. Cortical depth dependence of the BOLD initial dip and poststimulus undershoot in human visual cortex at 7 Tesla. Magn Reson Med. 2015; 73(6):2283–2295

[136] Norman KA, Polyn SM, Detre GJ, Haxby JV. Beyond mind-reading: multivoxel pattern analysis of fMRI data. Trends Cogn Sci. 2006; 10(9):424–430

[137] Haxby JV. Multivariate pattern analysis of fMRI: the early beginnings. Neuroimage. 2012; 62(2):852–855

[138] Mitchell TM, Hutchinson R, Niculescu RS, et al. Learning to decode cognitive states from brain images. Mach Learn. 2004; 57(1–2):145–175

[139] Mitchell TM, Shinkareva SV, Carlson A, et al. Predicting human brain activity associated with the meanings of nouns. Science. 2008; 320(5880):1191–1195

[140] Naselaris T, Kay KN, Nishimoto S, Gallant JL. Encoding and decoding in fMRI. Neuroimage. 2011; 56(2):400–410

[141] Tong F, Pratte MS. Decoding patterns of human brain activity. Annu Rev Psychol. 2012; 63:483–509

[142] Haxby JV, Connolly AC, Guntupalli JS. Decoding neural representational spaces using multivariate pattern analysis. Annu Rev Neurosci. 2014; 37: 435–456

[143] Hansen LK, Larsen J, Nielsen FA, et al. Generalizable patterns in neuroimaging: how many principal components? Neuroimage. 1999; 9(5):534–544

[144] McKeown MJ, Sejnowski TJ. Independent component analysis of fMRI data: examining the assumptions. Hum Brain Mapp. 1998; 6(5–6):368–372

[145] Cox DD, Savoy RL. Functional magnetic resonance imaging (fMRI) "brain reading": detecting and classifying distributed patterns of fMRI activity in human visual cortex. Neuroimage. 2003; 19(2, Pt 1):261–270

[146] Haynes JD, Rees G. Predicting the orientation of invisible stimuli from activity in human primary visual cortex. Nat Neurosci. 2005; 8(5):686–691

[147] Kamitani Y, Tong F. Decoding the visual and subjective contents of the human brain. Nat Neurosci. 2005; 8(5):679–685

[148] Schrouff J, Rosa MJ, Rondina JM, et al. PRoNTo: pattern recognition for neuroimaging toolbox. Neuroinformatics. 2013; 11(3):319–337

[149] Kriegeskorte N, Goebel R, Bandettini P. Information-based functional brain mapping. Proc Natl Acad Sci U S A. 2006; 103(10):3863–3868

[150] De Martino F, Valente G, Staeren N, Ashburner J, Goebel R, Formisano E. Combining multivariate voxel selection and support vector machines for mapping and classification of fMRI spatial patterns. Neuroimage. 2008; 43 (1):44–58

[151] Pereira F, Mitchell T, Botvinick M. Machine learning classifiers and fMRI: a tutorial overview. Neuroimage. 2009; 45(1 Suppl):S199–S209

[152] Meier TB, Desphande AS, Vergun S, et al. Support vector machine classification and characterization of age-related reorganization of functional brain networks. Neuroimage. 2012; 60(1):601–613

[153] Salvatore C, Battista P, Castiglioni I. Frontiers for the early diagnosis of AD by means of MRI brain imaging and support vector machines. Curr Alzheimer Res. 2015

[154] Ku SP, Gretton A, Macke J, Logothetis NK. Comparison of pattern recognition methods in classifying high-resolution BOLD signals obtained at high magnetic field in monkeys. Magn Reson Imaging. 2008; 26(7):1007–1014

[155] Misaki M, Kim Y, Bandettini PA, Kriegeskorte N. Comparison of multivariate classifiers and response normalizations for pattern-information fMRI. Neuroimage. 2010; 53(1):103–118

[156] Mahmoudi A, Takerkart S, Regragui F, Boussaoud D, Brovelli A. Multivoxel pattern analysis for FMRI data: a review. Comput Math Methods Med. 2012; 2012:961257

[157] Bengio Y, Courville A, Vincent P. Representation learning: a review and new perspectives. IEEE Trans Pattern Anal Mach Intell. 2013; 35(8):1798–1828

[158] Hjelm RD, Calhoun VD, Salakhutdinov R, Allen EA, Adali T, Plis SM. Restricted Boltzmann machines for neuroimaging: an application in identifying intrinsic networks. Neuroimage. 2014; 96:245–260

[159] Koyamada S, Shikauchi Y, Nakae K, Koyama M, Ishii S. Deep learning of fMRI big data: a novel approach to subject-transfer decoding. Statistics Machine Learning 2015. Available at: https://arxiv.org/abs/1502.00093. Accessed July 22, 2019

22 Neuroplasticity and Rewiring of the Brain

Juan A. Barcia, María Pérez-Garoz, and Cristina Nombela

Abstract

Besides histology, the extent of the resection is the main prognostic factor in the surgery of intrinsic brain tumors.[1] However, preservation of neurological function is highly relevant for maintaining quality of life during survival. These two needs compete when a tumor contains functional brain areas. The possibility to artificially induce brain plasticity by continuous cortical stimulation plus prehabilitation permits other areas of the brain to take over the function and then maximize tumor removal. Here, we present the rationale, methodology, and experience of our group in this field.

Keywords: neuroplasticity, brain tumor, electrode grid, functional MRI, rehabilitation.

22.1 Introduction

The most important surgical factor in the prognosis of gliomas is the extent of resection. In the case of high-grade gliomas, gross total removal may improve overall prognosis (from a median survival of 12 to 18 months).[2,3] In low-grade gliomas, curative resection is possible.[4] However, this can be jeopardized when the tumor is close to or even contains functional brain areas. Most gliomas infiltrate the surrounding brain, making it difficult to decide where the tumor ends and where functional brain tissue starts. In the case of gut tumors, for example, the surgeon can remove the tumor and adjoining segments until pathology has confirmed negative margins in what is referred to as extended resection. This is not the case in brain tumors because extended resection could lead to removal of key functional structures such as those dedicated to the so-called eloquent functions (motor or speech functions). When this is the case, the surgeon, according to the patient's preferences, must decide where to stop the tumor resection in order to preserve function, thus impacting disease prognosis. Accordingly, tenets of glioma surgery are to achieve maximal resection to improve survival, while respecting functional areas to maintain quality of life.

But what would happen if we could be able to move these eloquent functions away from the tumor, allowing increased extent of resection by letting other cortical areas, distant from the original ones, take charge of these key functions? In principle, this would be possible because of the plastic nature of cerebral connections. However, this property needs to be harnessed and induced artificially in order to apply it to the needs of our particular patients.

22.2 The Concept of Brain Plasticity

Plasticity is a property of the brain that allows it to adapt continuously to the environment. It can occur by several mechanisms, from changing the strength with which neurons communicate to the possibility of increasing the size and number of dendritic branches in order to make new connections between neurons. The concept of brain plasticity was initially conceptualized as early as 1904 by Santiago Ramón y Cajal[5] and since then it has been identified under healthy and pathological conditions, both in animals and humans.

One of the properties of plasticity is topographic plasticity. This means that the location of functions in the brain cortex is not fixed and can vary due to different mechanisms. It that sense, when Paul Broca described the area bearing his name at the left inferior frontal cortex,[6] it was widely accepted that the expression of speech was always located at this site. The same occurred with Wernicke's area at the left upper superior temporal cortex, the motor areas on the primary motor cortex, or the sensory areas along the sensory motor cortex as Penfield and others have described.[7] Later on, researchers including Michael Merzenich have demonstrated that certain areas in the brain are able to be displaced or to increase its size in response to several challenges from the environment. For example, this group showed that the size of the area responding to a particular frequency in the auditory cortex of the owl monkey may suffer modifications depending on the stimuli received.[8] In humans, Álvaro Pascual-Leone's group, for example, showed an effect of intermodal plasticity in normal volunteers that, after being blinded for 6 days, processed auditory information in the occipital lobe.[9]

These plasticity mechanisms are not immediate, but require long-term training. In a study evaluating London taxi drivers, Maguire et al showed that there were changes in the size of the drivers' hippocampus after years of daily navigation training.[10] Accordingly, patients who undergo a sudden loss, such as in stroke or trauma, are not able to spontaneously recover the lost function located within the affected areas. However, when the damage occurs steadily during a long period, plasticity mechanisms may compensate for the damage. It is known that slowly growing brain tumors (such as low-grade ones) may induce changes in the cortical representation of the functions. Robles et al observed that in patients operated on for low-grade gliomas in whom a complete resection of the tumor was not possible due to the vicinity of eloquent areas, the location of the affected functions had been displaced when evaluated during a second operation between 4 and 5 years later.[4]

The rationale of our studies is based on the idea of artificially accelerating this natural plasticity process of the brain tissue in areas containing eloquent functions at danger due to tumor presence and infiltration. According to the available literature, this could be done by a progressive inhibition of the key areas, which provokes an artificial dysfunction susceptible of being recovered through personalized training. That is what we called "prehabilitation."

22.3 First Case: Functional Inhibition through Repetitive Transcranial Magnetic Stimulation

Our first attempt was done trying to use a noninvasive method, repetitive transcranial magnetic stimulation (rTMS), to produce inhibition on an eloquent area located at the tumor region. The first case was a 59-year-old woman who presented with a left inferior frontal gyrus tumor. She was operated awake and the resection was limited because of the presence of speech functional areas (the pathological diagnosis was anaplastic oligodendroglioma). Experimentally, we tried to provoke a virtual lesion using rTMS in "theta burst" (which was supposed to produce an inhibition in the area which lasted for about 20 minutes), at the frontal end where Broca's area is supposed to be located.[11] The experiments included 12 sessions followed by intense speech rehabilitation. A functional language evaluation was performed immediately before TMS, immediately after TMS, and 20 minutes after intense speech. The assessment was conducted using the Boston test for aphasia (BDAE) that provides scores of repetition, nomination, auditory language comprehension, oral expression, and writing.[12] While results indicated expected absence of effect of rTMS on comprehension and identification, it appeared that rTMS stimulation had gradually less impairing effect on nomination, indicating that the procedure changed the characteristics of production of speech.[13] However, the lack of changes in topographic location of the function did not allow us to increase the resection of the tumor, reducing the chances of function prevention during surgery. We hypothesized that the lack of topographic changes during that procedure was because the rehabilitation was done at different times as the inhibition, so we were reinforcing the function at the very same location. A new protocol needed to be designed.

22.4 Second Case: Functional Inhibition through Continuous Stimulation

The previous experience, where the rehabilitation had strengthened the patient's function, led us to hypothesize that a continuous inhibition of the functionally affected area was necessary, together with an intense and personalized rehabilitation program for promoting compensatory mechanisms in other brain areas, and, thus, reallocating the affected function. We proposed to use continuous electrical current delivered through a subdural electrode grid implanted over the cortex. That solution would solve the time stimulation limitation of TMS, which cannot be delivered 24/7 to the patient. Following that rationale, a 27-year-old male with an anaplastic astrocytoma in the inferior left temporal gyrus was operated for a second time. During the first surgery, 5 years earlier, no resection was conducted due to the location and finding of speech functions within the tumor. Since then, the patient underwent radiotherapy and chemotherapy, but temozolomide produced aplastic anemia. Then, chemotherapy was interrupted and the patient developed impairments in speech production. The surgical team then decided to reoperate on the patient. In that occasion, a complete neuropsychological assessment was conducted before and after the surgery, including Mini-Mental State examination (MMSE),[14] letter-cancellation task,[15] verbal fluency,[16] Token Test,[17] and Boston Naming Test (BNT)[18] that demonstrated impairments in attention, comprehension, and fluency.

Functional magnetic resonance imaging (fMRI) evaluating fluency and comprehension activation patterns confirmed that those functions were at risk since they were located within the tumor. The patient underwent an awake surgery with cortical stimulation and electrophysiological and speech function monitoring, using the standard criteria of resecting exclusively non-eloquent areas (▶ Fig. 22.3a), followed by the implantation of a grid for electrocorticography over the unresected tumor and surrounding cortex (▶ Fig. 22.3b). One week later, a mapping recording was performed using stimulation through the grid to test whether there were still active functions linked to the affected areas. Results indicated that most of the tumor still contained speech areas (▶ Fig. 22.3c). Consequently, we initiated the "prehabilitation" protocol. It consisted of continuously stimulating at 130 Hz and 1 ms of pulse width. The stimulation was bipolar and the threshold was based on causing a disabling but affordable defect in the patient's performance that could be counterbalanced with an intense rehabilitation plan conducted by a neuropsychologist. The next day, once the speech impairment had been overcome through the rehabilitation, the threshold of the stimulation was increased following the same criteria. After 7 days, the increased stimulation was exclusively accompanied by motor side effects and did not produce any effects on speech. After a second fMRI, it was verified that the function had shifted to the contralateral hemisphere. Finally, in a repeated operation, we verified the clearance of functional activity in the stimulated cortex (▶ Fig. 22.3d), and, using the same surgical criteria as earlier, we were able to perform a more extensive resection.[19]

22.5 Functional Inhibition through Continuous Stimulation in a Clinical Trial: The Research Protocol

The protocol (▶ Fig. 22.1) we designed from the previous patient (case 2) has been later used in seven more cases (▶ Fig. 22.2). Details of fMRI paradigms and MRI analysis are described in the supplementary methods of our published paper.[20]

Behavioral assessment: Neuropsychological assessment included Mini-Mental State Examination (MMSE),[14] BNT,[18] phonological and semantic fluency tasks,[21,22] Token Test,[17] Trail Making Test (TMT) A and B,[23] Zoo Map (Behavioral Assessment of the dysexecutive syndrome),[24] and Spain-Complutense Verbal Learning Test (TAVEC).[25] In case of motor symptoms, assessment of mobility was administered including the Tinetti Balance Assessment Tool,[26] Timed up and Go Test (TUG),[27] performance in activities of daily living,[28] and Barthel Index.[29]

Intraoperative stimulation mapping procedure (ISM): ISM was performed using cortical bipolar electrodes (ref.019–400888/ 408600/408700- Nicolet, San Carlos, CA) with tips separated by 5 mm delivering 200 pulse trains with 50 Hz, 1-ms pulse width, and intensity between 2 and 8 mA. Intensity was referenced to the threshold value for evoking motor activity at the precentral gyrus. Subcortical mapping with monopolar electrodes, using the same cortical stimulation parameters, was continuously performed while the tumor was removed.

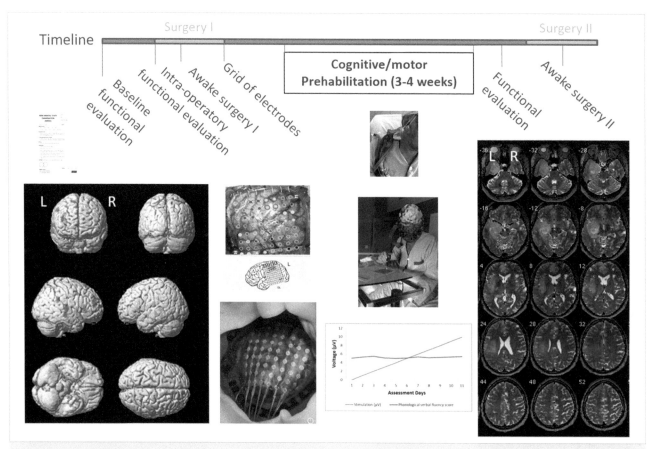

Fig. 22.1 Prehabilitation process schema.

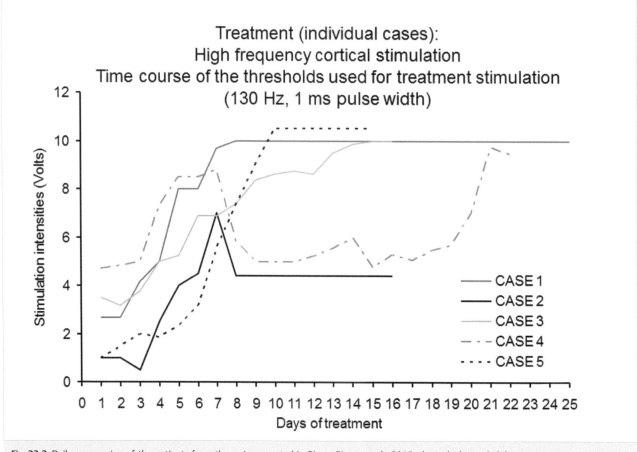

Fig. 22.2 Daily progression of the patients from the series reported in Rivera-Rivera et al., 2016, through the prehabilitation process.

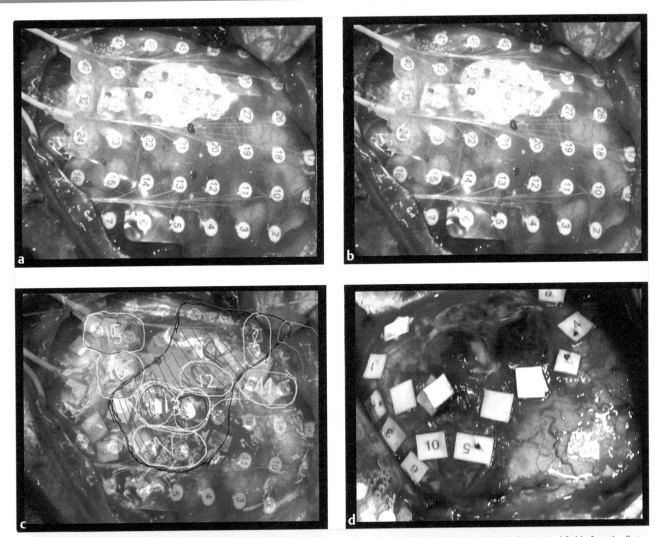

Fig. 22.3 Example of a patient who underwent the prehabilitation process. Pictures show the cortical mapping and the surgical field after the first resection (**a**), the placement of the electrode grid (**b**), the results of the cortical stimulation 1 week after grid implantation before the prehabilitation process (**c**), the cortical mapping after the second resection (**d**). Note that numbered tags are active functional points and blank tags are functionless points.

Continuous cortical electrical stimulation procedure: Grid's electrodes were 4.0 mm in diameter with 2.3-mm exposure, and 10-mm distance between contiguous electrodes. Electrodes were grouped in a bipolar montage with contact pairs located over the eloquent areas within the tumor. The stimulation intensity threshold increased in all subjects over time (▶ Fig. 22.2).

Prehabilitation process for language function: During a period of 30 days through the progressive increase of cortical stimulation, a slight deficit in naming and comprehension is produced as evaluated by neuropsychological tests such as Boston Naming Test, Token Test, and order comprehension. Once achieved, constant stimulation is maintained. For 2 hours a day, the patient performs language expression exercises with the neuropsychologist, such as naming objects and actions, reading, repetition, and comprehension of simple orders that are all adapted to his or her cognitive state. After the daily evaluation, the patient will perform rehabilitation exercises with his or her family member or therapist previously trained by the

neuropsychologist. Once the induced deficit is reversed, the stimulation will be increased following the same pattern.

Prehabilitation process of motor functions: The prehabilitation of motor functions requires a neurological physiotherapist. While the stimulation increases, the motor deficit caused is evaluated by direct observation of speed and motor coordination of the hand during tapping test. It will also be necessary to measure the strength of the hand movement and to attend to the sensory perceptions or paresthesia reported by the patient. Again, after producing a slight deficit with increase in stimulation, the patient performs rehabilitation exercises for coordination and strength of the hand for several hours every day until achieving functional recovery.

22.6 Results

This protocol was applied to an initial series of five patients (Rivera-Rivera et al., 2016). This series contains three males and two females, whose ages ranged from 27 to 52 years (median:

41 years). Initially, all patients except one were considered low-grade gliomas due to their radiological characteristics, but, on pathological diagnosis, two cases were grade II gliomas and three were grade III. Eloquent functions affected were speech production (three cases), speech comprehension (one case), and motor function (two cases, one in M1, the other case shared M1, SMA, and Broca's area invasion). Results indicated that the prehabilitation protocol managed to let other areas of the brain away from the tumor control eloquent functions, thus allowing for a more extended resection during a second surgery. Median residual volume after first surgery was 45.97%, and after second surgery 14.05%. In all cases, the final residual volume was less than 30 mL, which is considered a safe volume in regard to risk to malignant conversion.

Regarding the side effects, there were seizures in three cases during the increase in stimulation (controlled with modification of the stimulation and antiepileptic drugs), and a worsening in speech in three cases, all of them within a functional range. But the most important complication was infection that appeared in three cases. Two of them required surgery to drain abscesses.

22.7 Last Cases

After this series, we applied the method to three other more extreme cases, with poorer results. The first case was a 54-year-old male with a very extensive left temporal tumor extending from the hippocampus to the insula and a great part of the left temporal and frontal lobes. The first surgery permitted to remove the anterior third of the left temporal lobe, but this was limited by the presence of speech areas. After the first surgery and under an intense prehabilitation program (daily neuropsychological assessment and training with a neuropsychologist, plus individual training plan), the patient initiated to show reallocation of the verbal comprehension function to the contralateral side. Unfortunately, during the second surgery the patient suffered a choroidal artery stroke that led to mobility and speech sequelae. The pathological diagnosis was a grade IV glioma at the most medial areas of the tumor. The tumor continued to grow and the patient died 15 months later.

The second case was a left-handed 38-year-old woman with a tumor relapse at the right supplementary motor area. She had been successfully operated 4 years earlier. During the prehabilitation phase, the batteries ran out inadvertently, so the stimulation was ineffective during 1 week. During the reoperation, although a gross total resection of the mass was achieved, no evidence of a plastic change was obtained. The patient maintains a high quality of life, is professionally active, and is medically controlled for eventual recurrence.

The last case consisted of a reoperation of one of the cases of the first series. The patient was a 50-year-old man with a grade III astrocytoma that relapsed in the left primary motor area. After the second surgery, the patient presented with mobility problems, possibly due to a limitation of retrying, or an error during the selection of the area to resect. The pathological diagnosis was a grade IV glioma. Currently, the patient is under palliative treatment.

22.8 Prospective

To our knowledge, just one other medical team has put in practice our prehabilitation protocol. The group of Dr. Pedro Serrano, in Málaga, Spain, has initially achieved clinical success using this procedure, although the study is currently ongoing.[30]

The main inconveniencies of these methods are derived from the externalization of the stimulation generator during the prehabilitation phase. This, along with the lack of comfort for the patients, forces them to be hospitalized during the procedure (which may extend up to 2 months, including 3 weeks of prehabilitation) that increases the risk of infections. We have started a new clinical trial using implantable pulse generators instead of external stimulators. Although this is a phase IIa trial of feasibility and security, we expect that this will diminish the incidence of infection and make the procedure easier for the patient and for the healthcare system. Furthermore, it will give the patients the chance of doing outpatient rehabilitation, plus prehabilitating the functions they wish to conserve in a familiar and perhaps professional environment.

Another important step is to clarify the mechanisms that are involved in this process and the limitations of the technique. The use of connectivity models using magnetoencephalography, fMRI, and diffusion tensor imaging will possibly help us clarify these issues.

22.9 Conclusion

Besides histology, the extent of the resection is the main prognostic factor in the surgery of intrinsic brain tumors. However, preservation of neurological function is highly relevant for maintaining quality of life during survival. Extent of resection can therefore be limited by involvement of tumors in eloquent functions. We demonstrate a protocol for facilitating neuroplasticity to allow for more extensive resections of intrinsic tumors involving eloquent functions.

References

[1] Gil-Robles S, Duffau H. Surgical management of World Health Organization Grade II gliomas in eloquent areas: the necessity of preserving a margin around functional structures. Neurosurg Focus. 2010; 28(2):E8

[2] Keles GE, Lamborn KR, Berger MS. Low-grade hemispheric gliomas in adults: a critical review of extent of resection as a factor influencing outcome. J Neurosurg. 2001; 95(5):735–745

[3] Sanai N, Berger MS. Surgical oncology for gliomas: the state of the art. Nat Rev Clin Oncol. 2018; 15(2):112–125

[4] Robles SG, Gatignol P, Lehéricy S, Duffau H. Long-term brain plasticity allowing a multistage surgical approach to World Health Organization Grade II gliomas in eloquent areas. J Neurosurg. 2008; 109(4):615–624

[5] DeFelipe J. Brain plasticity and mental processes: Cajal again. Nat Rev Neurosci. 2006; 7(10):811–817

[6] Broca P. Perte de la parole, ramollissement chronique et destruction partielle du lobe antérieur gauche. Bulletin de la Société d. Anthropologie. 1861; 2: 235–238

[7] Penfield W, Boldrey E. Somatic motor and sensory representation in the cerebral cortex of man as studied by electrical stimulation. Brain. 1937(60):389–443

[8] Recanzone G, Schreiner C, Merzenich M. Plasticity in the frequency representation of primary auditory cortex following discrimination training in adult owl monkeys. J Neurosci. 2018(13):87–103

[9] Merabet LB, Hamilton R, Schlaug G, et al. Rapid and reversible recruitment of early visual cortex for touch. PLoS One. 2008(3). DOI: 10.1371/journal.pone.0003046

[10] Maguire EA, Gadian DG, Johnsrude IS, et al. Navigation-related structural change in the hippocampi of taxi drivers. Proc Natl Acad Sci U S A. 2000; 97 (8):4398–4403

[11] Huang YZ, Edwards MJ, Rounis E, Bhatia KP, Rothwell JC. Theta burst stimulation of the human motor cortex. Neuron. 2005; 45(2):201–206

[12] Goodglass H, Kaplan E. The Assessment of Aphasia and Related Disorders. 2nd ed. Philadelphia, PA: Lea & Febiger; 1996

[13] Barcia JA, Sanz A, González-Hidalgo M, et al. rTMS stimulation to induce plastic changes at the language motor area in a patient with a left recidivant brain tumor affecting Broca's area. Neurocase. 2012; 18(2):132–138

[14] Folstein MF, Folstein SE, McHugh PR. "Mini-mental state". A practical method for grading the cognitive state of patients for the clinician. J Psychiatr Res. 1975; 12(3):189–198

[15] Diller L. Studies of Cognition and Rehabilitation in Hemiplegia Rehabilitation Monograph. New York, NY: University Medical Center; 1974:50

[16] Spreen O, Strauss E. A Compendium of Neuropsychological Tests: Administration, Norms, and Commentary. 2nd ed. NY: Oxford University Press; 1998

[17] De Renzi E, Faglioni P. Normative data and screening power of a shortened version of the Token Test. Cortex. 1978; 14(1):41–49

[18] Kaplan E, Goodglass H, Weintraub S. Boston Naming Test. 2nd ed. Philadelphia, PA: Lippincott Williams & Wilkins; 2001

[19] Barcia JA, Sanz A, Balugo P, et al. High-frequency cortical subdural stimulation enhanced plasticity in surgery of a tumor in Broca's area. Neuroreport. 2012; 23(5):304–309

[20] Rivera-Rivera PA, Rios-Lago M, Sanchez-Casarrubios S, et al. Cortical plasticity catalyzed by prehabilitation enables extensive resection of brain tumors in eloquent areas. J Neurosurg. 2016; 126:1323–1333

[21] Goodglass H, Kaplan E. The assessment of aphasia and related disorders (rev. ed.). Philadelphia, PA; 1972

[22] Benton AL. Differential behavioral effects in frontal lobe disease. Neuropsychologia. 1968; 6:53–60

[23] Rabin LA, Barr WB, Burton LA. Assessment practices of clinical neuropsychologists in the United States and Canada: a survey of INS, NAN, and APA Division 40 members. Arch Clin Neuropsychol. 2005; 20(1):33–65

[24] Wilson B, Alderman N, Burgess P, et al. Behavioural Assessment of the Dysexecutive Syndrome (BADS). Manual. London: Harcourt Assessment; 1996

[25] Benedet MJ, Alejandre MA. Test de Aprendizaje Verbal España-Complutense. Madrid, Spain: TEA Ediciones; 1998

[26] Tinetti ME, Williams TF, Mayewski R. Fall risk index for elderly patients based on number of chronic disabilities. Am J Med. 1986; 80(3):429–434

[27] Bohannon RW. Reference values for the timed up and go test: a descriptive meta-analysis. J Geriatr Phys Ther. 2006; 29(2):64–68

[28] Gill TM. Assessment of function and disability in longitudinal studies. J Am Geriatr Soc. 2010; 58 Suppl 2:S308–S312

[29] Kwon S, Hartzema AG, Duncan PW, Min-Lai S. Disability measures in stroke relationship among the Barthel Index, the functional independence measure, and the Modified Rankin Scale. Stroke. 2004; 35(4):918–923

[30] Serrano-Castro PJ, Ros-Lopez B, Fernandez-Sanchez V, et al. Prehabilitación del lenguaje en cirugía de la Epilepsia: A propósito de un caso. V Reunión Anual de la Sociedad Española de Epilepsia. Málaga 25–27 de Octubre de 2018

23 Radiating in Eloquent Regions

Henry Ruiz-Garcia, Jennifer L. Peterson, and Daniel M. Trifiletti

Abstract

Radiating in eloquent regions requires a careful analysis of risk and benefit in order to prevent damage to adjacent tissues that serve important neurologic functions. Although a number of novel and precise techniques exist for microsurgical approaches to lesions located in eloquent regions, radiation therapy, and, more specifically, radiosurgery, is an effective noninvasive treatment option for the treatment of eloquently located lesions at excessive risk with surgery. In this chapter, we will describe the rationale and the trends in the management of the most common intracranial pathologies located in eloquent areas that benefit from radiotherapy and radiosurgery.

Keywords: stereotactic radiosurgery, Gamma Knife radiosurgery, eloquent brain regions, dose–volume histogram, tolerance

23.1 Introduction

Tumors located in eloquent intracranial regions can cause considerable morbidity and mortality and can pose a significant challenge during surgery. However, modern radiosurgical and radiotherapeutic techniques can extend the reach of local therapy both as adjuvant and definitive treatment, allowing for safe ablation of intracranial pathologies.

While any intracranial target could be considered high risk, sensorimotor, language, visual cortex, hypothalamus, thalamus, brainstem, cerebellar nuclei, optic pathways, and regions immediately adjacent to these structures are generally considered eloquent regions (organ-at-risk) for the purposes of this review. As in any other organ or specific region, the aims of irradiation in eloquent areas are to simultaneously achieve good local control and avoid normal tissue injury.

Quantitative Analysis of Normal Tissue Effects in the Clinic (QUANTEC) reports have set guidelines based on dose–volume histogram analysis (DVH) data to ensure maximizing the dose delivered to the target volume while providing limits for critical structures to minimize toxicity.[1] These guidelines have been subtly revised since their adoption in the 2000s.

In this chapter, we summarize the current evidence-based practice for radiation therapy and radiosurgery of lesions located in eloquent neurologic regions.

23.2 Critical Structures in Radiation Therapy

23.2.1 Brainstem

The brainstem is considered an eloquent area as it possesses highly condensed and critical neurologic functionality. Brainstem radiation injury can clinically manifest as cranial nerve palsies, focal motor or sensory deficits, or possibly death, most commonly when damage to the medulla oblongata occurs. QUANTEC recommends a maximal dose tolerance of 12.5 Gy to

limit the toxicity risk to less than 5% for single-session stereotactic radiosurgery (SRS)[2,3] and 54 to 59 Gy, depending on if a partial or total volume of brainstem is irradiated, with conventional fractionated radiotherapy. Some researchers suggest that the brainstem surface has a higher radiation tolerance than the brainstem "core," although data on this topic are generally limited.

Distinct anatomical regions of the brainstem have shown different radiosensitivity. Uh et al observed nonhomogeneous changes in substructures within the brainstem of pediatric patients[4]; in particular, the pontine transverse fibers were more susceptible to radiation when DTI parameters were analyzed. However, this has not yet translated into clinical practice and the same treatment is considered for any part of the brainstem.

23.2.2 Optic Pathway

In order to decrease the risk of radiation-induced optic neuropathy (RON), most studies and guidelines suggest a maximum point dose threshold of 8 Gy per single fraction to the optic nerves and optic chiasm. QUANTEC guidelines have recommended a maximum dose of 10 to 12 Gy for a single-fraction treatment, while Stafford et al from Mayo Clinic[5] reported the safety of 10 Gy as median point maximum dose and less than 2% of RON with ≤ 12 Gy based on DVH-toxicity analysis. This is in concordance with the most recent data from Milano et al that showed that there was a < 1% RON risk for 12, 20, and 25 Gy as maximum point doses for single-fraction, three-fraction, and five-fraction SRSs, respectively, where 10 Gy was their recommended dose for single-fraction SRS.[6] During conventionally fractionated radiation therapy, a maximum dose limit of 54 to 55 Gy is utilized, with a low risk of RON (< 2%), especially when the fractional dose is kept below 2 Gy.[6]

Patient-specific characteristics are associated with increased risk of RON. For instance, patients with pituitary neoplasms have increased radiosensitivity and a dose limit of 46 to 48 Gy at 1.8 Gy per day has been recommended in one series.[7]

23.2.3 Skull Base Structures

The majority of the patients who undergo SRS for skull base–located tumors usually carry benign neoplasms as meningioma, schwannomas, and pituitary adenomas (PA). Consequently, long-term tumor control in addition to a low-morbidity profile is the treatment goal.

Minimizing the radiation doses reaching tumor surroundings is particularly important as cranial nerves, pituitary, brainstem, blood vessels, venous sinuses, and the cochlea portray the organs at risk (OAR) in this anatomical region.

SRSs to lesions within the cavernous sinus (CS) and parasellar region have been focused on optic apparatus (OA) safety, and the previously described criteria apply in this regard. As new technologies such as Gamma Knife (GK) Perfexion and Icon allow for steep gradients that keep optic pathway doses way below 8 Gy, DVH of the others cranial nerves, sometimes even encased by the tumor, will guide therapy. Within the CS, the trigeminal nerve has been proven more sensitive to RON than oculomotor nerves,[8] which obtained safe and effective clinical alleviation and tumor control with upfront SRS delivering marginal doses of 12 to 14 Gy for small to medium size schwannomas.[9] For bigger tumors, surgical resection and adjuvant SRS can be offered. The same tumor margin dose ranges applied to vagal, glossopharyngeal, or hypoglossal nerves rarely lead to neurological deficits.

Dose tolerance of the cochlea should be considered in head and neck cancers as well as in vestibular schwannomas radiation planning. Mean dose tolerance of the cochlea to conventional radiotherapy is estimated from less than 35 to 45 Gy with different risk and severity of sensory neural hearing loss.[10] For SRS, marginal or maximum dose of 12 to 14 Gy to the cochlea and a mean dose of 4 to 6 Gy should be considered.

23.2.4 Spine

Advances in radiation delivery, including three-dimensional localization and intensity modulation, have resulted in high accuracy in achieving dose conformality, increasing the ability to deliver cytotoxic tumor doses while sparing normal tissue[11] and improving the response rate of radioresistant primary and metastatic spine tumors to external beam radiation.

Complications from spinal radiotherapy are usually mild and self-limited. These common toxicities include esophagitis, dysphagia, transient laryngitis, mucositis, diarrhea, paresthesia, and transient radiculitis.[12,13,14] However, radiating the spinal cord, a more compact continuation of the brainstem, with either fractionated radiation or SRS, can cause radiation myelopathy, a rare but feared complication. Careful planning is needed to prevent focal or segmental motor or sensory abnormalities, bowel or urinary incontinence, or Brown-Séquard syndrome, when high dose is delivered. If spinal cord injury occurs due to radiation, typical electromyography findings of myokymia and characteristic T2 abnormalities and gadolinium enhancement on magnetic resonance imaging (MRI) correspond to the level of injury. Symptoms of radiation myelopathy typically appear between 6 months and 3 years. Although there are no data supporting different radiosensitivity of various spinal cord segments, it is well known that the cauda equina is more tolerant to radiation injury, while the thoracic cord is the most sensitive.

Prior radiation increases the risk of myelopathy and cumulative dose limits have been proposed. Sahgal et al reported on the probability of developing radiation myelopathy for unirradiated and previously irradiated patients after a multicenter DVH-based analysis. For the unirradiated patients, a maximal single-fraction point dose of 12.4 Gy was recommended to the thecal sac or spinal cord planning organ-at-risk volume. For the second group, dose limits were based on the amount of prior conventional irradiation and at least a 5- to 6-month interval between prior conventional radiotherapy and spine SRS was suggested. For conventional fractionated radiation to the full circumference of the spinal cord in unirradiated patients, doses below 50 Gy are associated with a very low risk of radiation myelopathy (< 1%).

23.3 Treatment of Intracranial Pathologies in Eloquent Areas

23.3.1 Brain Metastases

Today, the most common indication for radiation therapy is brain metastases. In general, patients eligible for microsurgery should also be considered for radiosurgery, weighing the risks and benefits of these two approaches.[15,16] Moreover, even after gross total microsurgical resection, tumor progression within the tumor cavity occurs in over 50% of patients, and postoperative radiosurgery dramatically reduces this risk.[17] Additional data exist supporting favorable local control and survival[18,19] even in patients harboring up to 10 lesions.[20]

The utilization of radiosurgery for metastases located in eloquent regions of the brain has been studied by several researchers. Dea et al published a retrospective analysis of 164 metastases located in eloquent areas (primary motor, somatosensory, speech, and visual cortex; basal ganglia; thalamus; and brainstem) in 95 patients treated with Gamma Knife stereotactic radiosurgery (GKSR) in a single session. The median dose to the tumor margin was 18 Gy (range: 14–24 Gy) and the median maximal dose was 36 Gy (range: 22.5–48 Gy). This series showed radiosurgery to be safe and effective with a median time to tumor progression of 16 months and a median survival of 8.2 months. New neurological deficits occurred in a transient fashion resolving with steroids use in 5.7% of patients, seizures occurred in 5.7%, and biopsy-proven radiation necrosis in 1.4%.[21]

Hsu et al also reported on the use of GKRS for lesions located in eloquent areas in 24 patients: 11 in brainstem, 9 in thalamus, and 5 in basal ganglia. The median dose prescription to thalamus and basal ganglia was 18 Gy (range: 15–24 Gy) and 12 Gy to the brainstem (range: 12–18 Gy). In general, there was no difference in the overall survival when compared to the cohort harboring noneloquent lesions receiving a median prescription dose of 24 Gy.[22] The only symptomatic complication was grade 2 headaches, and asymptomatic radiation necrosis was present in 8.3%. An example of a metastatic tumor located in an eloquent region is shown in ▶ Fig. 23.1.

Our group published the results of radiosurgery in 161 patients harboring 189 metastases in the brainstem, where 52% of them had received whole brain radiotherapy (WBRT) prior to SRS. The median margin dose was 18 Gy prescribed to 50% isodose line. Overall local control was 87.3% at the last follow-up (95.2, 90.1, and 84.9% at 3, 6, and 12 months, respectively). Regression of tumor after SRS was found in 68% of patients and stable tumors in 19% of patients on follow-up imaging[23]. After controlling for other factors including number of brain metastases, Karnofsky Performance Status (KPS), WBRT, and brainstem tumor volume, a margin dose of at least 16 Gy was associated with superior local control on multivariate analysis.[23] Severe SRS-induced toxicity (grade ≥ 3) happened in 1.8% of treated tumors, and none of these received WBRT prior to SRS.

These results suggest that SRS can be safely administered after WBRT, even in eloquent locations. However, after this

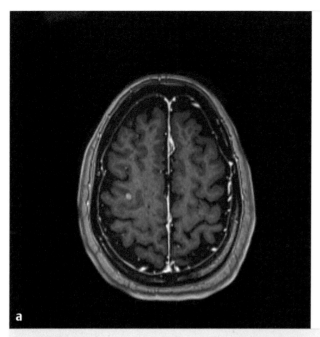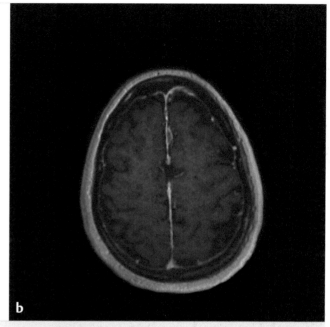

Fig. 23.1 MRI of a 74-year-old patient with metastatic non-small cell lung cancer. The patient was neurologically intact, but a small metastasis near the precentral gyrus was found in follow-up **(a)**. Gamma Knife radiosurgery with a dose of 20 Gy to the 50% isodose line with a maximum dose of 40 Gy in a single fraction was delivered. The lesion was not identifiable on the 3-month follow-up thin-slice MRI and no toxicities were presented **(b)**.

report, we conducted an international cooperative study to define response and toxicity in brainstem metastases and demonstrated an increased risk of injury when SRS is administered after WBRT. As the interval from SRS to WBRT grows, it is possible that sublethal damage recovery occurs and the risk of SRS decreases.[24] It is clear that previous intracranial therapies, specifically radiation, should be considered during treatment decision making.

This international study also demonstrated that, depending on tumor volume, margin doses of 16 to 24 Gy provide an adequate balance of the risks of severe toxicity while maintaining tumor control.[24] These data form the basis for our current practice, where we consider SRS for any patient with a brainstem metastasis who is otherwise fit for radiosurgery (KPS > 70, limited intracranial disease, etc.) and adjust margin dose based on tumor volume, location, and timing, as well as history of prior WBRT. We generally recommend a margin dose of 18 Gy. For patients who have received previous WBRT, we reduce the margin dose to 16 Gy. For larger brainstem tumors (> 2 cm diameter) or tumors adjacent to optic structures, fractionated SRS is considered. An example of a metastatic brain lesion within the brainstem is shown in ▶ Fig. 23.2.

In general, an experienced team can perform SRS to brain metastases located in eloquent areas. Of note, in these clinical scenarios, the target consists solely of tumor (i.e., nonneural tissue), and therefore accurate targeting rarely results in clinical toxicity. Moreover, patients with brain metastases have a generally poor prognosis, and may not live long enough to otherwise develop late toxicity. In patients with large metastases, particularly when located in eloquent areas, multisession SRS (i.e., fractionated radiosurgery) has been shown to improve tumor control and reduce radionecrosis.[25] Multisession radiosurgery for brain metastases is the topic of future prospective clinical research.

23.3.2 Arteriovenous Malformations

Patients with intracranial arteriovenous malformations (AVMs) have multiple treatment strategies. Microsurgery confers several advantages such as a high rate of obliteration and immediate protection against subsequent hemorrhage; however, radiosurgery is advantageous for AVMs located in eloquent regions of the brain which carry a high risk of morbidity with microsurgery and has been used for decades to safely and totally obliterate any nidus deemed to pose a high risk for hemorrhage and/or complication from microsurgical resection.[26,27,28] SRS typically results in obliteration within 2 to 4 years after treatment, eliminating any further risk of related hemorrhage.[29,30]

Flickinger et al analyzed 422 patients to create a scoring system that could predict the risk of symptomatic radionecrosis after radiosurgery for intracranial AVMs.[31] While tumor location (specifically brainstem and thalamus) predicted for symptomatic radionecrosis, the volume of normal brain receiving 12 Gy was also a key predictor in this toxicity, perhaps even more so than location.[31]

Additionally, Ding et al evaluated the outcomes of patients treated with GKRS for primary motor and sensory cortex AVMs and compared them to outcomes from a matched cohort of

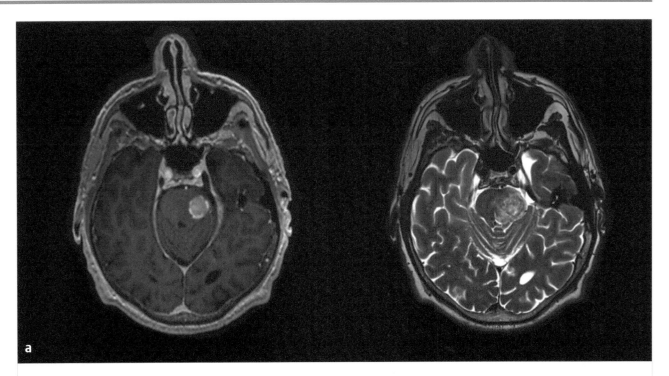

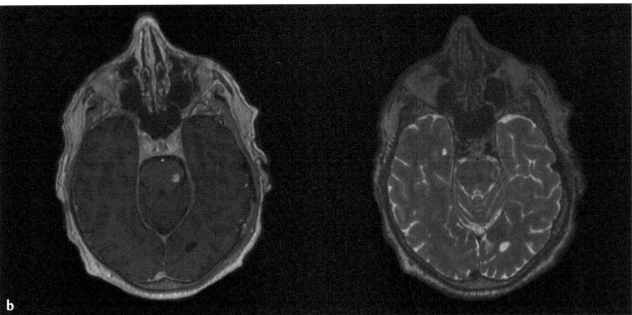

Fig. 23.2 MRI of a 78-year-old patient with a metastatic melanoma lesion in the pons (a). Gamma Knife radiosurgery with a total dose of 25 Gy in five fractions was delivered with a good radiographic response noted at 4 months of follow-up, without resultant clinical toxicity (b).

noneloquent AVMs. The median AVMs volume was 4.1 mL (range: 0.1–22.6 mL) and the prescription dose was 20 Gy (range: 7–30 Gy). The overall obliteration rate was 63% and the results failed to demonstrate that eloquent location impacted the effectiveness of radiosurgery.[32] Further research is needed to evaluate the impact of nidus location on radionecrosis risk after radiosurgery for AVMs. Example of an eloquent left occipital Spetzler-Martin grade 4 **AVM** abutting the optic radiations and inferior longitudinal fasciculus that was radiated is seen in ▶ Fig. 23.3.

Brainstem AVMs (bAVMs) constitute 2 to 6% of all intracranial AVMs and are more prone to rupture compared to AVMs located in other regions.[26,33] All treatment modalities carry potential morbidity. Cohen-Inbar et al[29] described the largest bAVMs SRS series. This multicenter study included 205 patients with bAVMs treated with a single session of GKRS. At a mean follow-up of 69 months (range: 6–269 months), the obliteration rate confirmed by MRI and/or cerebral angiography was 65.4%. None of the patients with obliteration confirmation by angiography developed hemorrhages. A margin dose of 21 to 24 Gy

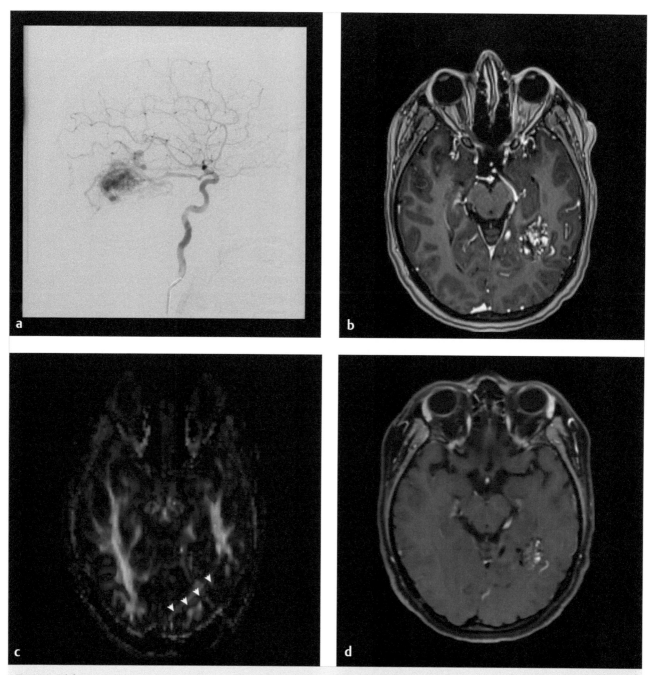

Fig. 23.3 A left occipital Spetzler-Martin grade 4 arteriovenous malformation abutting the optic radiations and inferior longitudinal fasciculus in a neurologically intact 24-year-old patient (**a, b, c**). Six months after radiosurgery to 20 Gy at the 50% isodose, reduction in nidus volume was evident and no treatment-related toxicity was observed (**d**).

was significantly more likely to obliterate the nidus while avoiding radiation-induced complications (RICs). Unlike RIC in non-bAVMs, complications were prolonged and not transient. Postsurgical hemorrhage was present in 8.8% of patients after SRS, with an annual latency period hemorrhage of 1.5%. Radiographic RICs were evident in 35.6% of patients, symptomatic RIC in 14.6%, and permanent RIC in 14.6% (which included long-tract signs and new cranial nerve deficits).[29] Radiographic RIC generally preceded nidal obliteration, which typically developed within 6 to 18 months after SRS.[34]

23.3.3 Skull Base Tumors

Cavernous sinus meningiomas have a higher rate of recurrence, as the risk of cranial nerve and vascular morbidity may represent a limitation during microsurgical dissection. After Duma et al[35] reported the first series of CS meningioma patients treated with SRS, it has gradually become accepted as standard of treatment for less than 3 cm tumors, while microsurgery plus adjuvant SRS became a therapeutic option for larger lesions.[36] Additionally, for patient with large and diffusely infiltrative tumors with suprasellar or brainstem extension, hypofractionated SRS or stereotactic radiotherapy (SRT) could be offered to minimize the risk of complications and optimize tumor therapy.[37]

Lee et al reported on the WHO grade 1 CS meningioma treated with SRS. Ranges of 86 to 99% and 69 to 97% were documented for 5- and 10-year progression-free survival (PFS), respectively. The median marginal dose for single-fraction SRS ranged from 11 to 19 Gy with more modern studies supporting doses of 12 Gy. Preserved neurological function was reported on 80 to 100% of patients.[36] A series from Mayo Clinic considering all types of meningiomas reported 16 Gy as effective in providing long-term local control (25 years of follow-up).[38]

While the aim of radiation for meningioma is long-term tumor control and preservation of neurological function, the success for PA radiation also requires achieving endocrine remission. Radiosurgery and radiotherapy should be reserved for postoperative residual, radiographically postsurgical persistent or recurrent, and/or endocrine active PA. In single-session SRS, margin doses vary from 12 to 18 Gy for nonfunctioning PA; tumor control rates of 83 to 100% and post-SRS hypopituitarism rates of 0 to 40% have been described in this group. For functioning PA, higher doses ranging from 15 to 30 Gy are required in order to obtain endocrinological control,[39,40] affording it in 17 to 70% of cases with rarely described cranial deficits (0–5%).[39] Although a distance of at least 3 mm between the PA and the OA is desirable, this is not a limiting factor but rather defines the steepness of the radiation gradient able to offer a safe dose to the optic pathway. In cases of functioning adenomas with radiographically evident CS invasion, shielding of normal stalk, gland, and OA could allow higher treatment doses.[40] Additionally, whole-sellar GKRS has proven to be effective in controlling adrenocorticotropic hormone secreting tumors when not clearly identified or invasive tumor receive a mean margin dose of 22.4 Gy (mean treatment volume of 2.6 cm).[41]

Vestibular schwannomas management relies primarily on clinical presentation, tumor growth rate, and tumor size. Although observation was recommended for small intracanalicular VS, growing data show that most of the tumors will grow and hearing will progressively decline in few years. As a result, GKRS was recommended when hearing is still useful at the time of diagnosis, and would offer an advantage of 73.3% over 35% on hearing preservation.[42] Recent CNS guidelines recommend observation if tinnitus is not present and the tumor is less than 2 cm.[43] SRS compares favorably with microsurgical resection for small to middle sized VS (Koss stages I–III) with lower rates of facial nerve neuropathy and higher rates of serviceable hearing preservation, where a dose of 13 Gy for single-fraction SRS has been recommended with this purpose.[43] GKRS series describe long-term tumor control range from 92 to 98% and trigeminal injury rates of 0 to 9% (3–10 years of follow-up).[44] As cochlear radiation doses have been associated with hearing preservation, previously described recommendation should be taken into consideration.

23.4 Conclusion

Radiosurgery and radiation therapy provide a means to extend the reach of traditional neurosurgery, and even modern microsurgery. This technique can be used to effectively treat tumors and other lesions in areas that are fraught with surgical risk. Future efforts will focus on creating and validating radiosurgical and radiotherapeutic techniques that further reduce these risks (i.e., proton and carbon ion therapy), as well as better defining genetic patient characteristics that predict for radiosensitivity.

References

[1] Siavash Jabbari LM, Lee YK, Lo SS, et al. Critical structures and tolerance of the central nervous system. In: Lunsford LD, Sheehan JP, eds. Intracranial Stereotactic Radiosurgery. 2nd ed. New York, NY: Thieme; 2016:266

[2] Levegrün S, Hof H, Essig M, Schlegel W, Debus J. Radiation-induced changes of brain tissue after radiosurgery in patients with arteriovenous malformations: correlation with dose distribution parameters. Int J Radiat Oncol Biol Phys. 2004; 59(3):796–808

[3] Kased N, Huang K, Nakamura JL, et al. Gamma knife radiosurgery for brainstem metastases: the UCSF experience. J Neurooncol. 2008; 86(2):195–205

[4] Uh J, Merchant TE, Li Y, et al. Differences in brainstem fiber tract response to radiation: a longitudinal diffusion tensor imaging study. Int J Radiat Oncol Biol Phys. 2013; 86(2):292–297

[5] Stafford SL, Pollock BE, Leavitt JA, et al. A study on the radiation tolerance of the optic nerves and chiasm after stereotactic radiosurgery. Int J Radiat Oncol Biol Phys. 2003; 55(5):1177–1181

[6] Milano MT, Grimm J, Soltys SG, et al. Single- and multi-fraction stereotactic radiosurgery dose tolerances of the optic pathways. Int J Radiat Oncol Biol Phys. 2018:[Epub ahead of print]

[7] Hirato M, Hirato J, Zama A, et al. Radiobiological effects of gamma knife radiosurgery on brain tumors studied in autopsy and surgical specimens. Stereotact Funct Neurosurg. 1996; 66 Suppl 1:4–16

[8] Kondziolka D, Flickinger JC, Lunsford LD. The principles of skull base radiosurgery. Neurosurg Focus. 2008; 24(5):E11

[9] Peciu-Florianu I, Tuleasca C, Comps JN, et al. Radiosurgery in trochlear and abducens nerve schwannomas: case series and systematic review. Acta Neurochir (Wien). 2017; 159(12):2409–2418

[10] Bhandare N, Jackson A, Eisbruch A, et al. Radiation therapy and hearing loss. Int J Radiat Oncol Biol Phys. 2010; 76(3) Suppl:S50–S57

[11] Bilsky MH, Angelov L, Rock J, et al. Spinal radiosurgery: a neurosurgical perspective. J Radiosurg SBRT. 2011; 1(1):47–54

[12] Jin JY, Chen Q, Jin R, et al. Technical and clinical experience with spine radiosurgery: a new technology for management of localized spine metastases. Technol Cancer Res Treat. 2007; 6(2):127–133

[13] Gerszten PC, Burton SA, Ozhasoglu C, Welch WC. Radiosurgery for spinal metastases: clinical experience in 500 cases from a single institution. Spine. 2007; 32(2):193–199

[14] Katagiri H, Takahashi M, Inagaki J, et al. Clinical results of nonsurgical treatment for spinal metastases. Int J Radiat Oncol Biol Phys. 1998; 42(5):1127–1132

[15] Flickinger JC, Lunsford LD, Somaza S, Kondziolka D. Radiosurgery: its role in brain metastasis management. Neurosurg Clin N Am. 1996; 7(3):497–504

[16] Gerosa M, Nicolato A, Foroni R, et al. Gamma knife radiosurgery for brain metastases: a primary therapeutic option. J Neurosurg. 2002; 97(5) Suppl: 515–524

[17] Mahajan A, Ahmed S, McAleer MF, et al. Post-operative stereotactic radiosurgery versus observation for completely resected brain metastases: a single-centre, randomised, controlled, phase 3 trial. Lancet Oncol. 2017; 18(8): 1040–1048

[18] Klironomos G, Bernstein M. Salvage stereotactic radiosurgery for brain metastases. Expert Rev Neurother. 2013; 13(11):1285–1295

[19] Kurtz G, Zadeh G, Gingras-Hill G, et al. Salvage radiosurgery for brain metastases: prognostic factors to consider in patient selection. Int J Radiat Oncol Biol Phys. 2014; 88(1):137–142

[20] Yamamoto M, Serizawa T, Shuto T, et al. Stereotactic radiosurgery for patients with multiple brain metastases (JLGK0901): a multi-institutional prospective observational study. Lancet Oncol. 2014; 15(4):387–395

[21] Dea N, Borduas M, Kenny B, Fortin D, Mathieu D. Safety and efficacy of Gamma Knife surgery for brain metastases in eloquent locations. J Neurosurg. 2010; 113 Suppl:79–83

[22] Hsu F, Nichol A, Ma R, Kouhestani P, Toyota B, McKenzie M. Stereotactic radiosurgery for metastases in eloquent central brain locations. Can J Neurol Sci. 2015; 42(5):333–337

[23] Trifiletti DM, Lee CC, Winardi W, et al. Brainstem metastases treated with stereotactic radiosurgery: safety, efficacy, and dose response. J Neurooncol. 2015; 125(2):385–392

[24] Trifiletti DM, Lee CC, Kano H, et al. Stereotactic radiosurgery for brainstem metastases: an international cooperative study to define response and toxicity. Int J Radiat Oncol Biol Phys. 2016; 96(2):280–288

[25] Minniti G, Scaringi C, Paolini S, et al. Single-fraction versus multifraction (3 × 9 Gy) stereotactic radiosurgery for large (> 2 cm) brain metastases: a comparative analysis of local control and risk of radiation-induced brain necrosis. Int J Radiat Oncol Biol Phys. 2016; 95(4):1142–1148

[26] Kurita H, Kawamoto S, Sasaki T, et al. Results of radiosurgery for brain stem arteriovenous malformations. J Neurol Neurosurg Psychiatry. 2000; 68(5): 563–570

[27] Kano H, Kondziolka D, Flickinger JC, et al. Stereotactic radiosurgery for arteriovenous malformations, Part 5: Management of brainstem arteriovenous malformations. J Neurosurg. 2012; 116(1):44–53

[28] Maruyama K, Kondziolka D, Niranjan A, Flickinger JC, Lunsford LD. Stereotactic radiosurgery for brainstem arteriovenous malformations: factors affecting outcome. J Neurosurg. 2004; 100(3):407–413

[29] Cohen-Inbar O, Starke RM, Lee CC, et al. Stereotactic radiosurgery for brainstem arteriovenous malformations: a multicenter study. Neurosurgery. 2017; 81(6):910–920

[30] Koga T, Shin M, Terahara A, Saito N. Outcomes of radiosurgery for brainstem arteriovenous malformations. Neurosurgery. 2011; 69(1):45–51, discussion 51–52

[31] Flickinger JC, Kondziolka D, Lunsford LD, et al. Arteriovenous Malformation Radiosurgery Study Group. Development of a model to predict permanent symptomatic postradiosurgery injury for arteriovenous malformation patients. Int J Radiat Oncol Biol Phys. 2000; 46(5):1143–1148

[32] Ding D, Yen CP, Xu Z, Starke RM, Sheehan JP. Radiosurgery for primary motor and sensory cortex arteriovenous malformations: outcomes and the effect of eloquent location. Neurosurgery. 2013; 73(5):816–824, 824

[33] Solomon RA, Stein BM. Management of arteriovenous malformations of the brain stem. J Neurosurg. 1986; 64(6):857–864

[34] Yen CP, Matsumoto JA, Wintermark M, et al. Radiation-induced imaging changes following Gamma Knife surgery for cerebral arteriovenous malformations. J Neurosurg. 2013; 118(1):63–73

[35] Duma CM, Lunsford LD, Kondziolka D, et al. Stereotactic radiosurgery of cavernous sinus meningiomas as an addition or alternative to microsurgery. Neurosurgery. 1993; 32(5):699–705

[36] Lee CC, Trifiletti DM, Sahgal A, et al. Stereotactic radiosurgery for benign (World Health Organization Grade I) Cavernous Sinus Meningiomas-International Stereotactic Radiosurgery Society (ISRS) Practice Guideline: a systematic review. Neurosurgery. 2018; 83(6):1128–1142

[37] De Salles AA, Frighetto L, Grande CV, et al. Radiosurgery and stereotactic radiation therapy of skull base meningiomas: proposal of a grading system. Stereotact Funct Neurosurg. 2001; 76(3–4):218–229

[38] Pollock BE, Stafford SL, Link MJ. Stereotactic radiosurgery of intracranial meningiomas. Neurosurg Clin N Am. 2013; 24(4):499–507

[39] Trifiletti DM, Xu Z, Dutta SW, et al. Endocrine remission after pituitary stereotactic radiosurgery: differences in rates of response for matched cohorts of Cushing disease and acromegaly patients. Int J Radiat Oncol Biol Phys. 2018; 101(3):610–617

[40] Chen-Chia Lee SJ. Stereotactic radiosurgery for pituitary adenomas. In: Lunsford LD, Sheehan JP, eds. Intracranial Stereotactic Radiosurgery. 2nd ed. New York, NY: Thieme; 2016:266

[41] Shepard MJ, Mehta GU, Xu Z, et al. Technique of whole-sellar stereotactic radiosurgery for Cushing disease: results from a multicenter, international cohort study. World Neurosurg. 2018; 116:e670–e679

[42] Régis J, Carron R, Park MC, et al. Wait-and-see strategy compared with proactive Gamma Knife surgery in patients with intracanalicular vestibular schwannomas: clinical article. J Neurosurg. 2013; 119 Suppl:105–111

[43] Olson JJ, Kalkanis SN, Ryken TC. Congress of Neurological Surgeons systematic review and evidence-based guidelines on the treatment of adults with vestibular schwannomas: executive summary. Neurosurgery. 2018; 82(2):129–134

[44] Rejis Jean CR, Christine D, Denis P, Jean-Marc T, Xavier M, Pierre-Huges R. Stereotactic radiosurgery for vestibular schwannoma. In: Lunsford LD, Sheehan JP, eds. Intracranial Stereotactic Radiosurgery. 2nd ed. New York: Thieme; 2016:266

Index

Note: Page numbers set **bold** or *italic* indicate headings or figures, respectively.